Rheumatology and the kidney

Other related titles

Analgesic and NSAID-induced kidney disease
Edited by J.H. Stewart

Dialysis amyloid
Edited by Charles van Ypersele and Tilman B. Drüeke

Infections of the kidney and urinary tract
Edited by W.R. Cattell

Polycystic kidney disease
Edited by Michael L. Watson and Vicente E. Torres

Treatment of primary glomerulonephritis
Edited by Claudio Ponticelli and Richard J. Glassock

Inherited disorders of the kidney
Edited by Stephen H. Morgan and Jean-Pierre Grünfeld

Complications of long-term dialysis
Edited by Edwina A. Brown and Patrick S. Parfrey

Lupus nephritis
Edited by E. Lewis, M. Schwartz, and S. Korbet

Nephropathy in type 2 diabetes
Edited by Eberhard Ritz and Ivan Rychlik

Hemodialysis vascular access
Edited by Peter J. Conlon, Michael Nicholson, and Steve Schwab

Mechanisms and clinical management of chronic renal failure (Second
edition; formerly *Prevention of progressive chronic renal failure*)
Edited by A. Meguid El Nahas with Kevin Harris and Sharon Anderson

Cardiovascular disease in end-stage renal failure
Edited by Joseph Loscalzo and Gérard M. London

Rheumatology and the kidney

Edited by

DWOMOA ADU
Consultant Physician
Department of Nephrology, Queen Elizabeth Hospital,
Birmingham, UK

PAUL EMERY
ARC Professor of Rheumatology
Academic Unit of Musculoskeletal Disease,
University of Leeds,
36 Clarendon Road,
UK

and

MICHAEL P. MADAIO
Penn Center for Molecular Studies of Kidney Diseases,
Department of Medicine, University of Pennsylvania,
Philadelphia, USA

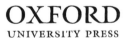

OXFORD
UNIVERSITY PRESS

OXFORD
UNIVERSITY PRESS

Great Clarendon Street, Oxford OX2 6DP
Oxford University Press is a department of the University of Oxford.
It furthers the University's objective of excellence in research, scholarship,
and education by publishing worldwide in
Oxford New York

Athens Auckland Bangkok Bogotá Buenos Aires Cape Town
Chennai Dar es Salaam Delhi Florence Hong Kong Istanbul Karachi
Kolkata Kuala Lumpur Madrid Melbourne Mexico City Mumbai Nairobi
Paris Sào Paulo Shanghai Singapore Taipei Tokyo Toronto Warsaw
with associated companies in Berlin Ibadan

Oxford is a registered trade mark of Oxford University Press
in the UK and in certain other countries

Published in the United States
By Oxford University Press Inc., New York

British Library Cataloguing in Publication Data

Data available

Library of Congress Cataloging in Publication Data
Rheumatology and the kidney / edited by Dwomoa Adu, Paul Emery and Micheal P. Madaio.
p. ; cm.
Includes bibliographical references and index.
1. Renal manifestations of general diseases. 2. Rheumatism—Complications. 3. Lupus
nephritis. 4. Autoimmune diseases. 5. Nephrotoxicology. I. Adu, Dwomoa. II. Emery,
Paul. III. Madaio, Michael P.
[DNLM: 1. Kidney Diseases—complications. 2. Lupus Nephritis. 3. Rheumatic
Diseases—complications. WJ 300 R472 2001]
RC903 .R488 2001   616.6'1—dc21   2001031170
ISBN 019 2631780 (Hbk)

1 3 5 7 9 10 8 6 4 2

Typeset by EXPO Holdings, Malaysia
Printed in Great Britain by
Antony Rowe Ltd, Chippenham, Wiltshire

PREFACE

This book provides up-to-date information on disorders that affect the kidneys as well as the joints. These disorders often affect several systems in the body and many have an immunological basis.

The majority of chapters focus on specific diseases and examine their aetiology, pathogenesis, immunological basis and pathology. In addition, the clinical features, current approaches to treatment and outcome are described.

Overall these chapters provide a balanced view of current understanding of these conditions. The major syndromes of rheumatologic diseases reviewed include systemic lupus erythematosus, the vasculitides (including Wegener's granulomatosis, polyarteritis nodosa, microscopic polyangiitis, Churg-Strauss syndrome, Takayasu's disease and Henoch-Schönlein purpura, and systemic sclerosis. Other chapters cover amyloidosis and hepatitis B and C associated systemic disease. Finally there are chapters on the nephrotoxicity of drugs used in the treatment of rheumatologic diseases and also on rheumatologic complications following renal transplantation.

The information in the book is up to date and brings together in a concise manner information that is otherwise widely scattered in the literature. This book should appeal to nephrologists and rheumatologists as well as all those interested in the care of patients with systemic autoimmune disorders.

CONTENTS

LIST OF CONTRIBUTORS

Dwomoa Adu MD FRCP
Department of Nephrology
Queen Elizabeth hospital
Edgbaston
Birmingham
B15 2TH
UK

Alessandro Amore MD
Nephrology, Dialysis and
Transplantation Unit
Regina Margherita University
Hospital
Torino
ITALY

William M Bennett
Professor of Medicine (Retired)
Oregon Health Sciences University
Medical Director, Solid Organ and
Cellular Transplantation
Legacy Good Samaritan Hospital
Portland
Oregon
USA

Dr Anne Ben-Smith PhD
Renal Immunobiology
MRC Centre for Immune Regulation,
The Medical School
University of Birmingham
Birmingham B15 2TT
UK

Dr Maria CM Bickerstatff PhD
MRCP
Centre for
Rheumatology/Bloomsbury
Rheumatology Unit
Department of Medicine
University College London
Arthur Stanley House
40–50 Tottenham Street
London W1P 9PG
UK

Sarah Bingham MA MRCP
(Specialist Registrar)
Academic Unit of
Musculoskeletal Disease
University of Leeds and Lead
Clinician
(Rheumatology) Leeds Teaching
Hospitals Trust
36 Clarendon Road
Leeds LS2 9NZ
UK

Dimitrios T Boumpas MD FACP
Professor of Medicine and
Rheumatology
Director
Division of Rheumatology
Allergy and Immunology
University of Crete
Medical School
715 00 Heraklion
GREECE

Dr Edwina Brown MD FRCP
Charing Cross Hospital
Fulham Palace Road
London W6 8RF
UK

J Stewart Cameron CBE MD BSc
FRCP
Emeritus Professor of Renal Medicine
Guys Campus
United Medical and Dental Schools
London
UK

Kirpal S Chugh
Professor Emeritus
Department of Nephrology
Postgraduate Institute of Medical
Education and Research
Chandigarh
INDIA

Rosanna Coppo MD
Nephrology, Dialysis and
Transplantation Unit
Regina Margherita University
Hospital
Torino
ITALY

Professor Giuseppe D'Amico MD
San Carlo Borromeo Hospital
Division of Nephrology
Via Pio III 3
20153 Milan
ITALY

Professor Marc E De Broe
Department of Nephrology
University of Antwerp
Wilrijkstraat 10
B-2650 Edegem
Antwerpen
BELGIUM

Paul Emery MA MD FRCP
ARC Professor of Rheumatology and
Head of Academic Unit of
Musculoskeletal Disease University of
Leeds and Lead Clinician
(Rheumatology) Leeds Teaching
Hospitals Trust
36 Clarendon Road
Leeds LS2 9NZ
UK

Ronald J Falk
Doe Thurston Professor and Chief
Division of Nephrology and
Hypertension
Department of Medicine
University of North Carolina
Chapel Hill,
NC 27599-7525
USA

Dr Franco Ferrario MD
Division of Nephrology
5 Carlo Borromeo Hospital
Via Pio III 3
20153 Milan
ITALY

Dr Alessandro Fornasieri MD
San Carlo Borrornco Hospital
Division of Nephrology
Via Pio III 3
20153 Milan
ITALY

Dr Megan Griffith MD MRCP
Charing Cross Hospital
Fulham Palace Road
London W6 8RF
UK

Loïc Guillevin MD
Professor of Medicine
Department of Internal Medicine
Hôpital Avicenne
Université Paris–Nord
Bobigny
FRANCE

PN Hawkins
Professor of Medicine
Centre for Amyloidosis & Acute
Phase Proteins and National
Amyloidosis Centre Department of
Medicine
Royal Free and University College
Medical School Royal Free Hospital
London
UK

Gabor G Illei MD
Senior Clinical Investigator
Office of the Clinical Director
National Institute of Arthritis and
Musculoskeletal and Skin Diseases
National Institutes of Health
Bethesda Maryland
USA

Professor David A Isenberg MD
FRCP
Centre for
Rheumatology/Bloomsbury
Rheumatology Unit Department of
Medicine
University College London
Arthur Stanley House
40–50 Tottenham Street
London W1P 9PG
UK

J Charles Jennette
Brinkhous Distinguished Professor
and Chair
Department of Pathology and
Laboratory Medicine
Professor Department of Medicine
University of North Carolina
Chapel Hill
NC 27599-7525
USA

Vivekanand Jha MD DM
Associate Professor of Nephrology
Postgraduate Institute of Medical
Education and Research and Director
National Kidney Clinic
Chandigarh
INDIA

Zunaid Karim MRCPI (Research
Fellow) Academic Unit of
Musculoskeletal Disease
University of Leeds
36 Clarendon Road
Leeds LS2 9NZ
UK

Joseph H Korn MD
Alan S Cohen Professor of Medicine
in Rheumatology
Director Section of Rheumatology
and Arthritis Center
Boston University School of Medicine
71 East Concord Street
Boston MA 02118
USA

RA Kyle MD
Professor of Medicine and Laboratory
Medicine
Division of Hematology and Internal
Medicine
Mayo Clinic Rochester
Minnesota 55905
USA

Wai Y Tse PhD MRCP
Consultant Physician
Department of Nephrology
Derriford Hospital
Plymouth
PL6 6DH
UK

Ihab M Wahba MD
Instructor in Medicine
Department of Medicine
Division of Nephrology Hypertension
and Clinical Pharmacology
Oregon Health Sciences University
Portland
Oregon
USA

Professor Mark Walport MA PhD
FRCP FRCPath FMedSci
Head Division of Medicine
Imperial College School of Medicine
Hammersmith Hospital
Du Cane Rd
London W12 0NN
UK

ABBREVIATIONS

anti ds DNA   anti double-stranded DNA antibodies
ACE   angiotensin-converting enzyme
ANA   anti-nuclear antibodies
BP   blood pressure
Clq Ab   autoantibodies to Clq
CT   computerised tomography
ENA   extractable nuclear antigens
ESR   erythrocyte sedimentation rate
FGF   fibroblast growth factor
GFR   glomerular filtration rate
GN   glomerulonephritis
HGF   hepatocyte growth factor
HLA   human lymphocyte antigen
HSP   heat shock protein
HSP   henoch-schoenlein purpura
ICAM   intercellular cell adhesion molecule
IgA-ANCA   IgA reacting with neutrophil cytoplasmic antigens
IgA/IgGIC   mixed IgA and IgG containing circulating immune complexes
IgAIC   circulating IgA containing immune complexes
IgAN   nephritis with prevalent IgA mesangial deposits
LFA   lymphocyte function-associated antigen
MASP   MBL-associated serine protease
MBL   mannose-binding lectin
MCGN   mesangiocapillery glomerulophritis
MHC   major histocompatibility complex
MRI   magnetic resonance imaging
PCR   polymerase chain reaction
PECAM   platelet-endothelial cell adhesion molecule
PTA   percutaneous transluminal angioplasty
TA   takayasu's arteritis
US   ultrasound
VEGF   vascular-endothelial growth factor

PART I
LUPUS NEPHRITIS

1

An overview of SLE

Maria C.M. Bickerstaff and David A. Isenberg

Introduction

Systemic lupus erythematosus (SLE, lupus) is a syndrome of multifactorial aetiology, characterized by widespread inflammation, most commonly affecting women during the childbearing years. Virtually every organ and/or system of the body may be involved, although the skin and the joints are the most frequently affected. The course of the disease is typically one of remissions and exacerbations. With good management this disease, which 50 years ago had a 50% mortality rate now has a 10-year survival figure of approximately 90%.

SLE is characterized serologically by autoantibodies to DNA, RNA, other nuclear antigens, cytoplasmic and cell surface antigens. The diversity of its clinical features is thus matched by an apparent diversity among the autoantibodies detectable in the serum. There are, in addition, a large number of other immunological abnormalities, which have been described in patients with SLE.

Much work has been done in the last 30 years to dissect and understand the complex array of immunological disturbances which culminate in the diverse clinical features which characterize the disease. A variety of murine and other animal models of lupus exist, which have been used extensively to investigate the immunogenetic and cellular abnormalities which are characteristic of human SLE.

Definition and classification

The American Rheumatism Association (now the American College of Rheumatology, ACR) initially published classification criteria in 1971 (Cohen *et al.* 1971), which were revised in 1982 (Tan *et al.* 1982). A further revision has recently been proposed (Hochberg 1997). The criteria are for the classification of the disease rather than for use as a diagnostic tool, although in practice there is a blurring of this distinction. The 1997 updated criteria are outlined in Table 1.1.

Table 1.1   Revised criteria of the American Rheumatism Assocation for the classification of SLE

1 Malar rash

2 Discoid rash

3 Photosensitivity

4 Oral ulcers

5 Arthritis

6 Serositis
   a. pleuritis, or b. pericarditis

7 Renal disorder
   a. proteinuria > 0.5g/24h or 3+, persistently, or b. cellular casts

8 Neurological discorder
   a. seizures or b. psychosis (having excluded other causes)

9 Haematological disorder
   a. haemolytic anaemia or
   b. leucopaenia or <4.0 × 10^9/1 on two or more occasions
   c. lymphopaenia or <1.5 × 10^9/1 on two or more occasions
   d. thrombocytopaenia <100 × 10^9/1

10 Immunological disorders
   a. raised anti-native DNA antibody binding or
   b. anti-Sm antibody or
   c. positive finding of antiphospholipid antibodies based on
       i. an abnormal serum level of IgG or IgM anticardiolipin antibodies
       ii. A positive test result for lupus anticoagulant using a standard method
       iii. A false–positive serological test for syphilis, present for at least 6 months

11 Anti-nuclear antibody in raised titre

'A person shall be said to have SLE if 4 or more of the 11 criteria are present, serially or simultaneously, during the interval of observation.'
From Tan *et al.* (1982) and modified by (Hochberg 1997).

Epidemiology and natural history

Lupus is found world-wide. It is, however, much more common amongst black females in the UK, the West Indies and the United States, although it curiously remains rare in Africa (Nived and Sturfeldt 1997). In a recent study from Birmingham, UK (Johnson *et al.* 1995), prevalence rates of 36.2, 90.6 and 206 per 100 000 amongst women of Caucasian, Asian and Afro-Caribbean origin, respectively were recorded. This study did not record the prevalence amongst Chinese women, although it is likely to be approximately 100 per 100 000 women.

It is widely agreed that lupus is between 10 and 20 times more common in women than men. The majority of patients will develop their disease between the ages of 15 and 40 years. It has been recognized, however, that in 10–15% of patients, the disease will begin after the age of 50, although in this subgroup, the female to male ratio falls to around 4:1.

The marked improvement in survival during the past 20 years is probably the consequence of greater awareness of the condition, increased availability of autoantibody testing to make the diagnosis earlier, the more judicious use of steroids and other immunosuppressive drugs, and undoubtedly the widespread availability of dialysis and renal transplantation. It does, however, remain a disease with the potential to cause considerable morbidity and increased mortality in a subset of patients.

Clinical features

SLE is characterized by a plethora of clinical features. Non-specific features such as severe fatigue, fever, anorexia, weight loss and lymphadenopathy are common and can form a major part of many patients' illness. Musculoskeletal features affect more than 90% of patients, with arthralgia predominating and a deforming arthritis, tenosynovitis or myositis occurring much more rarely. The classical butterfly rash found over the bridge of the nose and malar bones is actually found in only one-third of patients with the disease, although dermatological features as a whole are present in up to 85% of lupus patients (Pistiner *et al.* 1991). Many lupus rashes are exacerbated by ultraviolet light (occasionally leading to a generalized disease flare), this photosensitivity more commonly affecting white females. Diffuse non-scarring alopecia is common and hyperpigmentation, vasculitic skin lesions and livedo reticularis can also occur.

Pulmonary disease occurs in approximately 40% of patients, usually manifesting as breathlessness, pleurisy or small pleural effusions, although pulmonary function abnormalities can be found in up to 85% of patients with SLE. Parenchymal involvement is rare and has been reported in up to 18% of patients (Haupt *et al.* 1981), usually manifesting as interstitial fibrosis, pulmonary vasculitis or interstitial pneumonitis. Cardiac disease occurs less frequently, with pericardial disease being the most common component of heart involvement, although much is clinically silent (Mandell 1987). Myocardial disease occurs less often, usually as a myocarditis, although recent studies suggest that patients with SLE have a significant increase in atherosclerotic cardiac disease and death. The pathogenesis is probably multifactorial as patients with SLE have a high frequency of the traditional cardiac risk factors such as hypertension, diabetes and hyperlipidaemia, and complications that result from disease involvement, such as renal disease leading to hypertension and hyperlipidaemia, may also potentiate the atherosclerotic process. The classical endocarditis described by Libman and Sachs (1924), although identified in up to 50% of cases at autopsy, rarely causes significant lesions.

Gastrointestinal involvement is less common, with anorexia and abdominal pain occurring in approximately one-third of patients, and other features such as mouth ulcers, dysphagia, diarrhoea, hepato/splenomegaly and/or persistent liver function test abnormalities occurring infrequently (Sultan *et al.* 1999). A variety of haematological abnormalities can occur (Keeling and Isenberg 1993) such as a normochromic, normocytic anaemia (present in up to 70% of patients) and a Coombs positive haemolytic anaemia. Leucopaenia (less than 4×10^9 per litre white blood cells) and lymphopaenia (less than 1.5×10^9 Per litre) are the most frequent abnormalities of the white blood cell count in patients with lupus. There are at least three types of thrombocytopaenia associated with lupus, including a chronic thrombocytopaenia (rarely associated with bleeding disorders), an acute thrombocytopaenia, which may be both dramatic and life-threatening, or an 'idiopathic' thrombocytopaenia, i.e. patients who present solely with this feature who later develop further manifestation of the disease.

In perhaps no other system is the ability of lupus to mimic other disease more evident than in the nervous system. Virtually every feature of central nervous system disease from migraine to madness has been associated with lupus. Approximately 30% of patients with lupus suffer from migraine (Isenberg *et al.* 1982), but of much greater concern are the grand mal seizures which may be an initial manifestation of lupus in 5% of patients, although as many as 20% may develop them in due course. A variety of additional features can occur including hemiplegia, chorea, peripheral neuropathy and cranial nerve lesions, with non-specific features such as depression, anxiety and cognitive impairment being particularly common.

In most published series until very recently, renal disease has been the most common cause of death in patients with lupus and remains a cause of considerable morbidity in up to 30% of patients. The World Health Organisation (WHO) has subdivided renal lupus into five major categories based on renal biopsy results. In addition, end-stage renal disease with completely sclerosed glomeruli, tubular interstitial disease and the overlap of lupus nephritis and multiple small thrombi associated with antiphospholipid antibodies, can also occur.

Overall clinical assessment

In order to reflect the totality of effects of any disease upon a patient, it is necessary to distinguish disease activity (clinical features which are essentially reversible) from damage (irreversible features). In addition, an understanding of the disease from the patients' perspective is also important, i.e. the perceived disability. In the past 10 years there have been major developments in indices designed to assess each of these facets of disease, which are outlined below:

Disease activity

Several reliable and validated global activity scores have been developed to assess disease activity and, therefore, disease reversibility. These include the SLAM (Systemic Lupus Activity Measures, Liang *et al.* 1988) and SLEDAI (Systemic Lupus Erythematosus Disease Activity Index, Bombardier *et al.* 1992). Whilst robust and easy to use, these instruments remain relatively blunt tools and in order to provide a more detailed analysis, the BILAG (British Isles Lupus

Assessment Group, Hay *et al.* 1993) index was developed providing a more comprehensive approach based on the physician's intention to treat. This index provides an accurate means of grading disease activity from the most active (Grade A, requiring major immunosuppression) to inactive (Grade E, no evidence of disease activity currently or previously in an organ or system) in eight organ systems, namely; general, mucocutaneous, neurological, musculoskeletal, cardiovascular/respiratory, renal, haematological and vascular. Therefore, one can assess not only that a patient is flaring but in which particular system and over what period of time. For the purposes of comparison, the BILAG system can be converted into a global score (A grade = 9 points, B = 3, C = 1, D and E = 0) and the value of international collaboration has perhaps never been better demonstrated than in a long series of studies over the past decade which has shown strong correlations between the BILAG global score and the SLAM and SLEDAI scores.

Damage index

The Systemic Lupus International Collaborating Clinics group (SLICC) collectively devised a damage score for lupus to assess irreversible change, due either to disease or to therapy, that has been recognized by the American College of Rheumatology (Gladman *et al.* 1997). In this index, damage occurring since diagnosis of lupus is ascertained by clinical assessment and generally should be present for at least 6 months. Twelve systems are assessed, namely; ocular, neuropsychiatric, renal, pulmonary, cardiovascular, peripheral vascular, gastrointestinal, musculoskeletal, skin, premature gonadal failure, diabetes and malignancy. The same lesion cannot be scored twice and repeat episodes need to be at least 6 months apart to score. Therefore, this index gives a cumulative score of organ damage. It has now been used in a variety of studies and has gained international recognition.

Disability

Several health assessment questionnaires have been utilized in the study of disability in patients with lupus. John Ware and colleagues from the Rand Corporation developed a series of questionnaires designed to measure health attributes, using multi-item scales that are scored using a method of summated ratings (Ware 1987). The so-called Short-form (SF-20) was used initially but it was felt that it failed to capture certain important points and the slightly longer SF-36 is now regarded as preferable. It includes multi-item scales, measuring eight different health concepts and includes a further general health rating item which asks respondents to indicate a change in their health over a one-year period. It is now generally accepted and has been used to study a variety of chronic illnesses. A recent study (Stoll *et al.* 1997), demonstrated that there is little overlap between the BILAG disease activity index, the SLICC/ACR damage index and the SF20+ (SF-20 including a question related to fatigue), confirming the requirement for all three types of index to assess the full range of effects of lupus on a patient.

SLE in other situations

Systemic lupus erythematosus in children

Approximately 20% of all cases of lupus have an onset before the age of 18 (Tucker *et al.* 1995). The sex ratio of male to female differs between childhood onset and adult onset cases, with a relatively high number of boys with SLE presenting in childhood. Thus the boy:girl ratio in childhood lupus is probably about 1:5 (i.e. about half of that seen in adults). There is a lower frequency of arthritis and cardiopulmonary disease in childhood onset patients, with a higher frequency of renal disease and Coombs positivity in this group.

A neonatal lupus syndrome is well described. This disease of the new-born is defined by the demonstration of maternal autoantibodies to Ro and/or La, being detectable in the neonate (following transplacental passage) together with complete congenital heart block (Buyon *et al.* 1989), which may be permanent and sub-acute cutaneous lupus rashes which are transient. Much more rarely, haemolytic anaemia, thrombocytopaenia, urinary abnormalities and liver dysfunction have been described. Only 1:20 of mothers who have antibodies to Ro and/or La have children with the syndrome and it remains obscure as to why these 5% of children become affected but not the others.

Pregnancy and lupus

Most recent studies have concluded that fertility is little changed by lupus, although patients in renal failure are less likely to become pregnant. There is a diversity of opinion in the literature as to whether lupus patients who become pregnant are more likely to flare during pregnancy; however, in our experience they are not. In practice, most pregnant lupus patients need close observation throughout the duration of their pregnancy.

A combination of spontaneous abortion and still-birth causes a fetal mortality of around 20%. Furthermore, perhaps as many as a quarter of babies born to mothers with lupus are delivered prematurely. Despite the panoply of autoantibodies associated with lupus, only those binding phospholipids or the Ro antigen have an important effect during or just after pregnancy. Patients with the phospholipid variant of lupus are, like patients with the primary antiphospholipid syndrome, more prone to developing recurrent miscarriages, and anti-Ro/La antibodies are associated with the neonatal lupus syndrome.

Lupus in males

Lupus in males, especially Caucasian males, is relatively uncommon. Individuals with Klinefelter's syndrome, who have an XXY karyotype, are thought to be more susceptible to SLE (Isenberg and Malick 1994). Abnormalities in oestradiol metabolism in these patients may be linked to persistent oestrogenic stimulation, which might explain the predisposition.

The antiphospholipid antibody variant of lupus

The clinical features that are linked to the presence of antiphospholipid antibodies include venous and arterial thromboses, thrombocytopaenia, cerebral disease, recurrent fetal loss, pulmonary hypertension and livedo reticularis (Asherson *et al.* 1989). A meta-analysis undertaken by Love and Santoro (1990) of 29 published series estimated an average frequency of 34% of lupus patients having lupus anticoagulant and 44% having anticardiolipin antibodies. The anticardiolipin antibodies which appear to be linked to the presence of the above clinical features are probably binding a complex or a neo-epitope formed by phospholipid and a plasma cofactor β_2-glycoprotein I (Galli *et al.* 1990) and those that are pathogenic appear to be of the IgG isotype.

It has also been suggested that antibodies to the cofactor or even other cofactors may be better markers for the thrombotic tendency than antibodies to the phospholipid or the complex alone (Alarcon-Segovia and Cabral 1996).

Lupus and malignancy

A low frequency of malignancy has been noted in studies of SLE. Two recent large studies have demonstrated a link with non-Hodgkin's lymphoma (Abu-Shakra *et al.* 1996; Mellemkjaer *et al.* 1997) and an increased risk of cancers of the lung, liver and vagina/vulva has also been reported. A large multicentre study is needed to provide a definitive account of whether there is true increased prevalence of malignancy.

Drug induced lupus

Many drugs have been identified as inducing lupus-like features and/or anti-nuclear antibodies. In addition, other drugs such as antibiotics, non-steroidal anti-inflammatory drugs and gold salts may exacerbate the true systemic disease. The majority of new cases of drug-induced lupus are caused by minocycline, procainamide, isoniazid, chlorpromazine, hydralazine, methyldopa and D-penicillamine, the clinical features of which include arthralgia/arthritis, pleuritis, fever and weight loss, although glomerulonephritis and central nervous system disease are extremely rare.

Over 95% of these patients have an anti-nuclear antibody whose principal specificity is to histones and single-stranded DNA but not, unlike SLE, to double-stranded DNA. Genetic factors are likely to be important in the expression of drug-induced disease (Fritzler 1994) as the syndrome is rare in the black population, common in women, associated with HLA-DR4 and dependent on the acetylator phenotype of individual patients.

Immunogenetics

Many studies have described an increase in the incidence of HLA-DR2 and/or HLA-DR3 haplotypes in patients with SLE from a variety of ethnic backgrounds, although they are found in less than 50% of SLE patients, giving a modest relative risk in the range 2.0 to 3.0 (reviewed by Morrow *et al.* 1998). Some studies have suggested stronger HLA associations when SLE patients are categorized by clinical subsets, although the results are variable. DNA typing techniques have demonstrated strong linkage disequilibrium in the HLA class II region, particularly among certain DRB and DQ genes, so that particular combinations of alleles are often inherited as extended haploytpes found in patients from particular ethnic backgrounds. Studies have differed as to which allele has the strongest association; however, there is strong linkage disequilibrium among class II genes and it has generally been difficult to determine whether a particular locus is of primary importance. Although some class I antigen associations have been described in SLE patients, no specific class I gene has consistently been identified.

Genes encoding components of the complement system, however, have been shown to be important in SLE, with patients who lack various components of the complement system, particularly those in the classical pathway (C1q, C1r, C1s, C2), being predisposed to the development of SLE (reviewed in Walport *et al.* 1997). These deficiencies, therefore, function as independent risk factors for the development of SLE. The general consensus, however, is that SLE is a polygenic disease and that the genetic contributions are likely to be complex and multiple.

Immunopathology

Serology

A multitude of abnormalities can be found in the sera of patients with SLE (see Table 1.2).

Anti-nuclear antibodies

More than 95% of patients with SLE have a positive anti-nuclear antibody, detected by indirect immunofluorescence usually on nuclei from cell lines such as Hep-2 (human epithelial cell). Different staining patterns correlate with different antibody binding, such as the homogeneous pattern corresponding to the binding to double-stranded DNA and/or histones. Speckled or nucleolar patterns can also occur. ANA-negative patients generally have antibodies to Ro and/or La and tend to have less renal disease (Maddison *et al.* 1981).

Anti-DNA antibodies

Antibodies to dsDNA are found in between 40 and 90% of patients with SLE. Many studies have shown an association between anti-dsDNA antibodies, particularly IgG antibodies, and the occurrence and severity of renal disease

Table 1.2 Approximate prevalence of antibodies detectable in the serum of patients with SLE

Antibody specificity	Literature (%)	BRU (%)
ANA	>90	94
dsDNA	40–90	60
ssDNA	up to 70	–
Histone	30–80	–
Sm	5–30	9
RNP	20–35	21
Ro	30–40	32
La	10–15	12
Cardiolipin	20–50	25 (G), 13 (M)
LAC	10–20	14
Fc IgG (RF)	25	20
hsp 90	5–50	25 (G), 35 (M)
hsp 70	5–40	5
Thyroid Ags	up to 35	21
C1q	20–45	–

Taken from Morrow *et al.* 1998.
The 'literature' column refers to an approximate range from several published studies.
The BRU column is based on the first 300 patients with SLE under long-term follow-up in the Bloomsbury Rheumatology Unit.
LAC = lupus anticoagulant.
G = IgG; M = IgM; Ags = antigens.
ANA regarded as +ve if titre ≥ 1:80
RF regarded as +ve if titre ≥ 1:80

(Swaak *et al.* 1979; Lloyd and Schur 1981; ter Borg *et al.* 1990; Okamura *et al.* 1993). They have also been shown to correlate with cardio-pulmonary disease and global activity score as assessed by the BILAG index (Isenberg *et al.* 1997). Anti-dsDNA antibodies have been eluted from kidneys in murine models of SLE and antibodies showing anti-nuclear activity that could be partially inhibited by dsDNA have been eluted from the kidneys of patients that have died from renal lupus (Koffler *et al.* 1967).

Antibodies to extractable nuclear antigens

Antibodies to the extractable nuclear antigens (Ro, La, Sm, RNP) can be found in up to one-third of patients. Antibodies to La are particularly associated with the coincidence of Sjögren's syndrome and SLE. Anti-Ro antibodies are associated with photosensitivity, the sub-acute cutaneous form of lupus and possibly with glomerular inflammation, and both antigens are associated with the neonatal lupus syndrome. Antibodies to RNP are associated with undifferentiated autoimmune rheumatic disease, and anti-Sm antibodies, while being virtually diagnostic of SLE, are not associated with any particular disease feature, although they are found with an increased frequency in black lupus patients (30%) compared with Caucasians (5%).

Other autoantibodies

A variety of other autoantibodies have been described in patients with SLE. Antibodies to the nuclear polymer, poly(ADP-ribose) occur as often as anti-DNA antibodies and perhaps reflect clinical activity more accurately than antibodies to double-stranded or single-stranded DNA (Morrow *et al.* 1982). IgM lymphocytotoxic antibodies to both B and T cell populations can occur and appear to correlate with lymphopaenia. Antibodies to ribosomal P proteins occur commonly in Japanese and Malaysian Chinese ethnic groups (up to 35%) and although these antibodies appear relatively specific for lupus, they do not appear specific for neuropsychiatric disease as has been previously suggested (reviewed in Teh and Isenberg 1994). Anti-erythrocyte, anti-platelet and anti-cardiolipin antibodies and lupus anticoagulants can also be often detected. Approximately 25% of patients with lupus have rheumatoid factor, which are usually present in low titre and do not affect the course of the disease. Antibodies to C1q have been described in 20–45% of patients and have been shown to correlate with renal disease (reviewed in Walport *et al.* 1998). Antibodies to the heat shock protein hsp 90 are also present in about one-third of patients with SLE, notably those with central nervous system and cardiovascular involvement (Conroy *et al.* 1994).

Other factors

Immune complexes

The presence of circulating immune complexes in the sera of lupus patients is one of the most important immunopathological characteristics of the disorder. Deposition of immune complexes initiates tissue damage by a number of mechanisms. Patients with lupus have elevated levels of circulating immune complexes but there is not clear correlation with clinical disease and although anti-dsDNA antibodies are the serological hallmark of lupus, this antigen cannot consistently be demonstrated within circulating immune complexes. The study of patients with inherited complement deficiencies led to the suggestion that patients with lupus may have a failure of the physiological clearance mechanisms of immune complexes, perhaps by a reduction of the complement receptor CR1 on the surface of red blood cells, by which opsonized immune complexes are transported to the fixed mononuclear phagocyte system in the liver and spleen (Vaishnaw and Walport 1995).

Complement

The involvement of the complement system has been well studied in the context of SLE. Complement is fixed or consumed by immune complexes and localized in the tissues, particularly the kidney. The cleavage fragments C3a and C5a cause the release of vasoactive amines from mast cells and fragments of C2 can increase vascular permeability. These features allow the localization of immune complexes as well as causing acute inflammation per se. Levels of most of the major complement components are reduced in active disease, although the complement profile may be highly variable from patient to patient. The association of complement component deficiencies with the development of SLE has already been discussed.

Cellular dysregulation

Many functional defects have been identified in cells of the immune system in patients with SLE (reviewed in Morrow *et al.* 1998). These include changes in the number and cell surface expression of a variety of molecules in both B and T cells, utilizing both *in vitro* and *in vivo* experimental systems. Low production of TNF-α is found in DR2- and DQW1-positive donors and the DR-, DQW1 genotype in patients with SLE is associated with lupus nephritis in some populations. Altered levels of IL-1, IL-2, IL-4, IL-6, IL-10 and IFN-γ have also been described.

General management

The treatment of patients with lupus not only includes drug therapy but general advice, particularly in areas such as photoprotection, control of infection, pregnancy, diet and the use of hormone replacement. The pharmacological treatment of patients depends on the individual clinical manifestations, but generally includes combinations of NSAIDs, antimalarials and oral corticosteroids for mild/moderate disease, with the use of more powerful immunosuppressive drugs, such as azathioprine/cyclophosphamide, for the more serious manifestations such as renal or CNS disease, although treatment regimens can be controversial. Arterial and venous thromboses are treated conventionally with heparin/warfarin and patients with antiphospholipid antibodies are often treated prophylactically with aspirin instead of long-term anticoagulation.

Summary

SLE is a disease of great clinical diversity. Its precise aetiology is unknown, but hormonal, genetic, viral and environmental factors appear to interact and cause the disease. Disorders throughout all arms of the immune response are evident, with the presence of a wide range of autoantibodies and other serological abnormalities, such as circulating immune complexes, hypocomplementaemia and hypergammaglobulinaemia. Several independent defects are also found at the cellular level.

Improved management in recent years has led to a reduction in mortality, with a 10-year survival figure of 90%. The development of computerized data bases has aided clinical grading although treatment generally continues to comprise various degrees of immunosuppression, in addition to some other specific therapy.

References

Abu-Shakra, Gladman D.D. and Urowitz M. Malignancy in systemic lupus erythematosus. *Arthritis Rheum* 1996, 39: 1050–4.

Alarcon-Segovia D. and Cabral A.R. The antiphospholipid/cofactor syndromes. *J Rheum* 1996, 8: 1319–20.

Asherson R.A., Khamashta M.A., Ordi-Ros J., Derksen R.H., Machin S.J., Barquinero J., Outt H.H., Harris E.N., Vilardell-Torres M. and Hughes G.R. The 'primary' antiphospholipid syndrome: major clinical and serological features. *Medicine* (Baltimore) 1989, 68: 366–74.

Bombardier C., Gladman D.D., Urowitz M.B., Caron D. and Chang C.H. Derivation of the SLEDAI. A disease activity index for lupus patients. The Committee on Prognostic Studies in SLE. *Arthritis Rheum* 1992, 35: 630–40.

Buyon J.P., Ben-Chetrit E., Karp S., Roubey R.A., Pompeo L., Reeves W.H., Tan E.M. and Winchester R. Acquired congenital heart block. Pattern of maternal antibody response to biochemically defined antigens of the SSA/Ro-SSB/La system in neonatal lupus. *J Clin Invest* 1989, 84: 627–34.

Cohen A.S., Reynolds W.E. and Franklin E.C. Preliminary criteria for the classification of systemic lupus erythematosus. *Bull Rheum Dis* 1971, 21: 643–8.

Conroy S.E., Faulds G.B., Williams W., Latchman D.S. and Isenberg D.A. Detection of autoantibodies to the 90kD heat shock protein in SLE and other autoimmune diseases. *Br J Rheumatol* 1994, 33: 923–6.

Fritzler M.J. Drugs recently associated with lupus syndromes. *Lupus* 1994, 3: 445–9.

Galli M., Compurius P., Maassen C., Hemker H.C., de Baets M.H., van Breda-Vriesman P.J., Barbui T., Zwaal R.F. and Bevers E.M. Anticardiolipin antibodies (ACA) directed not to cardiolipin but to a plasma protein cofactor. *Lancet* 1990, 335: 1544–7.

Gladman D.D., Urowitz M.B. and Goldsmith C.H. The reliability of the Systemic Lupus International Collaborating Clinics/American College of Rheumatology damage index in patients with systemic lupus erythematosus. *Arthritis Rheum* 1997, 40: 809–13.

Haupt H.M., Moore W.G. and Hutchins G.M. The lung in systemic erythematosus. Analysis of the pathologic changes in 120 patients. *Am J Med* 1981, 71: 791–7.

Hay E.M., Bacon P.A., Gordon C., Isenberg D.A., Maddison P., Snaith M.L., Symmons D.P., Viner N. and Zoma A. The BILAG index: a reliable and valid instrument for measuring clinical disease activity in systemic lupus erythematosus. *Q J Med* 1993, 86: 447–58.

Hochberg M.C. Updating the American College of Rheumatology revised criteria for the classification of systemic lupus erythematosus. *Arthritis Rheum* 1997, 40: 1725.

Isenberg D.A., Meyrick-Thomas D., Snaith M.L., McKeran R.O. and Royston J.P. A study of migraine in systemic lupus erythematosus. *Ann Rheum Dis* 1982, 41: 30–2.

Isenberg D.A. and Malick J. Male lupus — the Loch Ness syndrome revisited. *Br J Rheumatol* 1994, 33: 307–8.

Isenberg D.A., Garton M., Reichlin M.W. and Reichlin M. Long-term follow-up of autoantibody profiles in black female lupus patients and clinical comparison with Caucasian and Asian patients. *Br J Rheumatol* 1997, 36: 229–33.

Johnson A.E., Gordon C., Palmer R.G. and Bacon P.A. The prevalence and incidence of systemic lupus erythematosus in Birmingham, England. Relationship to ethnicity and country of birth. *Arthritis Rheum* 1995, 38: 551–8.

Keeling D. and Isenberg D.A. Haematological manifestations of systemic lupus erythematosus. *Blood Rev* 1993, 7: 199–207.

Koffler D., Schur P.H. and Kunkel H.G. Immunological studies concerning the nephritis of systemic lupus erythematosus. *J Exp Med* 1967, 126: 607–24.

Liang M.H., Socher S.A., Roberts W.N. and Esdaile J.M. Measurement of systemic lupus erythematosus activity in clinical research. *Arthritis Rheum* 1988, 31: 817–25.

Libman E. and Sachs B. A hitherto undescribed form of valvular and mural endocarditis. *Arch Intern Med* 1924, 33: 701–38.

Lloyd W. and Schur P.H. Immune complexes, complement and anti-DNA in exacerbations of systemic lupus erythematosus (SLE). *Medicine* 1981, 60: 208–17.

Love P.E. and Santoro S.A. Anti-phospholipid antibodies: anti-cardiolipin and the lupus anticoagulant in systemic lupus erythematosus (SLE) and in non-SLE disorders. *Ann Intern Med* 1990, 112: 682–98.

Maddison P.J., Provost T.T. and Reichlin M. Serological findings in patients with 'ANA-negative' systemic lupus erythematosus. *Medicine* 1981, 60: 87–94.

Mandell B. Cardiovascular involvement in systemic lupus erythematosus. *Sem Arthritis Rheum* 1987, 17: 120–41.

Mellemkjaer L., Andersen V., Linet M.S., Gridley G., Hoover R. and Olsen J.H. Non-Hodgkin's lymphoma and other cancers among a cohort of patients with systemic lupus erythematosus. *Arthritis Rheum* 1997, 40: 761–8.

Morrow W.J.W., Isenberg D.A., Parry H.F., Shen L., Okalie E.E., Farzaneh F., Shall S. and Snaith M.L. Sutdies on autoantibodies to poly (adenosine diphosphate-ribose) in SLE and other autoimmune diseases. *Ann Rheum Dis* 1982, 41: 396–402.

Morrow W.J.W., Nelson J.L., Watts R. and Isenberg D.A. (eds). Systemic lupus erythematosus. In *Autoimmune Rheumatic Disease*, 2nd edn, Oxford Medical Publications, Oxford, 1998, pp. 56–103.

Nived O. and Sturfeldt G. Does the black population in Africa get SLE? If not, why not? In *Controversies in Rheumatology*, Isenberg D.A., Tucker L.B. (eds), Martin Dunitz Ltd, London, 1997, 65–75.

Okamura M., Kanayama Y., Amastu K., Negoro N., Kohda S., Takeda T. and Inoue T. Significance of enzyme linked immunosorbent assay (ELISA) for antibodies to double stranded and single stranded DNA in patients with lupus nephritis: correlation with severity of renal histology. *Ann Rheum Dis* 1993, 52: 14–20.

Pistiner M., Wallace D.J., Nessim S., Metzger A.L. and Klinenberg J.R. Lupus erythematosus in the 1980s: a survey of 570 patients. *Semin Arthritis Rheum* 1991, 21: 55–64.

Stoll T., Stucki G., Malik J., Pyke S. and Isenberg D.A. Association of the Systemic Lupus International Collaborating Clinics/American College of Rheumatology Damage Index with measures of disease activity and health status in patients with systemic lupus erythematosus. *J Rheumatol* 1997, 24: 309–13.

Sultan S.M., Ioannou Y. and Isenberg D.A. A review of gastrointestinal manifestations of systemic lupus erythematosus. *Rheumatology* 1999, 38: 917–32.

Swaak A.J.G., Aarden L.A., Statius van Eps L.W. and Feltkamp T.E. Anti-dsDNA and complement profiles as prognostic guides in systemic lupus erythematosus. *Arthritis Rheum* 1979, 22: 226–35.

Tan E.M., Cohne E.S., Fries S.F., Masi A.T., McShane D.J., Rothfield N.F., Schaller J.G., Talal N. and Winchester R.J. The 1982 revised criteria for the classification of systemic lupus erythematosus. *Arthritis Rheum* 1982, 25: 1271–7.

The L.S. and Isenberg D.A. Antiribosomal P protein antibodies in systemic lupus erythematosus. A reappraisal. *Arthritis Rheum* 1994, 37: 307–15.

ter Borg E.J., Horst G., Hummel E.J., Limburg P.C. and Kallenberg C.G. Measurement of increases in anti-double-stranded DNA antibody levels as a predictor of disease exacerbation in systemic lupus erythmatosus. A long-term, prospective study. *Arthritis Rheum* 1990, 33: 634–43.

Tucker L.B., Menon S., Schaller J.G. and Isenberg D.A. Adult- and childhood-onset systemic lupus erythematosus: a comparison of onset, clinical features, serology and outcome. *Br J Rheumatol* 1995, 34: 866–72.

Vaishnaw A.K. and Walport M.J. Systemic lupus erythematosus. In *Connective Tissue Diseases* eds J.F. Belch and R.B Zurier, Chapman and Hall, London, 1995, pp. 17–50.

Walport M.J., Davies K.A., Morley B.J. and Botto M. Complement deficiency and autoimmunity. *Ann N Y Acad Sci* 1997, 815: 267–81.

Walport M.J., Davies K.A.and Botto M. C1q and systemic lupus erythematosus. *Immunobiology* 1998, 199: 265–85.

Ware J.E. Standards for validating health measures: definition and content. *J Chronic Dis* 1987, 40: 473–80.

2

Clinical manifestations of lupus nephritis

J. Stewart Cameron

Age, sex and prevalence (1,2)

Lupus is not a common disease, but not so rare as sometimes supposed; it may affect individuals of any age race or sex, but is par excellence a disease affecting young black women. It is difficult to obtain prevalence or incidence data for lupus with clinically evident nephritis, which must be lower than that for lupus as a whole, but to which almost all the available data refer. However, the overall prevalence of lupus in the United States has varied in different series from 15 (3) to 51 (4) per 10^5 individuals (average ~40), being highest in black females (ca200/10^5). In predominantly Caucasian populations, prevalence varies from 12 and 28/10^5 in England (5) to 39/10^5 in Sweden) (1,2). The incidence of lupus varied from 1.8 to 7.6/10^5/y, again being highest in black females (8–11) and white females (2–3.5) than in males (1–5). Incidence is much lower in children (0.22/100 000/y) (6) commoner in girls (0.36) than boys (0.08), peaking in black women either from 15–44 years of age, but at a somewhat later amongst caucasians (45–64y) (7). Surprisingly, lupus is relatively rare in the black population of West Africa (8), although it is a little more common in east, south central and southern Africa. Data for Orientals are conflicting; some studies found a prevalence twice that of whites (9,10) but others noted no difference. There is a relatively low prevalence in mainland China, Taiwan, and Japan (1) despite reports of large series from small populations in both Singapore and Hong Kong.

Mortality data from the United States show 1–2 deaths/10^6/y for white males and up to 10–20/10^6/y for black females (1,11). As with incidence data, deaths attributed to lupus peaked at 30–60 years for blacks, whilst for caucasians the peak mortality was over 75 years of age. US data (12) from states with substantial oriental populations noted three times as many deaths amongst blacks and twice as many amongst Orientals as Europeans.

Thus *sex* is the major risk factor for the development of lupus. The female:male ratio rises from 2:1 in prepubertal children up to 4.5:1 throughout older childhood and adolescence to the 8–12:1 reported in most series of adult onset patients, falling back to 2:1 in patients presenting over 60 years of age. An onset of lupus before puberty is distinctly rare, although an onset in the first and second years of life (6,13,14) has been recorded. In females presentation is most commonly in the second and third decades of life (see above): in male patients, the age distribution is the mirror image of females, with peaks before puberty and in middle age.

Differential diagnosis (15)

The commonest other diagnoses made in patients who in fact suffer from lupus are *rheumatic fever, rheumatoid arthritis* and *haemolytic anaemia*. Overall, about 50% of patients with lupus are initially suspected of having a disease other than lupus. The presence of four or more of the ARA criteria (16) give a 96% sensitivity and specificity when applied to a population of patients seen in rheumatology clinics. These criteria have been used widely in situations outside their initial remit, although they do provide security in scientific studies that one is dealing with 'typical' patients. The problem is that in the real world of ward and clinic many patients fall outside this exclusive definition, but still need management and treatment.

Differentiation from *rheumatic fever* is relatively easy, but in a child or young adult with *chorea* is not so easy. Nephritis has been reported in a minority of patients with *mixed connective tissue disease (MCTD)* (17); the differential diagnosis can be difficult clinically, but analysis of the antinuclear antibody for the anti-Ro and anti-La antibodies and the absence of anti-dsDNA antibodies should make the diagnosis clear.

Lupus is often diagnosed to begin with as *rheumatoid arthritis*, but this disease does not usually show systemic features unless vasculitis is present, but on occasion proteinuria will be induced by one of the drugs used in its treatment and cause problems in diagnosis; in addition, rather rarely there may be associated glomerulonephritis other than vasculitic lesions, sometimes proliferative but also membranous in pattern. Some of these patients will go on to develop full clinical and immunological lupus later. The presence of erosions and a deforming arthritis makes lupus unlikely but does not exclude it.

Henoch-Schönlein purpura presents occasional difficulties since some lupus patients also show vasculitis, and others may have predominant IgA in their biopsies. Other forms of vasculitis also can be a source of uncertainty: it may be difficult to interpret ANCA in patients with lupus (18) but some patients do show these antibodies (usually p-ANCA) as well as anti-DNA antibodies (19). Sjögren's syndrome must be differentiated, especially in elderly patients. Patients with haemolytic uraemic syndromes and lupus are discussed below.

Clinical manifestations of lupus nephritis

Patients with lupus and nephritis do not constitute a clear subset with regard to other manifestations, although statistically they tend to have less rash, arthritis and Raynaud's syndrome and more alopecia and oral ulceration. Table 2.1 shows the data from the Eurolupus study (20) and Wallace (21). The main point to emerge is that only 16% of patients present with evident nephritis, raising to one-third later in the course. Nephritis is commoner in early onset and rarer in older patients (Table 2.2) the incidence is no different in males.

Table 2.1 Organ involvement at presentation and during the course of the disease in patients with systemic lupus

Manifestations	At onset No. (%)	During evolution No. (%)	8 Series 1956–1991 (%)
Malar rash	40	58	10–61
Discoid lesions	6	10	NA
Subacute cutaneous lesions	3	6	NA
Photosensitivity	29	45	11–48
Oral ulcers	11	24	7–36
Arthritis	69	84	53–95
Serositis	17	36	31–57
Nephropathy	**16**	**39**	**25–65**
Neurologic involvement	12	27	12–59
Thrombocytopenia	9	22	7–30
Haemolytic anaemia	4	8	2–18
Fever	36	52	41–86
Raynaud phenomenon	18	34	10–44
Livedo reticularis	5	14	NA
Thrombosis	4	14	NA
Myositis	4	9	42–79*
Lung involvement	3	7	1–22
Chorea	1	2	NA
Sicca syndrome	5	16	NA
Lymphadenopathy	7	12	10–59
Weight loss	NA	NA	31–71
Pericarditis	NA	NA	6–45
Hypertension	NA	NA	14–16
Alopecia	NA	NA	3–45

(Data of Cervera *et al.* 1993 (20) and Wallace 1993 (21)).
NA = Not available   * myalgia.

Table 2.2 Prevalence of nephritis in lupus of different ages

	n	% nephritis at onset	% nephritis at any time
Paediatric patients	76	28	46
Normal age patients	834	16	39
Older onset patients*	90	3	22

* Onset over 50 years of age.
(Data of Cervera *et al.* 1993) (20).

Renal lupus with 'normal' urine

Many patients with lupus but apparently without clinical nephritis will show abnormalities in renal biopsies (22–28), usually mild mesangial expansion with immune aggregates visible on immunohistology and/or electron microscopy. Membranous nephropathy may be seen also, and in occasional patients more severe diffuse patterns of nephritis (23). The zeal- and skill-with which the urine is examined, both chemically and by microscopy, will determine how many of such 'silent' nephritis patients are identified. If microalbuminuria is sought, it is usually present (29).

Should these patients with lupus and normal — or nearly normal — urine have renal biopsies? If no *action* is contemplated in the light of the biopsy findings, then the answer must be 'no'. Some observers disagree (26,27) because an occasional patient with more severe forms of nephritis is found. Does treating such patients with corticosteroids at this point prevent or ameliorate evolution into more severe overt disease? We do not know. What happens to such patients? Occasional cases have evolved into renal failure later (23) but the prognosis seems, in general, benign.

Lupus presenting as apparently idiopathic glomerulonephritis

Although multiple organ systems are involved from the onset in most patients with lupus, it is well-recognized that a minority of patients present initially with a single organ system affected. This is most commonly isolated arthralgia, but patients with apparently idiopathic thrombocytopenia are seen in haematology clinics who develop other symptoms and signs later in the disease. Similarly, isolated glomerulonephritis may be seen which 'evolves' later into immunologic and/or clinical lupus (16–30, 17–31, 32,33). The renal biopsy appearance found most frequently in these patients is membranous nephropathy, but a mesangiocapillary pattern is seen also (31). Histological pointers to the diagnosis of lupus nephritis are the presence in the biopsy of a 'full house' of all immunoglobulins and complement components (IgG, IgM, IgA, C3, C4, C1q), of mesangial deposits and irregular of extracapillary aggregates in epimembranous nephropathy, or a mixed pattern of membranous and mesangiocapillary glomerulonephritis (see Chapter 3).

Renal manifestations of clinical lupus nephritis

Thus about 20–50% of unselected patients with lupus have abnormalities of urine tests or renal function early in their course (34–36), and up to 60% of adults and 80% of children may develop overt renal abnormalities later.

Proteinuria (and its consequences) dominate the clinical presentation of lupus nephritis. It is present in almost every patient, often sufficient to be associated with some degree of *oedema*, that is, with a nephrotic syndrome, which is present in about half of lupus patients with nephritis (37,38) (Tables 2.3 and 2.4). The

Table 2.3 Incidence of abnormal urinary findings in unselected patients with lupus

	n = 193	n = 520	
	First test % positive	Any test % positive	First test % positive
Glycosuria	2	2	–
Proteinuria*	48 (2.0 g)	57 (2.9 g)	46
Haematuria	51	51	33
Granular casts	26	35	32
Red cell casts	3	6	8
Fatty casts	–	–	6
Oval fat bodies	–	–	4.4
Waxy casts	–	–	1.7

* Mean daily excretion shown in brackets.
(Data of Fries 1976 (49) and Dubois 1987 (51)).

Table 2.4 Prevalence of nephrotic syndrome in patients with clinically overt lupus nephritis

Author	Reference	Number of patients	% with nephrotic syndrome	Type of clinic
Estes	36	78	49	Rheumatology
Kellum	35	173	29	Rheumatology
Leaker	48	135	34	Nephrology
Adu and Cameron	38	102	59	Nephrology
Cameron	66	179	59	Nephrology
Baldwin	37	98	60	Nephrology

proteinuria of lupus may come and go spontaneously, as noted by Ropes many years ago (39). Today the true natural history is unobtainable, because almost all patients with proteinuria are treated with at least corticosteroids (see Chapters 6 and 7).

About one-quarter of all patients with lupus will show a *nephrotic syndrome* at some time in their course (Tables 2.4–2.6). In series based on renal units the proportion is of course higher, rising to 60% or more. In our data a full nephrotic syndrome was commoner in patients with WHO class III and IV renal biopsy appearances, but the differences were not sufficiently great to be clinically useful in predicting histology. Other observers have noted the same (37). Of 506 nephrotic adults from all causes seen in our unit 1963–86, 55 (10.8%) had lupus, but the proportion varies greatly with age, being highest in the 20s and almost negligible in the elderly. The clinical features of the nephrotic syndrome in patients with lupus do not differ from those with other renal biopsy appearances. It was suggested that *hypercholesterolaemia* is less common or absent in lupus patients with a nephrotic syndrome (40), but later studies (41) and our own unpublished data do not support this suggestion. The prognostic value (or lack of it) of the presence of a nephrotic syndrome at outset has been reviewed (42,43).

The *complications* of the nephrotic syndrome differ a little in patients with lupus. First, the question of accelerated atherogenesis seems much more important, young women or even children suffering myocardial infarcts. This is discussed further in Chapter 7. Second, patients with lupus, with or without anti-phospholipid antibody (Chapter 9) seem to suffer renal venous thrombosis more commonly than other nephrotics (44) with the exception of those with membranous nephropathy, and it is often those lupus patients with a WHO class V membranous pattern who show this complication (45). It may be associated with thrombosis of the vena cava (46); we (47) diagnosed 4/51 nephrotic lupus patients as having renal venous thrombosis in a systematic study, also using

Table 2.5   Renal manifestations of adults with systemic lupus at presentation of renal disease

	All		WHO biopsy Class IV	
Renal presentation	No.	%	No.	%
Nephrotic syndrome	30	37	18	38
Asymptomatic urinary abnormality	30	37	11	23
Rapidly progressive renal failure	20*	24	17*	35
Acute nephrotic syndrome	2	2	2	4
Total	82	100	48	100

* Seven of the patients had proteinuria in the nephrotic range.
(From S. O McLigeyo and J. S Cameron, unpublished data from patients presenting 1980–89 at Guy's Hospital).

Table 2.6   Presentation of children with lupus nephritis, collected from the literature

n	NS >3 g	Prot <3 g/24 h	hematuria Macro/micro	BPup	GFR <80/ P$_{creat}$up	ARF
208	114	89	4	125/159 48/121	103	3
	55%	43%	1.4% 79%	40%	50%	1.4%

NS = nephrotic syndrome, prot = proteinuria, BPup = blood pressure more than 2SD above normal for age, P$_{creat}$up = plasma creatinine of above 125 μmol/l, ARF = acute renal failure requiring dialysis, GFR = glomerular filtration rate or creatinine clearance of less than 80 ml/min. (For details of sources see Cameron (66)).

phlebography; all had class V nephropathy. Coagulation in lupus is discussed in more detail in Chapter 9.

Although persistent *microscopic haematuria* is common, it is never found in isolation, and macroscopic haematuria is very rare; we have seen it only in childhood lupus. Kincaid-Smith and her colleagues (48) have emphasised the prognostic value of quantitating haematuria, both in predicting the severity of renal biopsy appearances and the long-term outlook, a figure of more than 10 rbc/μl being associated with a poorer outlook. No other similar studies have been reported, however.

Urinary casts are present in about one-third of unselected patients (49,50) (Table 2.3) and the urinary sediment often contains *granular casts*, sometimes containing red cells, as well as red cells in excess of normal, depending upon the severity of the nephritis (Table 2.3). A higher proportion of red cell and white cell casts was reported in active lupus nephritis (35/43) by Hebert and colleagues (50), perhaps because the microscopy was performed in the unit on fresh urine.

About 20–50% of patients were assessed as *hypertensive* at presentation (Table 2.7), although these data are necessarily 'soft' given the nature and diversity of age, technique and normal ranges; but surprisingly this was not more common in those with clinical nephritis than those without. However, when the different histological grades of nephritis are examined those with more severe nephritis were more commonly hypertensive (class II, 17%; class IV, 55%) (37,38). The hypertension is not often of great severity; retinopathy is usually mild and accelerated hypertension rare, even in the presence of corticosteroid treatment. If retinopathy is present however, distinguishing which features may arise from the lupus and which from the increased blood pressure may be difficult. Usually retinopathy is a marker for active lupus with involvement of the central nervous system, and carries poor prognosis (52).

Table 2.7 Prevalence of hypertension in systemic lupus

Author	reference	n	% with hypertension
General series			
Dubois	51	520	25
Harvey	34	105	14
Kellum	35	275	43
Estes	36	150	46
Cervera	20	1000	?
Renal unit series			
Adu and Cameron	38	82	27
Leaker	48	135	36
Baldwin	37	98	51
Cameron*	66	79	41

* Collected series of children.

Clinical manifestations of lupus nephritis

Table 2.8 Prevalence of laboratory abnormalities at presentation (20)

| | Literature review | | | |
	Weighted average %	Range in different series %	1000 pts	onset any time
Haematological				
Anaemia	56	45–80	8*	13*
Leukopenia	47	33–66	NA	NA
Thrombocytopenia	25	7–33	16	32
Coombs positive	48	36–65	12	24
PT/PTT prolonged	27	16–70	14	15
IgG anti-cardiolipin antibody	NA	NA	24	26
Immunological				
ANF positive	97	94–100	96	97†
DNA binding raised	75	69–81	77	86†
Anti-Sm	NA		10	
Lupus cells present	84	69–100	NA	NA
C3 low	73	44–90	NA	NA
C4 low	70	65–75	NA	NA
Immune complexes present	70	55–100	NA	NA
Falsely positive Wasserman	21	15–28	NA	NA
CRP raised‡	5	0–10	NA	NA
ESR raised	94	89–100	NA	NA
IgG raised	64	44–67	NA	NA

* Haemolytic anaemia only   † biased by using positivity as a diagnostic feature   ‡ in the absence of infection NA = not available.

Over half of our patients had *reduced renal function* at diagnosis, as judged by a reduced GFR or a raised plasma creatinine (see below for details). Almost all studies report this as an adverse prognostic factor. Prevalence of laboratory test findings at presentation is given in Table 2.8.

Occasional patients with lupus glomerulonephritis present in *acute renal failure* (53), as in our own series, but this is rare. There are several circumstances in which this may be seen. First, there may a diffuse severe crescentic nephritis, but although smaller numbers of crescents frequently complicate class III and IV nephritis (see Chapter 3) this finding is unusual in lupus (54). Second, the glomeruli may show much more widespread capillary thrombi than usual (55), with or without clinical features of overlap with *haemolytic-uraemic syndromes or thrombotic thombocytopenic purpura* (56–60). Some of these patients have anti-phospholipid antibodies in high titre. Unlike those in whom the glomerular thrombi are an isolated feature, the outlook for these patients is bleak; both the patients in our own series in this category died.

Third, a pattern of intense, sometimes isolated *acute interstitial nephritis* may be seen (61–65). This does not seem to correlate with the presence of severe glomerular disease, or with immune aggregates along the tubular basement membrane. Diagnosis can only be made by renal biopsy, since proteinuria may be trivial and the urine findings unimpressive. With dialysis and immunosuppression, the majority of patients recover at least some renal function, but some have died.

Finally, as discussed above, renal vein and (much less commonly) renal arterial thrombosis occurs with some frequency in lupus nephritis, often in the presence but even in the absence of anti-phospholipid antibody, and may be associated with acute deteriorations in renal function (see Chapter 9).

Clinical presentations at different ages and in males

An analysis of more than 800 *children* with lupus from our own experience and the literature (66) showed few differences from the data in adults, and are shown in Tables 2.2 and 2.6. In the Europlupus study also (20) the only clinical differences between paediatric onset patients and adult onset cases were statistically less nephropathy and malar rash at onset. Different opinions have been expressed about presentation of lupus in *older patients*, but a lower incidence of proteinuria (Table 2.2) and a higher incidence of pleuropericarditis has been reported in general (67,68). The difficulties of diagnosis from Sjögren's syndrome in the elderly may account for some of this difference. There have been suggestions in the past that *male patients* differ in various ways from their more numerous female compatriots, but in the large Eurolupus study (20) there were no differences.

Both proximal and distal *renal tubular dysfunction* are present in many patients with lupus, which is not surprising in view of the presence of both tubular basement membrane immune aggregates and the interstitial infiltrate of monocytes and lymphocytes, more impressive and frequent in patients with class III and IV biopsy appearances. However, it is rarely of any clinical significance. In a high proportion of patients (69–73), urinary excretion of light chains and β_2-microglobulin are both increased. Urinary concentration is blunted (72) and hyperkalaemic renal tubular acidosis has been emphasised (73–77). The hyperkalaemia is common, affecting as many as 10% of patients with lupus nephritis (76) and may be a problem, requiring treatment with 9α-fluorohy drocortisone (78). Tubular disease appears to be less common in children with lupus than in adults (78a).

Patients with lupus nephritis may present with complications apparently or putatively associated with *anti-phospholipid antibodies* (Chapter 9). Renal venous thrombosis, renal arterial thrombosis with and without acute renal failure or renal infarction, renal glomerular capillary thrombosis, and thrombotic micro-angiopathy (see above) have all been reported. However the role (if any) of the antibody in precipitating these events in individual patients is often unclear.

Although not strictly a renal manifestation of lupus, nephrologists should be aware that SLE, with or without involvement of the kidney, occasionally may develop or present as a persistent severe *interstitial cystitis* (79–81) even if the patient has never received cyclophosphamide treatment. There is persistent severe dysuria with haematuria but (unless nephritis is present also) otherwise a normal sediment. The bladder wall becomes thickened and obstruction or reflux may develop. Vascular deposits of IgA and complement components may be present. Management is often unsatisfactory, perhaps because of delayed diagnosis in many cases, and despite aggressive immunosuppression urinary diversion may be necessary. In contrast to Wegener's granuloma, the ureters and prostate do not appear to be sites of disease in lupus.

Extra-renal manifestations of lupus

Nephrologists must remain aware of the fact that in treating someone with lupus they will be taking on a patient with actual or potential involvement of many other organ systems. In some patients, either to begin with or as the nephritis comes under control, these other manifestations may come to dominate the clinical picture and its management. Detailed accounts of these may be found in Wallace (21), Wallace and Dubois (82) and Boumpas *et al.* (83). The most common serious additional features are involvement of the central nervous system, and of the heart.

Clinicopathological correlations

This is discussed further in Chapter 3. Whilst it is well known that the more severe histological forms of nephritis tend to have more severe clinical manifestations (84) renal histology cannot be predicted with any certainty from the clinical picture (Table 2.5). For example, although not surprisingly patients with class IV biopsies are significantly more frequently nephrotic, hypertensive and show reduced renal function these do not allow prediction of histology, even between class I/II V and IV, whilst class III is particularly variable in presentation (84). In our own series from 1970–1989, 54 of 109 were hypertensive, but only 39 of these showed class IV biopsies, and 17 class IV patients were normotensive. Renal function is perhaps the best clinical guide: GFR (measured by a single injection isotopic method) averaged 39 ± 33 ml/min/1.73m^2 in 51 class IV patients, 91 ± 35 in 19 class V, and 87 ± 27 in 30 patients showing class II. Patients with class V biopsies often show nephrotic range proteinuria, but normal renal function. Interstitial changes correlate well with GFR at the time of biopsy, both cells (85) and interstitial volume (86), as well as with outcome.

In the great majority of patients by the time a renal biopsy is done, the patient will have received some immunosuppressive treatment, which alters the serological results. We could not show any correlations between titres of anti-dsDNA antibody and histology, as in a number of other published studies, but others (84,87,88) noted higher titres in grade IV biopsies. In our data there was no difference between concentration of complement components in different histological groups.

Amyloidosis and systemic lupus

It is a surprise to find how very rare amyloidosis is in patients suffering from lupus, with or without nephritis; renal amyloid in lupus is extremely uncommon (89–92). However, one of the characteristics of lupus, in contrast to almost all other chronic inflammatory disorders except perhaps ulcerative colitis, is that active lupus is rarely associated with any significant rise in C-reactive protein or serum amyloid A protein in the plasma, unless infection is present also.

Summing up

Thus systemic lupus with nephritis presents with features falling within the usual spectrum of renal syndromes, almost always with some added features of the systemic disease. Proteinuria dominates the presentation of lupus nephritis, and a haematuric presentation is rare.

References

1. Hochberg M.C. The epidemiology of systemic lupus erythematosus. In *Dubois' lupus erythematosus*, eds DJ Wallace and BH Hahn, Lea and Febiger, Philadelphia, 1993, pp. 49–57.
2. Citera G., Wilson W.A. Ethnic and geographic perspectives in SLE. *Lupus* 1993, 2: 351–3.
3. Siegel M., Lee S.L. The epidemiology of systemic lupus erythematosus. *Sem Arthritis Rheum* 1973, 3: 1–54.
4. Fessel W.J. Systemic lupus erythematosus in the community. Incidence, prevalence, outcome, and first symptoms; the high prevalence in black women. *Arch Intern Med* 1974, 134: 1027–35.
5. Johnson A.E., Gordon C., Palmer R.G., Bacon P.A. The prevalence and incidence of systemic lupus erythematosus in Birmingham, England. Relationship to ethnicity and country of birth. *Arthritis Rheum* 1995, 38: 551–8.
6. Lévy M., Montes de Oca M., Babron M.C. Lupus érythemateux disséminé chez l'enfant. Étude collaborative en région parisienne. *Journées Parisiennes de Pédiatrie*. Flammarion, Paris, 1989, pp. 52–58.
7. Nived O., Sturfelt G., Wollheim F. Systemic lupus erythematosus in an adult population in Southern Sweden: incidence, prevalence, and validity of the ARA revised classification criteria. *Br J Rheumatol* 1985, 24: 147–54.
8. Symmons D.P.M. Lupus around the world. Frequency of lupus in people of African origin. *Lupus* 1995, 4: 176–8.
9. Serdula M.K., Rhoads G.G. Frequency of systemic lupus erythematosus in different ethnic groups in Hawaii. *Arthritis Rheum* 1979, 22: 328–33.
10. Maskarinec G., Katz A.R. Prevalence of systemic lupus erythematosus in Hawaii: is there a difference between ethnic groups? *Hawaii Med J* 1995, 54: 406–9.
11. Lopez-Acuña D., Hochberg M.C., Gittelsohn A.M. Mortality from discoid and systemic lupus erythematosus in the United States 1968–78. *Arthritis Rheum* 1982, 25(suppl): S.80.
12. Kaslow R.A. High rate of death caused by systemic lupus erythematosus among US residents of Asian descent. *Arthritis Rheum* 1982, 25: 414–6.

13. Grossman J., Schwartz R.H., Callerame M.L., Condemi J.I. Systemic lupus erythematosus in a one year old child. *Am J Dis Child* 1975, 129: 123–5.
14. Lehman T.J.A., McCurdy D.K., Bernstein B.H., King K.K., Hanson V. Systemic lupus erythematosus in the first decade of life. *Pediatrics* 1989, 83: 235–9.
15. Wallace D.J. Differential diagnosis and disease associations. In *Dubois' lupus erythematosus* eds D.J. Wallace and B.H. Hahn Lea and Febiger, Philadelphia, 1993, pp. 473–84.
16. Tan E.M., Cohen A.S., Fries J.F., Masi A.T., McShane D.J., Rothfield N.F., Schaller J.G., Talal N., Winchester R.J. The 1982 revised criteria for the classification of systemic lupus erythematosus. *Arthritis Rheum* 1982, 25: 1271–7.
17. Cohen I.M., Swerdlin A.H.R., Steinberg S.M., Stone R.A. Mesangial proliferative glomerulonephritis in mixed connective tissue disease. *Clin Nephrol* 1980, 13: 93–6.
18. Schnabel A., Csemok E., Isenberg D.A., Mrowka C., Gross W.L. Antineutrophil cytoplasmic antibodies in systemic lupus erythematosus. Prevalence, specificities and clinical significance. *Arthritis Rheum* 1995, 38: 633–7.
19. Case records of the Massachusetts General Hospital. Case 20–1999. *New Engl J Med* 1999, 341: 110–16.
20. Cervera R., Khamashta M., Font J., Sebastaiani G.D., Gil A., Lavilla P., Doménech I., Aydintug A.O., Jedryka-Góral A., De Ramóh E., Galeazzi M., Haga H-J., Mathieu A., Houssiau F., Ingelmo M., Hughes G.R.V. and the European working party on systemic lupus erythematous. Systemic lupus erythematosus: clinical and immunologic patterns of disease expression in a cohort of 1000 patients. *Medicine* 1993, 72: 113–24.
21. Wallace D.J. The clinical presentation of SLE. In *Dubois' lupus erythematosus*, eds D.J., Wallace and B.H., Hahn, Lea and Febiger, Philadelphia, 1993, pp. 317–21.
22. Hollcraft R.M., Dubois E.L., Lundberg G.D. *et al.* Renal change in systemic lupus erythematosus with normal renal function. *J Rheumatol* 1976, 3: 251–61.
23. Mahajan S.K., Ordoñez N.G., Feitelson P.J., Lim V.S., Spargo B.H., Katz A.I. *Medicine (Baltimore)* 1977, 56: 493–501.
24. Cavallo T., Cameron W.R., Lapenas D. Immunopathology of early and clinically silent lupus nephropathy. *Am J Pathol* 1977, 87: 1–15.
25. Leehey D.J., Katz A.I., Azaran A.H., Aronson A.J., Spargo B.H. Silent diffuse lupus nephritis: longterm follow-up. *Am J Kidney Dis* 1982, 2(suppl 1): 188–96.
26. O'Dell J.R., Hays R.C., Guggenheim S.J., Steigerwald J.C. Systemic lupus erythematosus without clinical renal abnormalities: renal biopsy findings and clinical course. *Ann Rheum Dis* 1985, 44: 415–9.
27. Stamenkovic I., Favre H., Donath A., Assimacopoulos A., Chatelanat F. Renal biopsy in SLE irrespective of clinical findings: longterm follow-up. *Clin Nephrol* 1986, 26: 109–15.
28. Font J., Torras A., Cervera R., Darnell A., Revert L., Ingelmo M. Silent renal disease in systemic lupus erythematosus. *Clin Nephrol* 1987, 27: 283–8.
29. Terai C., Nojima Y., Takano K., Yamada A., Takaku F. Determination of urinary albumin excretion by radioimmunoassay in patients with subclinical lupus nephritis. *Clin Nephrol* 1987, 27: 79–83.
30. Cairns S.A., Acheson E.J., Corbett C.L., Dosa S., Mallick N.P., Lawler W., Williams G. The delayed appearance of an antinuclear factor and the diagnosis. *Postgrad Med J* 1979, 55: 723–7.

31. Adu D., Williams D.G., Taube D., Vilches A.R., Turner D.R., Cameron J.S., Ogg C.S. Late onset systemic lupus erythematosus and lupus-like disease in patients with apparent idiopathic glomerulonephritis. *Q J Med* 1983, 52: 471–87.

32. Simenhoff M.L., Merrill J.P. The spectrum of lupus nephritis. *Nephron* 1964, 1: 348–74.

33. Shearn M.A., Hopper J., Biava C.G. Membranous lupus nephropathy initially seen as idiopathic membranous nephropathy. *Arch Intern Med* 1980, 140: 1521–3.

34. Harvey A.M., Schulman L.E., Tumulty A., Lockard Conley C., Schonrich E.H. Systemic lupus erythematosus. Review of the literature and clinical analysis of 138 cases. *Medicine (Baltimore)* 1954, 33: 291–437.

35. Kellum R.E., Haserick J.R. Systemic lupus erythematosus. A statistical evaluation of mortality based upon a consecutive series of 299 patients. *Arch Intern Med* 1964, 113: 200–7.

36. Estes D., Christian C.L. The natural history of systemic lupus erythematosus by prospective analysis. *Medicine (Baltimore)* 1971, 50: 85–95.

37. Baldwin D.S., Gluck M.C., Lowenstein J., Gallo G.R. Clinical course as related to the morphologic forms and their transitions. *Am J Med* 1977, 62: 12–30.

38. Adu D., Cameron J.S. Lupus Nephritis. In GRV Hughes (ed.) *Systemic lupus erythematosus*. Clinics in Rheumatic Diseases, Vol. 8, No. 1. Philadelphia, Saunders 1982, pp. 153–83.

39. Ropes M.W. Observations on the natural course of disseminated lupus erythematosus. *Medicine (Baltimore)* 1964, 43: 387–91.

40. Shearn M.A. Normocholesterolemic nephrotic syndrome of systemic lupus erythematosus. *Am J Med* 1964, 36: 250–61.

41. Groggel G.C., Cheung A.K., Ellis-Benigni K., Wilson D.E. Treatment of nephrotic hyperlipoproteinemia with gemfibrozil *Kidney Int* 1989, 36: 266–71.

42. Gruppo Italiano per lo Studio della Nefrite del Lupus (GISNEL). Lupus nephritis: prognostic factors and probability of sustaining life-supporting renal function 10 years after diagnosis. *Am J Kidney Dis* 1992, 19: 473–79.

43. Donadio J.V. Jr, Hart G.M., Bergstralh E.J., Holley K.E. Prognostic determinants in lupus nephritis: a long term clinicopathologic study. *Lupus* 1995, 4: 109–15.

44. Hasselaar P., Derksen R.H.W.M., Blokzijl L., Hessing M., Niewwenhius H.K., Bouma B.N., De Groot P.G. Risk factors for thrombosis in lupus patients. *Ann Rheum Dis* 1989, 48: 933–40.

45. Appel G.B., Williams G.S., Melzer J.I., Pirani C.L. Renal vein thrombosis, nephrotic syndrome and systemic lupus erythematosus. *Ann Intern Med* 1976, 85: 310–7.

46. Mintz G., Acevedo-Vasquez E., Guterriez-Espinosa G., Avelar-Garnica F. Renal vein thrombosis and inferior vena cava thrombosis in systemic lupus erythematosus. *Arthritis Rheum* 1984, 27: 539–44.

47. Cameron J.S., Ogg C.S., Wass C.S. Complications of the nephrotic syndrome. In *The nephrotic syndrome*, eds J.S., Cameron, R.J., Glassock, Marcel Dekker, New York, 1988, pp. 849–920.

48. Leaker B., Fairley K.F., Dowling J., Kincaid-Smith P. Lupus nephritis: clinical and pathological correlation. *Q J Med* 1987, 62: 163–79.

49. Fries J.F., Holman H.R. *Systemic lupus erythematosus: a clinical analysis*. Saunders, Philadelphia, 1975.

50. Hebert L.A., Dillon J.J., Middendorf D.F., Lewis E.J., Peter J.B. Relationship between appearance of urinary red blood cell/white blood cell casts and the onset of renal relapse in systemic lupus erythematosus. *Am J Kidney Dis* 1995, 26: 432–8.

51. Wallace D.J., Dubois E.L. *Dubois' lupus erythematosus* Febiger, Philadelphia, 1987.

52. Stafford-Brady F.J., Urowitz M.B., Gladman D.D., Easterbrook M. Lupus retinopathy: patterns, associations and prognosis. *Arthritis Rheum* 1988, 31: 1105–10.

53. Phadke K., Trachtman H., Nicastri A., Chen C.K., Tejani A. Acute renal failure as the initial manifestation of systemic lupus erythematosus in children. *J Pediatr* 1984, 105: 38–41.

54. Yeung C.K., Wong K.L., Wong W.S., Ng M.T., Chan K.W., Ng W.L. Crescentic lupus glomerulonpehritis. *Clin Nephrol* 1984, 21: 251–8.

55. Ponticelli C., Imbasciati E., Brancaccio D., Tarantino A., Rivolta E. Acute renal failure in systemic lupus erythematosus. *Br Med J* 1979, 3: 716–9.

56. Cecere F.A., Yishinoya S., Pope R.M. Fatal thrombotic thrombocytopenic purpura in a patient with systemic lupus erythematosus. Relationship to circulating immune complexes. *Arthritis Rheum* 1981, 24: 550–3.

57. Finkelstein R., Carter A., Marel A., Brook J.G. Plasma infusions in thrombotic thrombocytopenic purpura complicating systemic lupus erythematosus. *Postgrad Med J* 1982, 58: 577–9.

58. Gelfand J., Truong L., Stem L., Pirani C.L., Appel G.B. Thrombotic thrombocytopenic purpura syndrome in systemic lupus erythematosus: treatment with plasma exchange. *Am J Kidney Dis* 1985, 6: 154–60.

59. Bridoux F., Vrtovsnik F., Noel C., Suanier P., Mougenot B., Lemaitre V., Dracon M., Lelievre G., Vanhille P. Renal thrombotic microangiopathy in systemic lupus erythematosus: clinical correlations and long-term renal survival. *Nephrol Dial Transplant* 1998, 13: 298–304.

60. Tuan Le, Nast C.C. Renal biopsy teaching case: TTP-like syndrome in a 44-year old woman with SLE and nephritis. *Am J Kidney Dis* 1999, 33: 1198–201.

61. Case records of the Massachusetts General Hospital. Case no 2-1976. Principal discussant: Epstein F.H. *N Engl J Med* 1976, 294: 100–5.

62. Cunningham E., Prevost J., Brentjens J., Reichlin M., Venuto C. Acute renal failure secondary to interstitial lupus nephritis. *Arch Intern Med* 1978, 138: 1560–1.

63. Tron F., Ganeval D., Droz D. Immunologically-mediated acute renal failure of non-glomerular origin in the course of systemic lupus erythematosus. (SLE). Report of two cases *Am J Med* 1979, 67: 529–32.

64. Cryer P.E., Kissane J.M. Washington University case conference. Interstitial nephritis in a patient with systemic lupus erythematosus. *Am J Med* 1980, 69: 775–81.

65. Gur H., Koplovic Y., Gross D.J. Chronic predominant interstitial nephritis in a patient with systemic lupus erythematosus. A follow-up of three years and review of the literature. *Ann Rheum Dis* 1987, 46: 617–23.

66. Cameron J.S. Lupus nephritis in childhood and adolescence. *Pediatr Nephrol* 1984, 8: 230–49.

67. Wilson H.A., Hamilton M.E., Spyker D.A., Brunner C.M., O'Brien W.M., Davis J.S. IV, Winfield J.B. Age influences the clinical and serological expression of systemic lupus erythematosus. *Arthritis Rheum* 1981, 24: 1230–5.

68. Ward M.M., Studenski S. Age associated clinical manifestations of systemic lupus erythematosus: a multivariate regression analysis. *J Rheumatol* 1990, 17: 476–81.

69. Tu W.H., Shearn M.A. Systemic lupus erythematosus and latent renal tubular dysfunction. *Ann Intern Med* 1967, 67: 100–9.

70. Spriggs B., Epstein W.V. Clinical and laboratory correlates of L-chain proteinuria in systemic lupus erythematosus. *J Rheumatol* 1974, 1: 287–92.
71. Parving H-H., Sorensen F., Mogensen C.E., Helin P. Urinary albumin and β_2-microglobulin excretion rates in patients with systemic lupus erythematosus. *Scand J Rheumatol* 1980, 9: 49–51.
72. Yeung C.K., Wong K.L., Ng R.P., Ng W.L., Tubular dysfunction in systemic lupus erythematosus. *Nephron* 1984, 36: 84–8.
73. Kozeny G.A., Barr W., Bansal V.K., Hano J.E. Occurrence of renal tubular dysfunction in lupus nephritis. *Arch Intern Med* 1987, 147: 891–5.
74. De Fronzo R.A., Cooke C.R., Goldberg M., Cox M., Myers A.R., Agus Z.S. Impaired renal potassium secretion in systemic lupus erythematosus. *Arch Intern Med* 1977, 86: 268–71.
75. Herrera Acosta J., Gurrero J., Erbessd M.L., Pez-Barahona M., Cheskal F., Alarcón Segovia D., Pena J.C. Normotensive hyperreninemia in systemic lupus erythematosus. An indicator of tubular dysfunction. *Nephron* 1978, 22: 128–37.
76. Kiley J., Zager P. Hyporeninemic hypoaldosternism in two patients with systemic lupus erythematosus. *Am J Kidney Dis* 1984, 4: 439–43.
77. Lee F.O., Quismorio F.P., Troum O.M., Anderson P.W., Do Y.S., Hsueh W.A. Mechanisms of hyperkalemia in systemic lupus erythematosus. *Arch Intern Med* 1989, 148: 397–401.
78. Dreyling K.W., Wanner C., Schollmeyer P. Control of hyperkalemia with fludrocortisone in a patient with systemic lupus erythematosus. *Clin Nephrol* 1980, 33: 179–83.
78a. Hataya H., Ikeda M., Ide Y., Kobayashi Y., Kuramochi S., Awazu M. Distal tubular dysfunction in lupus nephritis of childhood and adolescence. *Pediatr Nephrol* 1999, 13: 846–9.
79. De Arriba G., Velo M., Barrio V., Garcia-Martin F., Hernando L. Association of interstitial lupus cystitis with systemic lupus erythematosus. *Clin Nephrol* 1992, 39: 287–8.
80. Koike T., Takabayashi K. Lupus cystitis in the Japanese. *Intern Med* 1996, 35: 87–8.
81. Benghanem Gharbi M., Hachim K., Ramdani B., Fatihi El M., Jabrane A., Zaïd D. Cystite interstitielle lupique. A propos d'un cas. *Néphrologie* 1998, 19: 117–9.
82. Wallace D.J., Dubois E.L. *Dubois' lupus erythematosus*, Lea and Febiger, Philadelphia, 1993.
83. Boumpas D.T., Austin H.A., III, Fessler B.J., Balow J.E., Klippel J.H., Lockshin M.D. Systemic lupus erythematosus: emerging concepts. Part 1: Renal, neuropsychiatric, cardiovascular, pulmonary and hematologic disease. *Ann Intern Med* 1995, 122: 940–50.
84. Hill G.S., Hinglais N., Tron F., Bach J-F. Systemic lupus erythematosus. Morphologic correlations with immunologic and clinical data at the time of biopsy. *Am J Med* 1978, 64: 61–79.
85. Schwartz M.M., Kawala, K.S., Corwin H.L., Lewis, E.J. The prognosis of segmental glomerulonephritis in systemic lupus erythematosus. *Kidney Int* 1987, 52: 274–9.
86. Alexopoulos E., Cameron J.S., Hartley B.H. Lupus Nephritis: correlation of interstitial cells with glomerular function. *Kidney Int* 1990, 37: 100–9.
87. Magil A.B., Ballon, H.S., Chan V., Lirenman D.S., Rae A., Sutton R.A.L. Diffuse proliferative glomerulonephritis. Determination of prognostic significance of clinical, laboratory and pathologic factors. *Medicine* 1984, 63: 210–20.

88. Okamura M., Kanayama Y., Amatsu K., Negoro M., Kohda S., Takeda T., Inoue T. Significance of enzyme-linked immunosorbent assay (ELISA) for antibodies to double stranded and single stranded DNA in patients with lupus nephritis: correlation with severity of renal histology. *Ann Rheum Dis* 1993, 52: 14–20.

89. Klein M.H., Thomer P.S., Yoon S-J., Poucell S., Baumal R. Determination of circulating immune complexes, C3 and C4 complement components and anti-DNA antibody in different classes of lupus nephritis. *Int J Pediatr Nephrol* 1984, 5: 75–82.

90. Huston D.P., McAdam K.P.W.J., Balow J.E., Bass R., De Lellis R.A. Amyloidosis in systemic lupus erythematosus. *Am J Med* 1981, 70: 320–3.

91. Orellana C., Collado A., Hernandez M.V., Font J., Del Olmo J.A., Muñoz-Gomez J. When does amyloidosis complicate systemic lupus erythematosus? *Lupus* 1995, 4: 415–7.

92. Queffelou G., Berentbaum F., Michel C., Mougenot B., Mignon F. AA amyloidosis in systemic lupus erythematosus: an unusual complication. *Nephrol Dial Transplant* 1998, 13: 1846–8.

3

Lupus nephritis: histology

Melvin M. Schwartz

Introduction

The renal biopsy answers critical questions concerning the current status and the long-term prognosis of the kidney in a patient with systemic lupus erythematosus (SLE). To pose the questions, the clinician must understand the limitations imposed on a renal biopsy by sample size considerations. Because SLE glomerular pathology is characteristically focal (only a proportion of the glomeruli are involved), larger samples are more accurate in defining the presence and extent of glomerular involvement. If 10% of glomeruli are actually involved, there is a 35% probability that no abnormal glomeruli will be seen in a biopsy containing only 10 glomeruli. The probability of missing a focal lesion falls to 12% in a biopsy containing 20 glomeruli.[1] The clinician must articulate the critical questions and understand the terms that the pathologist uses to describe the pathology. In turn, the pathologist determines the adequacy of the specimen, describes and quantitates the pathology, and makes a diagnosis that allows comparison between the patient and others with similar histopathology. The biopsy report should contain the diagnosis and the findings that support the diagnosis and, in the end, the clinician should review the biopsy with the pathologist to ensure that he/she understands the pathological diagnosis and its implications.

Renal dysfunction is frequent in SLE,[2] and despite improved survival attributed to therapy, renal involvement remains a significant cause of morbidity and mortality.[3-5] Although broad correlations have been shown between glomerular pathology and the renal manifestations of lupus nephritis, individual patients may show disparity between the clinical presentation and the class of glomerular disease.[6,7] Also, renal dysfunction may be unrelated to SLE: elevated serum creatinine, the most reliable prognosticator in SLE nephritis (reviewed in[7]), may also result from tubular damage due to hemodynamic injury or drug toxicity. The renal biopsy allows an evaluation that is independent of the clinical findings: it distinguishes SLE from non-SLE renal diseases; it identifies which part of the kidney (glomeruli, tubulo-interstitum, blood vessels) is involved; and in SLE glomerulonephritis (GN), the WHO classification[8] allows assignment of lesion specific therapy and prognostication.

This chapter has three goals: to describe the renal pathology of lupus nephritis and the classification of the lesions; to review the prognosis of the WHO classes of glomerular pathology; and to identify the critical questions that may be answered by the renal biopsy.

SLE GN

Pathology

The pathological features of SLE (Table 3.1) denote either 'active lesions' (potentially reversible acute inflammation) or inactive lesions' (irreversible scarring).

Hypercellularity

Proliferation of intrinsic glomerular cells (endothelial, epithelial and mesangial) and infiltration of leukocytes is the most frequent histological finding in SLE GN. Isolated mesangial hypercellularity may be the only sign of inflammation in mild forms of SLE GN, but endocapillary proliferation (endothelial cell proliferation and leukocyte infiltration that occlude the capillary lumen) (Fig. 3.1) and crescent formation (epithelial cell proliferation and leukocyte infiltration in Bowman's space-extracapillary proliferation) (Fig. 3.2) indicate more serious forms of GN.

Wire loop

Wire loops are segmental areas of refractile, eosinophilic, thickening of the glomerular basement membranes seen by light microscopy[9] (Fig. 3.3). They correspond to massive, subendothelial, electron-dense deposits, and to preserve their significance as a sign of severe GN, small subendothelial deposits seen by electron microscopy should not be diagnosed as wire loops.

Table 3.1 Histologic findings considered to reflect the presence or absence of activity of the renal lesions in patients with SLE (modified from[27])

Active lesions	Inactive lesions
Glomeruli	
Local necrosis	Basement membrane thickening
Cellular proliferation	Fibrosis
Karyorrhexis	Adhesions
Fibrinoid	
Wire loops	
Hematoxyphil bodies	
Hyaline thrombi (rare)	
Tubulo-interstitium	
Inflammatory infiltrates	Fibrosis
Tubular necrosis	Tubular atrophy
Edema	
Arteries and arterioles	
Fibrinoid	Arterial sclerosis
Fibrin/Platelet thrombi	Arteriolar hyalinosis
Necrosis	

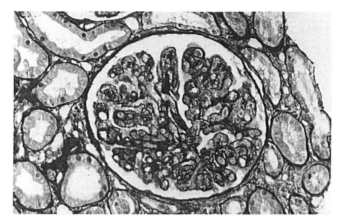

Fig. 3.1 Endocapillary proliferation. Glomerular hypercellularity in SLE GN is usually due to proliferation of cells normally found within the basement membrane (endothelial and mesangial cells) and infiltrating leukocytes (monocytes and neutrophils). In the figure the basement membranes are stained black and the capillary lumens are occluded by the proliferating cells. Jones stain (methenamine silver periodic acid Schiff), ×165.

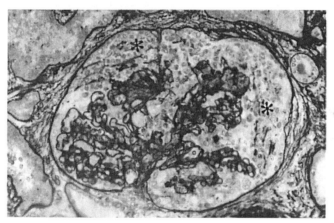

Fig. 3.2 Extracapillary proliferation is synonymous with crescent formation, and it represents a severe form of glomerulonephritis with a poor prognosis when it is widely distributed among the glomeruli. The cells of the crescent are derived from the parietal epithelium of Bowman's capsule and infiltrating monocytes. In this figure the crescent is seen outside the black stained, partially collapsed glomerular capillaries, and it is marked by an asterisk. Jones stain, ×158.

Fibrinoid

Fibrinoid is a reactive extracellular inflammatory exudate (fibrin, serum proteins, immune aggregates, and extracellular matrix proteins such as fibronectin) seen in areas of severe glomerular inflammation that stain purple-red with

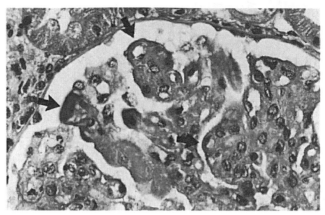

Fig. 3.3 Wire loop. This histological sign of activity is a light microscopic finding. As illustrated in this figure, it comprises a segmental thickening of the glomerular basement membrane by intensely eosinophilic and refractile material (arrow). It represents a large subendothelial electron-dense deposit composed of immune complexes. Hematoxylin and eosin, ×317.

hematoxylin and eosin in contrast to the red-orange colour of normal extracellular matrix.

Necrosis

Necrosis implies a destructive inflammatory lesion that heals with scarring and is frequently associated with crescent formation. The histological diagnosis of necrosis is established by the triad of neutrophilic infiltrates with karyorrhexis, fibrin exudates, and discontinuities (breaks) in the glomerular basement membrane.

Hyalin thrombi

Hyalin thrombi are acellular, eosinophilic, PAS positive masses which occlude the glomerular capillary lumens. They are an infrequent finding in lupus nephritis, and they consist of immune reactants without significant amounts of fibrin.[10–12] They may be distinguished by fluorescence microscopy from fibrin/platelet thrombi (see Vasculitis Chapter 12)

Hematoxylin body

Hematoxylin bodies are smaller than a nucleus and are composed of degenerate nuclear material. They are ill-defined, purple or lilac stained masses seen in foci of severe inflammation. They are distinguished from nuclear dust (karyorrhexis) and apoptotic bodies (dead cells containing fragmented nuclei) by their characteristic staining reaction, size, and appearance. Although hematoxylin bodies are the only pathological finding that is diagnostic of SLE, they are seen in less than 25% of biopsies.

Ultrastructural findings

There are several features visible only with the electron microscope: they are characteristic but not diagnostic of SLE; they may be seen in any WHO class of

SLE GN; and they do not distinguish among the classes. These include tubular reticular structures in endothelial cells[13] and organized electron-dense deposits (fingerprints).

Glomerular scars

Global or segmental glomerular scars are seen either alone or in association with signs of 'active' inflammation. Although glomerular scars imply loss of function, they do not correlate well with glomerular filtration rate or serum creatinine.

WHO classification of glomerular pathology in SLE

Qualitative and quantitative differences in the glomerular lesions in SLE are related to patient and renal outcomes, and the demonstration of acute, potentially reversible pathology provides a therapeutic focus.[14-19] Clinicopathological studies culminated in the detailed classification of the International Study of Kidney Disease in Childhood (ISKDC) (reviewed in[20]) that was subsequently adopted and modified as the World Health Organization Classification (Table 3.2).[8,21] This classification has guided the discourse between clinicians and pathologists and has provided a 'gold standard' for clinical trials. Note that Categories III,

Table 3.2 WHO Classification of SLE GN (modified from[8])

I   Normal Glomeruli
(a) Nil (by all techniques)
(b) Normal by light microscopy, but deposits by electron or immunofluorescence microscopy
II Pure Mesangial Alterations (Mesangiopathy)
(a) Mesangial widening and/or mild hypercellularity (+)
(b) Moderate hypercellularity (++)
III Focal Segmental Glomerulonephritis (associated with mild or moderate mesangial alterations and limited to active segmental lesions in <50% of the glomeruli)
(a) 'Active' necrotizing lesions
(b) 'Active' and sclerosing lesions
(c) Sclerosing lesions
IV Diffuse Glomerulonephritis (severe mesangial, endocapillary or mesangio-capillary proliferation and/or extensive subendothelial deposits; segmental GN involving ≥50% of glomeruli; and membranous GN with Class III or IV proliferative lesions)
(a) Without segmental lesions
(b) With 'active' necrotizing lesions
(c) With 'active' and sclerosing lesions
(d) With sclerosing lesions
V   Diffuse membranous Glomerulonephritis
(a) Pure membranous glomerulonephritis
(b) Associated with lesions of Category II (a or b)
VI Advanced Glomerular Sclerosis

words, biopsies with WHO Class IV have proliferation and/or necrosis in more than 50% of the glomeruli with or without membranous changes.[3] These three patterns of glomerular disease are all included in Class IV because they have similar responses to therapy, and, as a group they have the worst prognosis of all the forms of lupus GN[30,31,35]. The glomeruli contain large amounts of immunoglobulin and complement in the mesangium and capillary walls. Electron microscopy confirms light and fluorescence microscopy findings: electron-dense deposits are seen in the mesangium and on both sides of the glomerular basement membrane.

Class IV patients usually have evidence of active systemic disease, and renal disease frequently dominates the clinical picture.[15,22,23,25,31,36] Despite the overall improved survival for SLE patients,[30,37] Class IV patients continue to have a poor prognosis despite optimal treatment.[3,31] Although *heterogeneous* morphologically, Class IV patients have similar clinical presentations, and 40% have an adverse outcome within five years of biopsy.[3] The poor prognosis of patients with WHO Class IV GN relative to patients with less widely distributed classes of SLE GN makes it imperative to recognize these quantitative differences in the extent of glomerular pathology among patients, and in evaluating therapeutic trials it is critical to note the proportion of Class IV patients because this aspect of study design will directly affect outcome.

Membranous GN (WHO class V)

Class V is characterized by thickened basement membranes seen by light microscopy, but the Jones' stain (methenamine silver periodic acid Schiff) is required to demonstrate the characteristic spikes, holes, and thickening of membranous transformation[38] (Fig. 3.6). The *sine qua non* of Class V is diffuse,

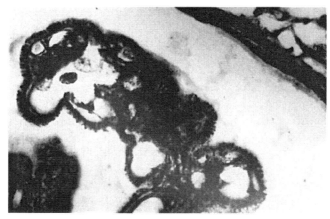

Fig. 3.6 Membranous glomerulonephritis (WHO Class V). This high power photomicrograph shows diffuse thickening of the glomerular basement membrane and 'spikes' projecting from the basement membrane into the subepithelial space. In the WHO classification biopsies qualify for this category only if they have relatively pure membranous changes with mild or moderate mesangial hypercellularity. Segmental or diffuse endocapillary proliferation superimposed upon membranous changes place the biopsy in another class (see text). Jones stain, ×648.

granular, immune aggregates and subepithelial electron-dense deposits that are identical to the deposits seen in idiopathic membranous GN.[39] The granular deposits occur with or without mesangial deposits. Although subepithelial granular deposits may also be seen in Class IV (see above — Diffuse GN), they are segmental and involve a smaller proportion of the capillaries.[40]

Class V patients usually have proteinuria or the nephrotic syndrome, limited evidence of nephritis and renal insufficiency, and mild serologic abnormalities.[15,16,22,24,25,41–43]

Class V occurs in a pure form with no associated glomerular proliferation (Va), and it may also be associated with mild or moderate mesangial proliferation (Vb). When membranous glomerulonephritis is associated with the glomerular pathology of Class IV and/or significant subendothelial deposits, it is included in Class IV.[8] The rationale is that patients with membranous GN and proliferative changes in ≥50% of glomeruli have similar presenting findings, serology, renal function, urinary sediment, levels of protein excretion and adverse clinical outcomes as patients in Class IV.[31,35] Membranous GN associated with proliferative changes in <50% of glomeruli also has a poor prognosis,[42] and these patients should also be included with the proliferative forms of SLE GN for therapeutic purposes.[41]

Chronic GN (WHO class VI)

Glomerular scarring may follow active GN, and after repeated episodes, the glomeruli may show widespread scars. When scarring involves more than 80% of the glomeruli, the biopsy is classified as chronic GN.

Interstitial nephritis

The incidence of interstitial nephritis increases from 14% in Class II to 50% in Class IV.[44] The infiltrates contain lymphocytes, plasma cells, neutrophils and macrophages with tubular injury suggested by atrophy and regeneration, and the extent of interstitial nephritis inversely correlates with renal function.[45] The tubular interstitial lesions may be secondary to glomerular sclerosis and ischemia, but in 50% the presence of extraglomerular immunoglobulin deposits suggest direct tubular injury by immune complex mechanisms.[44–46] Similar histologic findings are seen with drug induced interstitial nephritis and acute tubular necrosis. Because the therapeutic implications are different, deciding whether the tubulo-interstitial lesions are due to SLE or secondary to some other process is critical (see Questions p. 43).

Vasculitis

SLE renal vascular disease may be divided into two categories: lesions accompanying GN that are extensions of immune complex injury to blood vessels, and fibrin and/or platelet thrombi that are renal manifestations of local or systemic hypercoaguable states.

Lupus vasculitis with fibrinoid necrosis, neutrophilic infiltrates and karyorrhexis is an unusual renal biopsy finding, but if the definition of vasculitis is

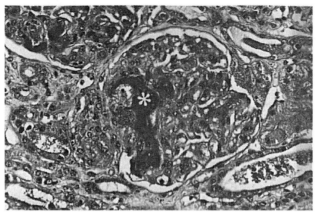

Fig. 3.7 Glomerular thrombus. There is a large thrombus (asterisk) near the glomerular hilum. Thrombotic lesions can be seen in the lupus patients with severe glomerulonephritis, the anticoagulant/antiphospholipid syndrome, hemolytic uremic syndrome, and TTP. Periodic acid Schiff stain, ×226.

expanded to include glomerular necrosis (capillaritis), fibrinoid changes in blood vessels and vascular immune deposits, the prevalence is much higher.[47] Glomerular capillary fibrin thrombi seen in association with severe SLE GN (WHO III and IV) may be caused by the same immunopathologic mechanisms responsible for glomerular inflammation and necrosis.[15]

In addition, there are three coagulopathic syndromes associated with renal vascular and glomerular thrombi: lupus anticoagulant/anti-phospholipid syndrome, hemolytic uremic syndrome (HUS), and thrombotic thrombocytopenic purpura (TTP). The glomerular capillary thrombi are present in variable numbers from occasional capillary thrombi to glomerular casts (Fig. 3.7). They comprise eosinophilic, acellular material that occludes the vessel, and their inconsistent staining for fibrin suggests that they are sometimes principally composed of platelets. Arterial thrombi undergo organization with recanalization of the lumen and reactive mucoid subintimal thickening in the wall of the vessel. The clinical differentiation of the syndromes and their therapeutic implications have been reviewed recently.[48] Although the pathogenesis of thrombus formation is apparently different in TTP and HUS with systemic platelet aggregation caused by an autoantibody to von Willebrand factor metalloproteinase in the former and by localized, renal endothelial damage in the latter,[49] there is considerable morphological overlap, and the pathological features do not distinguish between the two processes.

Histological indices of renal pathology in SLE

Several studies have reported a lack of correlation between the WHO class and outcome[36,50,51] leading to a search for better prognostic and therapeutic guides.

Pathological indices, derived from semi-quantitative scoring of the histological signs of activity and inactivity (Table 3.1), have been proposed, and the National Institutes of Health[52] activity (AI) and chronicity (CI) indices are the most popular examples of this approach. The CI has been used to predict outcome[52,53] and assess therapy.[54] However, the generation and interpretation of the indices has been criticized.[20]

In brief, because numerous studies have failed to show a relation between the AI and outcome, its role as a therapeutic or prognostic guide appears to be unwarranted. When methodological problems are combined with a critique of the interpretation and implications of the chronicity index, its validity is also compromised. Thus, the use of either the AI or the CI as a prognostic or therapeutic guide is problematic. However, as a summary of the active (potentially responsive) and chronic (irreversible) lesions of lupus nephritis, the numerical score(s) of the indices may help the pathologist to communicate the character of the renal pathology to the clinician.

Transformations

Transformations among the WHO classes are frequent.[55] Although they have been documented between all WHO classes,[15] transformations to diffuse GN (WHO IV) from the lesser forms of GN are obviously the most significant. Transformation and glomerular scarring can lead to complex lesions, and the renal pathology in these cases will be a combination of accumulated acute injury and scarring. It should be noted that the WHO classification allows classification of even these complex patterns. In the presence of scarring, the proportion of unscarred glomeruli with 'active' lesions can still serve as a therapeutic guide by providing a quantitative assessment of the extent of inflammatory activity.

Questions to be answered by the renal biopsy

Does the patient have SLE?

The diagnosis of SLE is based upon clinical criteria.[56] Although the biopsy findings are non-diagnostic with the exception of the hematoxylin body, the pathology may be used to support the clinical diagnosis if it establishes the presence of SLE renal disease.

Is renal dysfunction caused by lupus or a non-SLE renal lesion?

Renal insufficiency in SLE may be caused by SLE related glomerular pathology or non-SLE complications such as prerenal hemodynamic factors or a drug related tubulo-interstitial nephritis. In general, if the biopsy shows active SLE GN (Class III or IV), renal insufficiency may be attributed to the glomerular disease. If the biopsy shows one of the less inflammatory forms of glomerular involvement (Class I, II, or V), and there is acute tubulo-interstitial nephritis, a non-lupus etiology of the renal dysfunction should be excluded, clinically. The presence of both lupus GN and tubulo-interstitial damage requires treatment of the glomerular lesion and removal of potentially damaging drugs from the therapeutic regimen.

How severe is the glomerular pathology?

The renal biopsy documents the presence and distribution of pathology among the glomeruli. Using these observations, the pathologist makes a diagnosis based upon the WHO classification. The prognosis (and severity) of the lesion is implicit in the class of the glomerular pathology.

Is the pathology reversible?

Whether the pathology seen on renal biopsy is reversible depends upon the relative contribution of lesions that can be expected to heal with and without scarring. By its nature, SLE GN can heal with scarring, and a glomerular scar implies a loss of function. Although the extent of glomerular scarring does not correlate well with function, the associated tubular atrophy and interstitial fibrosis directly correlate with the creatinine clearance. Thus, the pathology indicates reversibility of the lesion by describing the nature and the extent of glomerular inflammation (potentially reversible in the absence of necrosis) and the extent of glomerular scarring, interstitial fibrosis, and tubular atrophy (irreversible lesions).

How should the patient be treated?

The renal pathology makes a major contribution to the answer of this critical question. Once it has been determined that the patient has lupus nephritis, the biopsy is placed into one of the WHO classes. The glomerular pathology of Class I and II lesions receive limited treatment in the absence of systemic disease activity. The lesion specific treatment of proliferative (Classes III and IV)[57] and membranous (Class V)[58] forms of SLE GN have been recently reviewed. When renal insufficiency results from extensive, irreversible lesions (WHO VI), the renal biopsy may be used to support a decision not to treat.

References

1. Corwin H.L., Schwartz M.M., Lewis E.J. (1988). The importance of sample size in the interpretation of renal biopsy. *Am J Nephrol*, 85–9.
2. Harvey A.M., Shulman L.E., Tumulty P.A., Conley C.L., Schoenrich E.H. (1954). Systemic lupus erythematosus: review of the literature and clinical analysis of 138 cases. *Medicine*, 291–330.
3. Lewis E.J., Hunsicker L.G., Rohde R.D., Lachin J.M. for the Lupus Nephritis Collaborative Study Group (1992). A controlled trial of plasmapheresis therapy in

severe lupus nephritis. The Lupus Nephritis Collaborative Study Group. *N Engl J Med*, 1373–9.

4. Abu-Shakra M., Urowitz M.B., Gladman D.D., Gough J. (1995). Mortality studies in systemic lupus erythematosus. Results from a single center. I. Causes of death. *J Rheumatol*, 1259–64.

5. Rubin L.A., Urowitz M.B., Gladman D.D. (1985). Mortality in systemic lupus erythematosus: the bimodal pattern revisited. *Q J Med*, 87–98.

6. Mahajan S.K., Ordonez, N.G., Feitelson P.J., Lim V.S., Spargo B.H., Katz A.I. (1997). Lupus nephropathy without clinical renal involvement. *Medicine* (Baltimore), 493–501.

7. Esdaile J.M., Levinton C., Federgreen W., Hayslett J.P., Kashgarian M. (1989). The clinical and renal biopsy predictors of long-term outcome in lupus nephritis: A study of 87 patients and review of the literature. *Q J Med*, 779–833.

8. Churg J., Bernstein J., Glassock R.J. (1995). Lupus Nephritis. In *Renal Disease. Classification and Atlas of Glomerular Diseases* Igaku-Shoin, pp. 151–80.

9. Klemperer P., Pollack A.D., Baehr G. (1941). Pathology of disseminated lupus erythematosus. *Arch Pathol*, 569–631.

10. McPhaul J.J. Jr (1978). Cryoimmunoglobulinemia in patients with primary renal disease and systemic lupus erythematosus. *Clin Exp Immunol*, 131–40.

11. Conte J., Blanc M., Mignon-Conte M., Aubal M., Orfila C. (1974). Cryoglobulinemie au cours des glomerulonephrites: Etude de 130 cas. *J Urol Nephrol*, 773–85.

12. Druet P., Letonturier P., Contet A., Mandet C. (1973). Cryoglobulinemia in human renal disease; A study of seventy-six cases. *Clin Exp Immunol*, 483–96.

13. Rich S.A. (1981). Human lupus inclusions and interferon. *Science*, 772–5.

14. Muehrcke R.C., Kark R.M., Pirani C.L., Pollak V.E. (1957). Lupus nephritis: A clinical and pathologic study based on renal biopsies. *Medicine*, 1–146.

15. Baldwin D.S., Gluck M.C., Lowenstein J., Gallo G.R. (1977). Lupus nephritis. Clinical course as related to morphologic forms and their transitions. *Am J Med*, 12–30.

16. Baldwin D.S., Lowenstein J., Rothfield N.F., Gallo G., McCluskey R.T. (1970). The clinical course of the proliferative and membranous forms of lupus nephritis. *Ann Intern Med*, 929–942.

17. Striker G.E., Kelly M.R., Quadracci L.J., Scribner B.H. (1973). The Course of Lupus Nephritis. A Clinical-Pathological Correlation. In *Glomerulonephritis* eds P. Kincaid-Smith, T.H. Mathew, E.L. Becker, John Wiley and Sons, pp. 1141–1166.

18. Cameron J.S., Ogg C.S., Boulton Jones M. (1973). Lupus Nephritis: Long-Term Follow-up. In *Glomerulonephritis* eds P. Kincaid-Smith, T.H. Mathew, E.L. Becker, John Wiley and Sons, pp. 1187–1192.

19. Pollak V.E., Pirani C.L., Dujovne I., Dillard M.G. (1973). The Clinical Course of Lupus Nephritis: Relationship to the Renal Histologic Findings. In *Glomerulonephritis* eds P. Kincaid-Smith, T.H. Mathew, E.L. Becker, John Wiley and Sons, pp. 1167–1182.

20. Schwartz M.M. (1999). The pathological classification of lupus nephritis. In *Lupus nephritis* eds E.J. Lewis, M.M., Schwartz, S.M. Korbet Oxford University Press, pp. 126–158.

21. Churg J. and Sobin L.H. (1982). Lupus Nephritis. In *Renal disease, classification and atlas of glomerular diseases* Igaku-Shoin, pp. 127–149.

22. Pollak V.E., Pirani C.L., Schwartz F.D. (1964). The natural history of the renal manifestations of systemic lupus erythematosus. *J Lab Clin Med*, 537–550.
23. Morel-Maroger L., Mery J.P., Droz D., Godin M., Verroust P., Kourilsky O., Richet G. (1976). The course of lupus nephritis: contribution of serial renal biopsies. *Adv Nephrol Necker Hosp*, 79–118.
24. Hill G.S., Hinglais N., Tron F., Bach J.F. (1978). Systemic lupus erthematosus. Morphologic correlations with immunologic and clinical data at the time of biopsy. *Am J Med*, 61–79.
25. Sinniah R. and Feng P.H. (1976). Lupus nephritis: correlation between light, electron microscopic and immunofluorescent findings and renal function. *Clin Nephrol*, 340–351.
26. Appel G.B., Silva F.G., Pirani C.L., Meltzer J.I., Estes D. (1978). Renal involvement is systemic lupus erythematosus (SLE): A study of fifty-six patients emphasizing histologic classification. *Medicine*, 371–410.
27. Pirani C.L., Pollak V.E., Schwartz F.D. (1964). The reproducibility of semiquantitative analyses of renal histology. *Nephron*, 230–237.
28. Dujovne I., Pollak V.E., Pirani C.L., Dillard M.G. (1972). The distribution and character of glomerular deposits in systemic lupus erythematosus. *Kidney Int*, 33–50.
29. Dillard M.G., Tillman R.L., Sampson C.C. (1975). Lupus Nephritis. Correlations between the clinical course and presence of electron-dense deposits. *Lab Invest*, 261–269.
30. Schwartz M.M., Kawala K.S., Corwin H.L., Lewis E.J. (1987). The prognosis of segmental glomerulonephritis in systemic lupus erythematosus. *Kidney Int*, 274–279.
31. Schwartz M.M., Lan S.P., Bonsib, S.M., Gephadt G.N., Sharma H.M. and the Lupus Nephritis Collaborative Study Group (1989). Clinical outcome of three discrete histologic patterns of injury in severe lupus glomerulonephritis. *Am J Kidney Dis*, 273–283.
32. Grishman E. and Churg J. (1982). Focal segmental lupus nephritis. *Clin Nephrol*, 5–13.
33. Gourley M.F., Austin H.A. III, Scott D., Yarboro C.H., Vaughan E.M., Muir J., Boumpas D.T., Klippel J.H., Balow, J.E., Steinberg A.D. (1996). Methylprednisolone and cyclophosphamide, alone or in combination, in patients with lupus nephritis. A randomized, controlled trial. *Ann Intern Med*, 549–557.
34. Austin H.A. and Balow J.E. (1999). Natural history and treatment of lupus nphriti. *Semin Nephrol*, 2–11.
35. Schwartz M.M., Bernstein J., Hill G.S., Holley K., Phillips E.A., The Lupus Nephritis Collaborative Study Group (1989). Predictive value of renal pathology in diffuse proliferative lupus glomerulonephritis. *Kidney Int*, 891–896.
36. Magil A.B., Ballon H.S., Rae A. (1982). Focal proliferative lupus nephritis. A clinicopathologic study using the W.H.O. classification. *Am J Med*, 620–630.
37. Gladman D.D. (1995). Prognosis and treatment of systemic lupus erythematosus. *Curr Opin Rheumatol*, 402–408.
38. Ehrenreich T. and Churg J. (1968). Pathology of membranous nephropathy. In *Pathology Annual* ed. W.C. Sommers, pp. 145–186.
39. Jennette J.C., Iskandar S.S., Dalldorf F.G. (1983). Pathologic differentiation between lupus and nonlupus membranous glomerulopathy. *Kidney Int*, 377–385.
40. Schwartz M.M., Roberts J.L., Lewis E.J. (1982). Subepithelial electron-dense deposits in proliferative glomerulonephritis of systemic lupus erythematosus. *Ultrastruct Pathol*, 105–118.

41. Schwartz M.M., Kawala K., Roberts J.L., Humes C., Lewis E.J. (1984). Clinical and pathological features of membranous glomerulonephritis of systemic lupus erythematosus. *Am J Nephrol*, 301–311.
42. Sloan R.P., Schwartz M.M., Korbet S.M., Borok R.Z. The Lupus Nephritis Collaborative Study Group (1996). Long-Term Outcome in Systemic Lupus Erythematosus Membranous Glomerulonephritis. *J Am Soc Nephrol*, 299–305.
43. Pasquali S., Banfi G., Zucchelli A., Moroni G., Ponticelli C., Zucchelli, P. (1993). Lupus membranous nephropathy: long-term outcome. *Clin. Nephrol*, 175–182.
44. Park M.H., D'Agati V., Appel G.B., Pirani C.L. (1986). Tubulointerstitial disease in lupus nephritis: relationship to immune deposits, interstitial inflammation, glomerular changes, renal function, and prognosis. *Nephron*, 309–319.
45. Schwartz M.M., Fennell J.S., Lewis E.J. (1982). Pathologic changes in the renal tubule in systemic lupus erythematosus. *Hum Pathol*, 534–547.
46. Magil A.B. and Tyler M. (1984). Tubulo-interstitial disease in lupus nephritis. A morphometric study. *Histopathology*, 81–87.
47. Appel G.B., Pirani C.L., D'Agati, V. (1994). Renal vascular complications of systemic lupus erythematosus. *J Am Soc Nephrol*, 1499–1515.
48. Appel G.B. (1999). Renal vascular involvement in SLE. In *Lupus Nephritis* eds E.J. Lewis, M.M. Schwartz S.M., Korbet, Oxford University Press, pp. 241–261.
49. Moake J.L. (1998). von Willebrand factor in the pathophysiology of thrombotic thrombocytopenic purpura. *Clin Lab Sci*, 362–364.
50. Appel G.B., Cohen D.J., Pirani C.L., Meltzer J.I., Estes D. (1987). Long-term follow-up of patients with lupus nephritis. A study based on the classification of the World Health Organization. *Am J Med*, 877–885.
51. Ponticelli C., Zucchelli P., Moroni G., Cagnoli L., Banfi G., Pasquali, S. (1987). Long-term prognosis of diffuse lupus nephritis. *Clin Nephrol*, 263–271.
52. Austin H.A., III, Muenz L.R., Joyce K.M., Antonovych T.A., Kullick M.E., Klippel J.H., Decker J.L., Balow J.E. (1983). Prognostic factors in lupus nephritis. Contribution of renal histologic data. *Am J Med*, 382–391.
53. Austin H.A.I., Muenz L.R., Joyce K.M., Antonovych T.A., Balow J.E. (1984). Diffuse proliferative lupus nephritis: Identification of specific pathologic features affecting renal outcome. *Kidney Int*, 689–695.
54. Austin H.A.I., Klippel J.H., Balow J.E., le Riche N.G., Steinberg A.D., Plotz P.H., Decker J.L. (1986). Therapy of lupus nephritis. Controlled trial of prednisone and cytotoxic drugs. *N Engl J Med*, 614–619.
55. Hill G.S. (1992). Systemic lupus erythematosus. In *Pathology of the Kidney* ed. R.H. Heptinstall, Little Brown and Company, pp. 871–950.
56. Tan E.M., Cohen A.S., Fries J.F., Masi A.T., McShane D.J. Rothfield N., Talal N., Winchester R.J. (1982). The 1982 revised criteria for the classification of systemic lupus erythematosus. *Arthritis Rheum*, 1271–1277.
57. Lewis E.J. (1999). The natural history and treatment of lupus nephritis. In *Lupus nephritis* eds E.J. Lewis, M.M. Schwartz S.M. Korbet, Oxford University Press, pp. 185–218.
58. Korbet S.M. (1999). Membranous lupus glomerulonephritis. In *Lupus nephritis* eds E.J. Lewis, M.M. Schwartz, S.M. Korbet, Oxford University Press, pp. 219–240.

4

Lupus nephritis: complement in lupus

Michael G. Robson and Mark J. Walport

Introduction

Complement is a system of proteins with activities that include the recruitment of inflammatory cells, cellular activation, cell lysis, antimicrobial defence, clearance of immune complexes, and amplification of the humoral immune response (1, 2). There are three pathways of activation of complement. The classical pathway is activated by immune complexes, initiated by the binding of C1q to the Fc portion of immunoglobulin (3). The alternative pathway is activated by C3 either spontaneously, in the fluid phase, or by 'activator' surfaces on microorganisms or damaged cells lacking control mechanisms expressed on normal host tissues (4). The mannose-binding lectin (MBL) pathway is initiated by mannose-binding lectin and its MBL-associated serine proteases MASP1 and MASP2 (5). These have homology with C1q and C1r/s respectively. MBL binds to carbohydrate residues on bacteria, and activates C4 by a pathway analogous to the classical pathway. The cleavage of C3 is the central event in complement activation by all three pathways. This generates C3b and C3a, as well as the formation of the C5 convertases, allowing terminal pathway activation (6). A simplified diagram of the complement system is shown in Figure 4.1. The complement system is tightly regulated by a range of control proteins (7). Although there is evidence that immune complexes can activate the alternative pathway of complement in some situations, they initiate the classical pathway far more readily. Classical pathway activation is a feature of systemic lupus erythematosus because immune complexes containing autoantibodies and nuclear components cause much of the pathogenesis of this disease. This classical pathway activation is reflected in the fact that C1q, C4 and C3 are depleted from serum, and deposited in the tissues.

This chapter is divided into three parts. First, the serological abnormalities of the complement system that are seen in patients with lupus will be described, with a discussion of the aetiology and clinical utility of these findings. Second, the localization of complement components in tissue samples of patients with lupus using immunohistochemical or immunofluorescent techniques will be reviewed, followed by some comments on the evidence that this complement activation contributes to tissue injury. The third section discusses the association of homozygous genetic deficiencies of complement proteins with SLE that is seen in a small minority of patients. This is followed by an account of the theories that may explain this link.

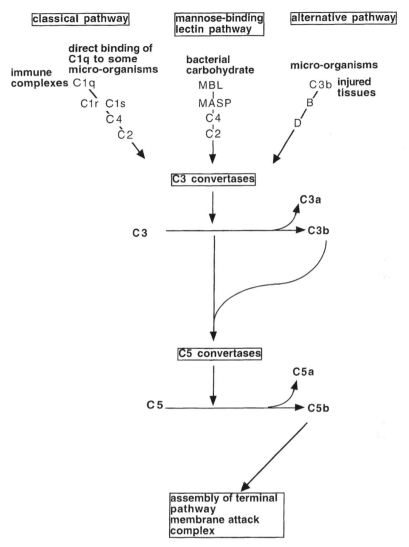

Fig. 4.1 Overview of the complement system showing formation of C3 and C5 convertases by the classical, lectin and alternative pathways.

Serological abnormalities of the complement system

There are two categories of serological abnormalities of complement that are commonly seen in patients with lupus. These are: hypocomplementaemia due to activation and consumption of complement components; and autoantibodies to complement proteins. This section will discuss these in turn. Primary genetic deficiency of classical pathway components, although strongly associated with

62. Albert M.L., Sauter B. and Bhardwaj N. Dendritic cells acquire antigen from apoptotic cells and induce class I- restricted CTLs. *Nature* 1998, 392: 86–9.
63. Mevorach D., Zhou J.L., Song X. and Elkon K.B. Systemic exposure to irradiated apoptotic cells induces autoantibody production. *J Exp Med* 1998, 188: 387–92.

5

Pathogenesis of lupus nephritis for rheumatology and the kidney

Michael P. Madaio

Introduction

Renal involvement occurs in the majority of patients with lupus sometime during their lifetime (Chapter 2). Many variable aspects of nephritis among patients (e.g. the severity of initial inflammation, response to therapy, relapse rate, recurrence following renal transplant) indicate that multiple immunologic and non-immunologic parameters influence both the initial clinical presentation and the subsequent course. In general, breakdown in immunologic tolerance leads to the production of autoreactive cells that either through direct infiltration (e.g. T cells, macrophages) and/or through their secretory products (e.g. autoantibodies, cytokines) initiate inflammation. The degree of inflammation is determined by the extent of this invasion along with both the systemic and local response to the assault. The intensity of inflammation coupled with the renal response to these events influences both disease severity and the extent of fibrosis. Immunosuppressive therapy improves renal outcome (Chapters 2 and 3), although some patients progress to renal failure despite aggressive treatment. When caring for patients with lupus nephritis, it is essential to realize that non-immunologic factors (e.g. systemic hypertension, the propensity to develop fibrosis) influence outcome regardless of the initiating events, and therefore, recognition of the contribution of these parameters is essential for effective therapy (1–3). Thus, individuals with apparently similar immunologic and pathologic profiles may progress to renal failure at different rates, despite similar therapeutic interventions. This chapter focuses mainly on the immunologic factors that contribute to disease.

Genetic contributions

Much has been learned from both the study of families with lupus and inbred strains of mice that spontaneously develop disease. Overall, the results indicate that there is a genetic susceptibility to develop lupus (4–15). A few points are worth emphasizing. First multiple genes are operative. They influence both susceptibility to lupus in general (Chapter 1) and susceptibility to nephritis among lupus patients. MHC and Fc receptor genes have been most extensively studied, and some have been linked to autoantibody production and disease, although the associations vary with the populations studied (4–15) (6). Inherited deficiencies of

Table 5.1 Evidence for participation of antibodies, cells and inflammatory mediators in lupus nephritis (selected*)

AutoAb/ IgG	– Type and severity of disease associated with immunoglobulin deposition, isotype of deposited Ig, location and quantity of immune deposits.
	– Autoantibodies (some, but not all) produce nephritis after transfer to normal animals.
	– Lupus-prone mice without B cells do not develop glomerulonephritis, interstitial nephritis or vasculitis; however lupus prone mice with B cells that express surface Ig but do not secrete Ig develop lesions.
	– Lupus-prone mice without CD40L do not get nephritis.
FcR	– FcR phenotype associated with lupus and lupus in some populations but not others.
	– Lupus-prone mice without FcR have reduced nephritis, despite Ig deposition.
	– Treatment of lupus-prone mice with high dose GCSF results in decreased FcR γIII expression and less disease.
T cells	– Prognosis associated with severity of interstitial nephritis, in part due to cellular infiltration.
	– Interstitial infiltrates in human lupus consist of macrophages and T cells.
Macrophages/ Co-stim mol.	– Immunosuppressive therapy that limits T cell activation, reduces nephritis.
	– Lupus-prone mice without $\alpha\beta$T cells have less disease, despite presence of immune deposits;
	– Lupus prone mice without either class II molecules or β2M have less nephritis.
	– Activated macrophages are present within interstitial lesions, where they express proinflammatory and fibrogenic cytokines;
	– Transfer of macrophages exacerbates disease.
	– In lupus-prone mice, therapy directed at interruption of cellular interactions involving T cells reduces disease activity (e.g. CD40-CD40L; CTLA4 Ig; anti-LFA 1; anti-ICAM).
	– Either cyclosporine or thymectomy prevents disease in some lupus prone strain.
	– Lupus-prone mice without class II molecules have reduced autoantibodies and nephritis.
	– Treatment of lupus prone mice with either anti-LFA 1 or anti-ICAM attenuates nephritis.
	– Class II, CD40 increased in renal tubular epithelial cells lupus nephritis.

Table 5.1 Evidence for participation of antibodies, cells and inflammatory mediators in lupus nephritis (selected*) *continued*

Cytokines/ Chemokines	– Cytokine and chemokine overexpression/suppression in lupus-prone mice alters disease by influencing both systemic autoimmunity and local inflammation. – In sclerotic areas, TGF-β receptors are increased in mesangial cells and epithelial cells. – Interferon γ, MIP-1, MCP 1, CSF-1 TGF-β, PDGF and TNF-α implicated in lupus nephritis, whereas Rantes, IL-8 and others have mediate inflammation and fibrosis in other models of nephritis. – Perforin is decreased in murine lupus nephritis. – MIP-1 and MCP 1 are upregulated in human nephritis via CCR5. – Proinflammatory cytokines (e.g. TNF, sVCAM) increased in urine of patients with lupus nephritis. – Procoagulants (e.g. plasminogen) upregulated in lupus nephritis.

* See text for references.

Cellular contributions: T cells, B cells macrophages, renal cells and inflammatory mediators

There is a complex interplay among these constituents that occurs through both cell–cell contact and secretion of soluble mediators. Evidence for participation is derived from demonstration of their presence within tissue, correlation of levels with disease activity, extrapolation from other inflammatory diseases, and experiments in lupus-prone mice where individual factors and cells have been either eliminated or suppressed. Regarding the latter, although elimination of the individual participants in experimental animal models of lupus nephritis prior to disease onset often prevents disease, elimination/suppression of established disease by targeted therapy is more difficult. Application to patients with lupus nephritis has been even more trying. Nevertheless, further definition of the pathophysiological events that leads to nephritis, perpetuate inflammation and foster fibrosis should provide the basis for more rationale therapy in the future. A summary of recent studies, where contributions of individual components were evaluated, is indicated in Table 5.1 (13,43,45,47,48,65, 75–99,100).

Conclusions

Multiple cells and soluble factors participate in the initiation and perpetuation of lupus nephritis. Variable disease expression, responsiveness to therapy, and disease progression commonly observed among patients is typical: this is both genetically determined and under the influence of environmental and exogenous factors. In human lupus, T cell dependent, autoantibody production leads pression in lupus nephritis and other glomerulonephritides. *Arthritis Rheum* 40: 124–34, 1997.

99. Zavala F., Masson A., Hadaya K., Ezine S., Schneider E., Babin O., Bach J.F. - conver Granulocyte-colony stimulating factor treatment of lupus autoimmune disease in MRL-1pr/1pr mice. *J Immunol* 163: 5125–32, 1999.

100. Tesch G.H., Maifert S., Schwarting A., Rollins B.J., Kelley V.R. Monocyte chemoattractant protein 1-dependent leukocytic infiltrates are responsible for autoimmune disease in MRL-Fas(1pr) mice. *J Exp Med* 190: 1813–24, 1999.

6

Lupus nephritis: Treatment – pulse cyclophosphamide

Kazuki Takada, Dimitrios T. Brumpas, and Gabor G. Illei

Historical background

Before the discovery of cortisone and its introduction into clinical practice, lupus nephritis was a leading cause of mortality in patients with SLE with a mean survival of less than two years after diagnosis (Muehrccke *et al.* 1957; Pollak *et al.* 1961). The use of corticosteroids and better control of comorbid conditions improved survival in lupus patients. Improved longevity revealed the true incidence of kidney involvement by SLE and led to increases in the proportion of patients that succumbed to renal failure. Corticosteroid treatment resulted in modest benefits (Pollak *et al.* 1961; Kagan and Christian 1966) but was frequently associated with debilitating and life-threatening toxicities, and the prognosis of lupus nephritis remained poor.

Immunosuppressive drug therapy for lupus nephritis was initially based on responses seen in animal models, and case reports and small series published in humans (Fox and McCune 1994). An early study on azathioprine with corticosteroid showed improvement in survival rate, fewer hospitalizations, and decreasing corticosteroid requirement (Sztejnbok *et al.* 1971). The benefit of azathioprine, however, may have been overestimated in this study (Steinberg 1986), and subsequent trials demonstrated modest benefits, at best (Decker *et al.* 1975; Steinberg and Decker 1974; Donadio *et al.* 1974; Donadio *et al.* 1972). Nitrogen mustard was the first alkylating agent to be studied in patients with lupus nephritis (Dubois 1954). Severe side effects, including local tissue injury, vascular damage, and nausea and vomiting, rendered it undesirable for long-term administration (Fox and McCune 1994), and over the last few decades cyclophosphamide became the most widely used alkylating agent.

Cyclophosphamide is metabolized to 4-hydroxycyclophosphamide by P450 isoenzymes in the liver. 4-hydroxycyclophosphamide is in steady state with its acyclic tautomer, aldophosphamide, which cleaves non-enzymatically to generate phosphoramide mustard and acrolein (Chabner *et al.* 1995). Phosphoramide mustard is the therapeutically active compound and is believed to be responsible for alkylation and crosslinking of DNA, while the acrolein is responsible for bladder toxicity. Besides depleting B and T lymphocytes, cyclophosphamide was also shown to modulate T-cell activation responses and B-cell antibody production (Aisenberg 1973; Cupps *et al.* 1982; Varkila and Hurme 1983). Based on its effectiveness in the treatment of murine lupus (Russell and Hicks 1968; Steinberg *et al.* 1983; Steinberg *et al.* 1975; Miller and Steinberg 1983; Steinberg *et al.* 1972), as well as anecdotal reports in humans (Cameron *et al.* 1970; Feng *et al.* 1973; Hadidi 1970), controlled clinical trials were started in the late 1960s both at the National Institutes of Health (NIH) and the Mayo Clinic.

Overview of clinical trials

Thirty-eight patients with diffuse glomerulonephritis were randomized by Steinberg and colleagues at the NIH to maintenance dose prednisone with daily oral cyclophosphamide (for at least six months), azathioprine, or placebo (Steinberg and Decker 1974). Donadio and colleagues at Mayo Clinic randomized 50 patients with progressive lupus glomerulonephritis to daily oral cyclophosphamide (six months), or placebo both with maintenance dose prednisone (Donadio *et al.* 1974; Donadio *et al.* 1972). Both studies showed favourable short-term results of continuous oral cyclophosphamide. The superiority of cyclophosphamide in controlling renal disease over azathioprine or prednisone, however, became less obvious after an extended follow-up (Donadio *et al.* 1978; Decker *et al.* 1975). Furthermore, daily oral cyclophosphamide was restricted to short-term use due to anticipated toxicities such as bladder complications (Elliott *et al.* 1982), infections and neoplasias (Calabresi 1983; Puri and Campbell 1977).

To reduce the toxicity and increase the efficacy, alternative means of administration of cyclophosphamide were explored. Intermittent bolus administration of cyclophosphamide was shown to be at least as effective as daily treatment in murine models of lupus nephritis (Steinberg *et al.* 1972). This method limits the exposure to cyclophosphamide to only a fraction of the time, and its risk/benefit advantage over daily oral cyclophosphamide was demonstrated in oncology studies.

Proof of comparable advantage of pulse cyclophosphamide over corticosteroids alone in human lupus nephritis was realized stepwise, in long-term studies. In the first of a series of clinical trials at the NIH, Dinant *et al.* (1982) randomized 41 patients with lupus nephritis to prednisone alone, daily oral cyclophosphamide and oral azathioprine, or quarterly intravenous bolus cyclophosphamide. To minimize bladder toxicity, all doses of intravenous bolus cyclophosphamide were followed by vigorous hydration. Both regimens containing cyclophosphamide were superior to prednisone alone in controlling renal function (Dinant *et al.* 1982) and in attenuating renal pathologic changes over time (Balow *et al.* 1984). An extended follow-up of the study showed that only intermittent bolus cyclophosphamide had a statistically significant benefit over prednisone alone in maintaining renal function (Austin *et al.* 1986). In a landmark study, Austin *et al.* (1986) compared high dose prednisone to four different immunosuppressive regimens. Of these, only pulse intravenous cyclophosphamide reduced the risk of end-stage renal disease significantly; 1/21 (5%) patient treated with cyclophosphamide progressed to end-stage renal disease compared to 10/28 (35%) treated with high doses of corticosteroids. The study also supported the relative safety of pulse cyclophosphamide over continuous daily administration. Although herpes zoster infections and premature ovarian failure were more common in patients receiving any cyclophosphamide-containing regimen, the frequency of these complications was significantly reduced with pulse therapy. Moreover, no patient in the intermittent bolus cyclophosphamide group had hemorrhagic cystitis compared to 17% in the oral cyclophosphamide group (Austin *et al.* 1986). The demonstrated efficacy of intermittent bolus cyclophosphamide and the greater risks for cumulative side effects with daily cyclophosphamide has rendered the former the preferable approach. Patients in this study were treated with cytotoxic drugs until clinical remission had been sustained for at least 18 months or until approximately four years of protocol treatment had been completed.

In an attempt to define the optimal length of therapy and compare the efficacy of high dose pulse corticosteroids to pulse cyclophosphamide Boumpas *et al.* compared a six month course of monthly methylprednisolone boluses to a shorter (six months) and a longer ($\geq$18 months) course of cyclophosphamide (Boumpas *et al.* 1992). Patients treated with the long course of cyclophosphamide were significantly less likely to double their serum creatinine or progress to end-stage renal disease. The rate of exacerbation of lupus nephritis was also lower in patients who were treated with a long course compared to a six-month course of cyclophosphamide.

To evaluate the possibility that the superior outcome seen in this trial with the long course of cyclophosphamide was solely due to the shorter duration of pulse methylprednisolone treatment, a longer course of methylprednisolone was compared to cyclophosphamide by Gourley *et al.* (1996). In this study, patients randomized to monthly boluses of methylprednisolone received at least one year and up to a maximum of three years of therapy. Based on animal experiments and anecdotal experience in humans suggesting that cyclophosphamide may be more effective when given with substantial doses of corticosteroids, a third group was assigned to receive both methylprednisolone and cyclophosphamide boluses. The primary outcome in this study was the rate of renal remission, defined as proteinuria < 1 gram/day, inactive urinary sediment and stable serum creatinine. Compared to the methylprednisolone group, remission was achieved in significantly higher number of patients treated with cyclophosphamide alone or in combination. The probability of doubling of serum creatinine was lower in the cyclophosphamide groups, with the combination group achieving and the cyclophosphamide group approaching statistical significance. Although renal outcomes did not differ significantly between the cyclophosphamide and combination groups at the end of the five-year follow-up, a trend towards higher rate of remission and lower rate of relapses was noted in the combination group compared to cyclophosphamide alone. Compared to methylprednisolone, patients receiving cyclophosphamide had a higher rate of premature amenorrhea, serious infections, herpes zoster infection and cervical dysplasia. The addition of methylprednisolone to cyclophosphamide resulted in a marginal increase in the numbers of avascular necrosis (5/28 vs. 3/27) and herpes zoster infections (6/28 vs. 4/27).

An extended follow-up (median follow-up 11 years) of the study cohort demonstrated persistent benefit of cyclophosphamide and the combination of cyclophosphamide and methylprednisolone compared to methylprednisolone alone (Illei *et al.* 2000). Although no overall difference was seen in mortality or the rate of progression to end-stage renal disease among the three groups in an intention to treat analysis, the majority of the patients who received methylprednisolone initially, required cyclophosphamide eventually for the control of continuous renal activity or renal flare. To further evaluate treatment effectiveness, we used a composite end-point to capture all important aspects of treatment failure, including death, doubling of serum creatinine, or the need for additional immunosuppressive therapy not specified in the protocol. All patients were included, regardless of the length of therapy or whether they completed the protocol. In this analysis, patients receiving cyclophosphamide or combination therapy were significantly less likely to experience treatment failure than those in the methylprednisolone group. Although no statistical difference was seen between the cyclophosphamide and the combination groups in this analysis, the number of patients reaching the composite end-point was lower in the combination group (8/28, 28%) than in the cyclophosphamide group (13/27, 48%). Among patients who had completed the protocol, the rate of 50% increase or doubling of creatinine was significantly lower in the combination group compared to the cyclophosphamide group. No patient who completed protocol treatment in the combination group experienced doubling of serum creatinine after a median follow-up of 11 years. The addition of methylprednisolone boluses to cyclophosphamide did not result in added toxicity. It is of interest that the rates of adverse events frequently seen with corticosteroids, such as avascular necrosis of the bone and osteoporosis, were not higher when methylprednisolone was added to cyclophosphamide. On the other hand, using methylprednisolone alone as initial therapy did not result in lower rates of premature amenorrhea, a predictable complication of cyclophosphamide (Illei *et al.* 2000).

The effectiveness of pulse cyclophosphamide was also evaluated in a number of small, open label prospective or retrospective studies in adults (Belmont *et al.* 1995; Chu *et al.* 1994; Ciruelo *et al.* 1996; Dooley *et al.* 1997; Eiser *et al.* 1993; Ioannidis *et al.* 2000; Lehman *et al.* 1989; Martinelli *et al.* 1996; Sesso *et al.* 1994; Yan *et al.* 1995) and children (Baqi *et al.* 1996). The largest prospective study by Dooley *et al.* (1997) showed an overall five-year renal survival similar to the NIH trials. Moreover, the toxicities of the regimen, employed in diverse clinical settings outside the confines of a rigorous clinical study, were not different from reported clinical trials. Renal survival was significantly worse in blacks compared with non-black patients, a finding supported by others (Bakir *et al.* 1994; Belmont *et al.* 1995; Baqi *et al.* 1996; Conlon *et al.* 1996). Among white patients, renal survival was 95% at five years whereas black patients showed a progressive yearly decline to 58% at five years. The factors that predispose black patients to more aggressive and treatment-resistant lupus nephritis were not apparent. Racial differences in renal outcome were independent of age, duration of lupus, control of hypertension and activity or chronicity indices on renal biopsy.

Other investigators have attempted to maximize the efficacy of cyclophosphamide pulses by combining it with plasmapheresis (Euler *et al.* 1994), a strategy termed by some investigators 'stimulation and deletion' or 'synchronization' (Lewis *et al.* 1992). This strategy is based on the assumption that high dose cyclophosphamide administration after a series of plasmapheresis increases the deletion of pathogenic clones activated by the removal of autoantibodies. In a multicentre clinical trial 151 patients were randomized to receive three daily plasmapheresis followed by intravenous pulse cyclophosphamide every month or pulse cyclophosphamide alone. After six cycles of treatment, the reduction of disease activity was almost identical in both arms with a higher incidence of adverse effects in the plasmapheresis group (Schroeder *et al.* 1997). Similar conclusions were reached by Wallace *et al.* (1998) who randomized 18 patients with proliferative lupus nephritis to either synchronized plasmapheresis or cyclophosphamide boluses for six months. No significant differences between the two groups were found during the two-year follow up (Wallace *et al.* 1998). Moreover, Aringer *et al.* (1998) noticed more frequent life-threatening bacterial and viral infections among patients treated with plasmapheresis and pulse cyclophosphamide when compared to carefully matched patients treated with cyclophosphamide alone.

Administration of pulse cyclophosphamide

Based on these studies we suggest the following algorithm for pulse cyclophosphamide therapy. Patients with focal or diffuse proliferative glomerulonephritis without other risk factors (Table 6.1) could be treated with a limited trial of oral prednisone (1 mg/kg/day) first. If a complete response occurs within eight weeks, prednisone should be tapered to alternate day (0.25 mg/kg) and patients should be monitored for flares. If patients have incomplete or no response, they should be treated with monthly pulse cyclophosphamide. For those with diffuse proliferative and severe focal proliferative glomerulonephritis, we recommend monthly pulse cyclophosphamide in combination with prednisone 1.0 mg/kg/day, as initial treatment. Patients with rapidly progressive disease or multiple adverse prognostic factors are best treated with the combination of pulse cyclophosphamide and methylprednisolone (1 gm intravenously before each dose of cyclophosphamide) for the first six months. Prednisone should be tapered after the first month to 0.25 mg/kg every other day by the end of the third month. After the first six months, most patients receive maintenance therapy with quarterly cyclophosphamide boluses. If preservation of fertility is high priority, one could consider alternative maintenance therapies (e.g. azathioprine-2 mg/kg/d, mycophenolate mofetil-2 g/d, alternate day prednisone-0.25 mg/kg/d or cyclosporine- less than 5 mg/kg/d) in patients who responded to the cyclophosphamide induction regimen with complete or partial remission (proteinuria less than 1 gm/day, clearing of cellular casts, normalization of complement and stable or improved renal function). These patients should be monitored closely for flares.

Table 6.1   Features of severe lupus nephritis

Demographic
Black race
Male gender

*Clinical and laboratory**
Failure to achieve or marked delay, i.e. >3 months, to renal remission
Multiple relapses of lupus nephritis
Renal insufficiency
Anemia (i.e. Hct ≤26)

*Renal pathology**
Mixed membranous and proliferative glomerulonephritis
Proliferative glomerulonephritis (focal or diffuse) with fibrinoid necrosis and/
   or cellular crescents
Very high activity index
Moderate-to-high chronicity index (especially tubular atrophy and/or interstitial fibrosis)
Combinations of active (e.g. cellular crescents or fibrinoid necrosis) and chronic
   histologic features (e.g. tubular atrophy or interstitial fibrosis)

---

* These features, when present alone or in combination, are indications for cytotoxic therapy.

Daily oral cyclophosphamide, 2 mg/kg/d for 2–6 months is uncommonly being used to induce remission because of its increased toxicity. Controlled, randomized studies are in progress in Europe to compare the efficacy of cyclosporine versus azathioprine to decrease renal flares after remission with a short course of oral cyclophosphamide. In the USA a controlled study is comparing pulses of cyclophosphamide to mycophenolate mofetil as initial therapy for proliferative lupus nephritis.

Table 6.2 describes our protocol for pulse cyclophosphamide therapy. Pulse cyclophosphamide is usually administered in an outpatient setting as intravenous infusion. Alternatively, equivalent dose of cyclophosphamide can be taken orally in highly motivated patients (Dawisha *et al.* 1996). It is critically important to adjust the dose of cyclophosphamide to renal function. Decreased glomerular filtration rate prolongs the half-life of cyclophosphamide and its metabolites; inappropriately high doses can be associated with life-threatening bone marrow suppression. We recommend that doses of cyclophosphamide should be increased gradually to achieve moderate leukopenia at the expected 10–14 day nadir. Use of low doses of cyclophosphamide which do not affect white blood cell counts has been advocated by some investigators (Martin-Suarez *et al.* 1997), but this may lead to ambiguity whether the expected clinical response is due to cyclophosphamide resistance or to inadequate dosing. Protection of the urinary bladder against toxicity of cyclophosphamide metabolites is accomplished by forced diuresis, mesna treatment, frequent voidings and diuretics (as needed) for at least 12 hours after pulse cyclophosphamide. Newer antiemetic drugs (serotonin receptor antagonists) have greatly improved the tolerability of pulse cyclophosphamide (Yarboro *et al.* 1996).

Table 6.2 Recommendation for administration of pulse cyclophosphamide therapy

- Estimate glomerular filtration rate (GFR) by standard methods.
- Calculate body surface area (m²):

$$BSA = \sqrt{\frac{\text{height (cm)} \times \text{weight (kg)}}{3600}}$$

- Cyclophosphamide (Cytoxan) (CY) dosing and administration:
  Initial dose CY is 0.75 g/m² (*important note*: start with 0.5 g/m² of CY if
    glomerular filtration rate is less than one-third of expected normal).
  Administer CY is 150 ml normal saline IV over 30–60 minutes (*alternative*:
    equivalent dose of pulse CY may be taken orally in highly motivated and
    compliant patients).
- Obtain WBC at days 10 and 14 after each CY treatment (*note*: advise patient to delay
  taking prednisone until after blood tests are drawn to avoid transient steroid-induced
  leukocytosis).
- Adjust subsequent doses of CY to keep nadir WBC above 1,500/ µL (escalate CY to
  maximum dose of 1.0 g/m² unless WBC nadir falls below 1,500/µL).
- Repeat CY doses monthly (every 3 weeks in patients with extremely aggressive
  disease) for 6 months, then quarterly for one year *after* remission is achieved;
  remission is defined by inactive urine sediment, proteinuria <1 g/day, and a state of
  minimal or no activity of extrarenal lupus (also, ideally, normalization of serum
  complement and anti-DNA).
- Protect bladder against CY-induced hemorrhagic cystitis.
  Induce diuresis with 5% dextrose and 0.45% saline (e.g. 2 litres at 250 ml/hr) and
    encourage frequent voiding; continue high dose oral fluids through 24 hours;
    counsel patients to return to clinic if they cannot sustain ingestion of enteral
    fluids.
  Give mesna (Mesnex) (each dose 20% of total CY dose) intravenously or orally at
    0, 2, 4, and 6 hours after CY dosing (*note*: use of mesna strongly urged
    whenever sustained diuresis may be difficult to achieve, or if pulse CY is given
    in outpatient setting).
  If patients anticipated to have difficulty with sustaining diuresis (e.g. severe
    nephrotic syndrome) or with voiding, insert a 3-way Foley catheter with
    continuous bladder flushing with standard antibiotic irrigating solution (e.g.
    3 litres) for 24 hours to minimize risk of hemorrhagic cystitis.
- Antiemetics (usually administered orally)
  Dexamethasone (Decadron) 10 mg single dose *plus*:
  Serotonin receptor antagonists: granisetron (Kytril) 2 mg with CY dose;
    alternative: ondansetron (Zofran) 8 mg tid for 1–2 days (more expensive)
- Monitor fluid balance during diuresis: if patient develops progressive fluid
  accumulation, use diuretics to re-establish fluid balance.

From Balow *et al.* (1998), with permission.

Although there are no established guidelines in general we consider discontinuing cyclophosphamide for failure to achieve remission. This is defined as continuous activity after a protracted period (e.g. 3–5 years) of treatment with
adequate doses of cyclophosphamide. A renal biopsy in these cases may help to

resolve any ambiguity, i.e. whether there is a residual active disease or whether there are fixed non-reversible lesions. It is important to realize that lupus nephritis can have a slow response to immunosuppressive therapy and that cyclophosphamide can have delayed effects. Therefore, one should not abandon therapy if renal disease is active after 6–12 months, unless there is a definite worsening of the disease. In these cases, exclusion of non-lupus related causes of deterioration of renal function (hypertension, dehydration, nephrotoxic drugs) is essential. Complete renal remission can also be delayed by more than two years. Patients failing pulse cyclophosphamide could be treated with mycophenolate mofetil (2 g/d) alone or in combination with low-dose cyclosporine (2–3 mg/kg/d). However, experience with these regimens is limited to small case series with relatively short-follow-up (Dooley *et al.* 1999; Glicklich and Acharya 1998).

Development of irreversible chronic renal insufficiency is another indication for discontinuing treatment. This category includes patients with prolonged (≥3 months) dialysis-dependent renal failure, not explained by other factors; steadily rising serum creatinine ≥6 mg/dl; inactive urinary sediment with broad and/or waxy casts; contracted kidney size (<3/4 of expected normal) or renal biopsy showing exclusively scarring, atrophy, and fibrosis.

Adverse effects of pulse cyclophosphamide

Pulse cyclophosphamide is associated with short-term and long-term adverse effects. Common short-term adverse effects include reversible alopecia, nausea and vomiting, and bone marrow suppression. Alopecia is less common than with oncologic doses; however, it is unpredictable and patients should be warned about the possibility before the treatment. Nausea and vomiting used to be a dose-limiting side effect of cyclophosphamide but is less of a problem now with the use of the newer serotonin receptor antagonist antiemetics (Yarboro *et al.* 1996).

Bone marrow suppression and infection

Transient bone marrow suppression after pulse cyclophosphamide administration is dose-dependent. Leukopenia is the first to appear as cyclophosphamide dose is increased, and often is dose limiting in order to keep its efficacy and toxicity from infection well balanced. In the NIH studies the dose of cyclophosphamide was adjusted to keep nadir leukocyte counts on days 10–14 after treatment above 1,500/μl.

An increased rate of herpes zoster infections has been associated with cyclophosphamide in most studies. No significant difference in the incidence of major infections was observed in patients treated with pulse cyclophosphamide compared to other immunosuppressive agents or corticosteroids in most studies (Austin *et al.* 1986; Boumpas *et al.* 1993). Cyclophosphamide boluses alone or in combination with methylprednisolone were associated with a higher rate of major infections at five years in another study (Gourley *et al.* 1996). Long-term follow-up of this study, however, showed no difference in the cumulative rates of major infections after a median of 11 years of follow-up.

Bladder toxicity

Urotoxicity caused by acrolein, a breakdown product of cyclophosphamide (Brock *et al.* 1981a; Brock *et al.* 1982; Brock *et al.* 1981b), was of great concern with the use of cyclophosphamide and other oxazaphosphorines. Hemorrhagic cystitis was seen frequently with high doses and long-term daily administration of cyclophosphamide, and often limited dose and duration of treatment (Klein and Smith 1983). Moreover, the appearance of bladder cancer long after oxazaphosphorine therapy has also been reported (Talar-Williams *et al.* 1996). Hyperhydration with forced diuresis was shown to be effective in reducing the incidence and severity of this complication (Droller *et al.* 1982). Cyclophosphamide doses used in the pulse treatment of lupus nephritis are much smaller, and these bladder complications were essentially eliminated with vigorous hydration (Dinant *et al.* 1982). In 1978 Brock *et al.* discovered the protective effect of sodium 2-mercaptoethane-sulfonate (mesna). The uroprotective effect of mesna is due to its unique pharmacokinetics. After parenteral or oral administration, mesna is rapidly oxidized to an inactive disulfide, which remains in the intravascular space. After glomerular filtration, mesna disulfide permeates into the kidney epithelium and is reduced to the free active mercapto compound which reacts with and detoxifies acrolein in urine (Brock 1996). Its relative efficacy over hyperhydration with forced diuresis is uncertain (Hows *et al.* 1984; Shepherd *et al.* 1991; Vose *et al.* 1993). Maintaining adequate diuresis is the best and only proven intervention in preventing bladder toxicity. It may be prudent, however, to administer mesna with modest amount of hydration when vigorous hydration is not possible due to renal, cardiac, or other reasons. Using this protocol we have only seen one case of hemorrhagic cystitis after several years of treatment in a patient who refused to take mesna and was not complaint with directions for hydration and voiding. Studies in patients receiving oral cyclophosphamide therapy have suggested that urine cytology is not useful in screening for bladder carcinoma (Talar-Williams *et al.* 1996). Although the risk for bladder carcinoma is very small after pulse cyclophosphamide therapy, development of unexplained non-glomerular hematuria in these patients after pulse cyclophosphamide therapy should probably include cystoscopy in the diagnostic work-up.

Malignancy

The concern about drug-induced neoplasias has limited the use of cyclophosphamide in various rheumatic diseases. Long-term studies of daily oral cyclophosphamide in patients with rheumatoid arthritis found that approximately 10% of patients developed cyclophosphamide-induced malignancies involving the urinary tract, bone marrow, or skin (Baker *et al.* 1987; Baltus *et al.* 1983; Radis *et al.* 1995). Incidence of treatment-induced malignancy seems to be related to high cumulative dose (Gmelig-Meyling *et al.* 1992). In the 20-year follow-up study of Radis *et al.* the mean total dose of cyclophosphamide in those who developed malignancy was 79.0 gm compared with 41.2 gm in those without malignancy, with 53% risk of malignancy in patients receiving more than 80 gm (Radis *et al.* 1995). In fact, the controlled studies of pulse cyclophosphamide for lupus nephritis did not report increased incidence of malignancy except for increased incidence of cervical dysplasia (Austin *et al.* 1986; Boumpas *et al.* 1992). Increased vigilance in monitoring for gynecologic malignancies is therefore essential.

Gonadal failure

Gonadal failure occurs in both women and men who receive alkylating agents. This is of significant concern in the treatment of lupus nephritis since the majority of patients are women of reproductive age. Cyclophosphamide leads to follicular death by damaging rapidly dividing granulosa cells, which produce estrogen and progesterone to nurse developing follicles. Decreased production of gonadal steroids stimulates pituitary gonadotropin production, which further enhances recruitment of follicles into the pool of maturing follicles susceptible to cyclophosphamide. The resultant vicious cycle results in hypergonadotropic hypogonadism and accelerated irreversible depletion of ovarian oocytes (approximately 300,000–400,000 at menarche) (Slater *et al.* 1999). A study of women treated for breast cancer reported that the average dose of cyclophosphamide administered before the onset of amenorrhea in women in their twenties, thirties, and forties were 20.4 g, 9.3 g, and 5.2 g (Koyama *et al.* 1977). In their retrospective analysis of women treated with intermittent pulse cyclophosphamide for lupus nephritis, Boumpas *et al.* reported an age and dose-dependent relationship between cyclophosphamide and the rate of sustained amenorrhea. Treatment with a short course (≤ 7 pulses) of cyclophosphamide resulted in sustained amenorrhea in 0% of patients under 25 years of age, 12% of patients aged 26–30 years, and 25% of patients aged 31 years or over. On the other hand, 17% of patients under 25 years of age, 43% of patients aged 26–30 years, and 100% of patients aged 31 years or over experienced sustained amenorrhea after a long course (≥ 15 pulses) of cyclophosphamide (Boumpas *et al.* 1993). Several other retrospective studies in lupus nephritis also showed that sustained amenorrhea was dependent on route of administration, age of patient at the initiation of cyclophosphamide therapy, cumulative dose, and duration of therapy (Wang *et al.* 1995; Belmont *et al.* 1995; Boumpas *et al.* 1993; Langevitz *et al.* 1992; Bermas and Hill 1995; Rivkees and Crawford 1988).

Recent animal and human studies suggest that gonadotropin-releasing hormone agonist (GnRH-a) may prevent accelerated recruitment and depletion of ovarian follicles via suppression of FSH and LH production in the pituitary gland, and therefore protect against premature ovarian failure (Blumenfeld and Haim 1997). Further clinical trials, however, are needed to better demonstrate its efficacy and to balance it against its deleterious effect on bone mineral metabolism (Dlugi *et al.* 1990; Fogelman 1992; Scialli *et al.* 1993; Johansen *et al.* 1988; Dawood *et al.* 1995; Fogelman *et al.* 1994). Its use in cyclophosphamide therapy for lupus nephritis should be considered with caution since patients often require treatment for a few years or longer. 'Add-back' use of estrogen alone or in combination with progesterone with GnRH-a for prevention of bone mineral loss is another point of controversy (Arden *et al.* 1994; Buyon *et al.* 1995) because of the prothrombotic events and potential risk for exacerbating SLE itself.

The mechanism for transient or permanent azoospermia observed in men is less clear, but it is implied that cyclophosphamide damages germinal cells with increased mitotic activity. Masala *et al.* reported the efficacy of testosterone in preserving fertility in patients with nephrotic syndrome treated with a short course of cyclophosphamide (Masala *et al.* 1997). Fifteen patients were treated with either daily oral cyclophosphamide, monthly intravenous cyclophosphamide, or monthly intravenous cyclophosphamide with testosterone (100 mg intramuscularly every 15 days) for a total of 6–8 months, and all 15 patients became azoospermic during cyclophosphamide therapy. Six months after the discontinuation of therapy, all five patients who received testosterone recovered normal sperm count compared to only one of 10 patients without testosterone. Further investigations are needed to evaluate the effect of GnRH-a and testosterone on the preservation of fertility in patients treated with cyclophosphamide.

Future directions

Although aggressive immunosuppressive therapy with cyclophosphamide has improved renal survival in lupus nephritis, it is not uniformly effective and is associated with potentially serious toxicities. Investigators continue to explore new treatments for lupus nephritis, searching for agents or their combinations with equal or improved efficacy and reduced toxicities. Some of the novel approaches include cyclophosphamide in immuno-ablative doses with or without bone marrow transplantation, or combinations of cyclophosphamide with nucleoside analogues or with biological response modifiers. Another approach includes short-course use (3–6 months) of oral (3 months) or intravenous (6 months) cyclophosphamide to induce substantial improvement or remission followed by maintenance therapy with other agents such as azathioprine, cyclosporin A, or mycophenolate mofetil to prevent relapse.

High dose cyclophosphamide without bone marrow transplantation

Improvement or prolonged remission of autoimmune diseases after bone marrow ablation and allogeneic transplantation in animal models (Knaan-Shanzer *et al.* 1991; Karussis *et al.* 1992; Karussis *et al.* 1995) and in humans with concurrent malignancies prompted investigators to evaluate this procedure as a potentially effective and possibly curable therapy for various autoimmune diseases with poor prognosis. High-dose cyclophosphamide therapy without bone marrow transplantation has emerged as an alternative to this approach. Preliminary clinical results in patients with refractory autoimmune diseases, including lupus, were published by Brodsky *et al.* Patients in this study were able to recover from cyclophosphamide-induced pancytopenia without bone marrow transplantation, demonstrating that hematopoietic stem cells survive high-dose cyclophosphamide (Brodsky *et al.* 1997), in part due to their high level expression of aldehyde dehydrogenase (Jones *et al.* 1996; Gordon *et al.* 1985), an enzyme responsible for cellular resistance to cyclophosphamide. The short-term clinical response of the underlying diseases was cautiously encouraging. Further studies with longer follow-up are necessary, however, to better evaluate the risk-benefit ratio of high-dose cyclophosphamide.

Combination of cyclophosphamide with fludarabine

Fludarabine is a halogenated adenosine analogue with a high specificity for lymphoid cells. Based on in vitro studies showing synergistic effect of nucleoside analogues with cyclophosphamide (Plunkett and Gandhi 1997), a combination of fludarabine and cyclophosphamide has been used in chronic lymphocytic leukemia with encouraging preliminary results (O'Brien *et al.* 1994). Since both B and T lymphocytes are thought to be pathogenic in lupus, lymphocyte depletion is a theoretically useful approach to treat lupus nephritis. Fludarabine causes a profound lymphopenia (B>T cells), but B cell counts return to pretreatment levels within 3–6 months after discontinuation of therapy. In contrast, regeneration of T cells is slower and may take more than 1–2 years. Low lymphocyte counts and decreased T cell function after fludarabine require increased vigilance in monitoring for infections (Davis *et al.* 1998). A Phase I/II study combining monthly low-dose oral cyclophosphamide boluses with fludarabine in lupus nephritis is in progress at the NIH.

Biological response modifiers alone or in combination with cyclophosphamide

Costimulatory molecules such as B7-CD28 and CD40-CD40L pairs of cell surface molecules play an important role in the pathogenesis of lupus nephritis. Inhibitors of these pathways such as the CTLA4-Ig fusion molecule and anti-CD40L antibodies alone may ameliorate lupus nephritis in animals and are being evaluated in humans (Daikh and Wofsy 1998). Combination of biologic response modifiers and cyclophosphamide may have a synergistic effect and are being considered in human lupus nephritis.

Summary

Lupus nephritis is the most common major organ manifestation of SLE. Aggressive immunosuppressive therapy has improved renal survival with only a minority of patients reaching end-stage renal disease. Intermittent pulse cyclophosphamide has been shown to be the most effective treatment of proliferative lupus nephritis and should be considered as the treatment of choice for moderate to severe proliferative lupus nephritis. Those patients who have aggressive proliferative glomerulonephritis, especially those with additional adverse demographic, clinical, and histologic prognostic factors, should be treated with the combination of pulse methylprednisolone and pulse cyclophosphamide for six months and continued on quarterly cyclophosphamide thereafter. This approach leads to preservation of renal function in the majority of patients. Pulse cyclophosphamide is associated with an increased risk of herpes zoster infections on the short term, but there is no evidence of any association with an increased risk of long-term adverse events, with the exception of infertility in susceptible age-groups.

References

Aisenberg A.C. (1973) Immunosuppression by alkylating agents – tolerance induction. *Transplant Proc* 5, 1221–6.

Arden N.K., Lloyd M.E., Spector T.D. and Hughes G.R.V. (1994) Safety of hormone replacement therapy (HRT) in systemic lupus erythematosus (SLE). *Lupus* 3, 11–3.

Aringer M., Smolen J.S. and Graninger W.B. (1998) Severe infections in plasmapheresis-treated systemic lupus erythematosus. *Arthritis Rheum* 41, 414–20.

Austin H.A.I., Klippel J.H. and Balow J.E. (1986) Therapy of lupus nephritis: controlled trial of prednisone and cytotoxic drugs. *N Eng J Med* 314, 614–9.

Baker G.L., Kahl L.E., Zee B.C. *et al.* (1987) Malignancy following treatment of rheumatoid arthritis with cyclophosphamide. Long-term case-control follow-up study. *Am J Med* 83, 1–9.

Bakir A.A., Levy P.S. and Dunea G. (1994) The prognosis of lupus nephritis in African-Americans: a retrospective analysis. *Am J Kidney Dis* 24, 159–71.

Balow J.E., Austin H.A.I. and Muenz L.R. (1984) Effect of treatment on the evolution of renal abnormalities in lupus nephritis. *N Eng J Med* 311, 491–5.

Balow J.E., Boumpas D.T. and Austin H.A.I. (1998) Lupus Nephritis. In H.R. Brady and C.S. Wilcox (eds) *Therapy in Nephrology and Hypertension*, pp. 130–137. Philadelphia: W.B. Saunders Company.

Baltus J.A., Boersma J.W., Hartman A.P. *et al.* (1983) The occurrence of malignancies in patients with rheumatoid arthritis treated with cyclophosphamide: A controlled retrospective follow-up. *Ann Rheum Dis* 42, 368–73.

Baqi N., Moazami S., Singh A., Ahmad H., Balachandra S. and Tejani A. (1996) Lupus nephritis in children: a longitudinal study of prognostic factors and therapy. *J Am Soc Nephrol* 7, 924–9.

Belmont H.M., Storch M., Buyon J. and Abramson S. (1995) New York University/Hospital for Joint Diseases experience with intravenous cyclophosphamide treatment: efficacy in steroid unresponsive lupus nephritis. *Lupus* 4, 104–8.

Bermas B.L. and Hill J.A. (1995) Effects of immunosuppressive drugs during pregnancy. *Arthritis Rheum* 38, 1722–32.

Blumenfeld Z. and Haim N. (1997) Prevention of gonadal damage during cytotoxic therapy. *Ann Med* 29, 199–206.

Boumpas D.T., Austin H.A.I., Vaughan E.M., Klippel J.H., Steinberg A.D., Yarboro C.H. and Balow J.E. (1992) Controlled trial of pulse methylprednisolone versus two regimens of pulse cyclophosphamide in severe lupus nephritis. *Lancet* 340, 741–5.

Boumpas D.T., Austin H.A.I., Vaughan E.M., Yarboro C.H., Klippel J.H. and Balow J.E. (1993) Risk for sustained amenorrhea in patients with systemic lupus erythematosus receiving intermittent pulse cyclophosphamide therapy. *Ann Intern Med* 119 (5), 366–9.

Brock N. (1996) The history of the oxazaphosphorine cytostatics. *Cancer* 78, 541–7.

Brock N., Pohl J. and Stekar J. (1981a) Studies on the urotoxicity of oxazaphosphorine cytostatics and its prevention – Comparative study on the uroprotective efficacy of thiols and other sulfur compounds. *Eur J Cancer* 17, 1155–63.

Brock N., Pohl J. and Stekar J. (1981b) Studies on the urotoxicity of oxazaphosphorine cytostatics and its prevention–Experimental studies on the urotoxicity of alkylating compounds. *Eur J Cancer* 17, 596–607.

Brock N., Pohl J. and Stekar J. (1982) Studies on the urotoxicity of oxazaphosphorine cytostatics and its prevention–Profile of action of sodium 2-mercaptoethane sulfonate (mesna). *Eur J Cancer* 18, 1377–87.

Brodsky R.A., Sensenbrenner L.L. and Jones R.J. (1997) Complete remission in severe aplastic anemia after high-dose cyclophosphamide without bone marrow transplantation. *Blood* 87, 491–4.

Buyon J.P. *et al.* (1995) Can women with systemic lupus erythematosus safely use exogenous estrogens? *J Clin Rheumatol* 1, 205–12.

Calabresi P. (1983) Leukemia after cytotoxic chemotherapy–a pyrrhic victory? *N Eng J Med* 309, 1118–9.

Cameron J.S., Boulton-Jones M., Robinson R. and Ogg C. (1970) Treatment of lupus nephritis with cyclophosphamide. *Lancet* 2, 846–9.

Chabner B.A., Allegra C.J., Curt G.A. and Calabresi P. (1995) Antineoplastic agents. In J.G. Hardman A. Gilman and L.E. Limbird (eds) *Goodman & Gillman's The Pharmacological Basis of Therapeutics*, 9 edn. pp. 1233–87. New York: McGraw-Hill.

Chu S.J., Chang D.M., Kuo S.Y., Hsu C.M., Chen C.M. and Chang M.L. (1994) Intermittent intravenous treatment of lupus nephritis with cyclophosphamide: a four-year experience with twenty-four patients. *Chung Hua I Hsueh Tsa Chih (Taipei)* 53, 325–30.

Ciruelo E., de la Cruz J., Lopez I. and Gomez-Reino J.J. (1996) Cumulative rate of relapse of lupus nephritis after successful treatment with cyclophosphamide. *Arthritis Rheum* 39, 2028–34.

Conlon P.J., Fischer C.A., Levesque M.C., Smith S.R., St Clair E.W., Allen N.B. *et al.* (1996) Clinical, biochemical and pathological predictors of poor response to intravenous cyclophosphamide in patients with proliferative lupus nephritis. *Clin Nephrol* 46, 170–5.

Cupps T.R., Edgar L.C. and Fauci A.S. (1982) Suppression of human B lymphocyte function by cyclophosphamide. *J Immunol* 128, 2453–7.

Daikh D.I. and Wofsy D. (1998) Reversal of advanced murine lupus nephritis with combined CTLA4Ig and cyclophosphamide. *Arthritis Rheum* 41, S140.

Davis J.C. Jr., Fessler B.J., Tassiulas I.O., McInnes I.B., Yarboro C.H., Pillemer S., Wilder R., Fleisher T.A., Klippel J.H. and Boumpas D.T. (1998) High dose versus low dose fludarabine in the treatment of patients with severe refractory rheumatoid arthritis. *J Rheumatol* 25, 1694–1704.

Dawisha S.M., Yarboro C.H., Vaughan E.M., Austin H.A.I., Balow J.E. and Klippel J.H. (1996) Outpatient monthly oral bolus cyclophosphamide therapy in systemic lupus erythematosus. *J Rheumatol* 23, 273–8.

Dawood M.Y., Ramos J. and Khan-Dawood F.S. (1995) Depot Leuprolide acetate versus danazol for treatment of pelvic endometriosis: changes in vertebral bone mass and serum estradiol and calcitonin. *Fertil Steril* 63, 1177–83.

Decker J.L., Klippel J.H., Plotz P.H. and Steinberg A.D. (1975) Cyclophosphamide or azathioprine in lupus glomerulonephritis: A controlled trial: Results at 28 months. *Ann Intern Med* 83(5), 606–15.

Dinant H.J., Decker J.L., Klippel J.H., Balow J.E., Plotz P.H. and Steinberg A.D. (1982) Alternative modes of cyclophosphamide and azatioprine therapy in lupus nephritis. *Ann Rheum Dis* 96(1), 728–36.

Dlugi A.M., Miller J.D. and Knittle J. (1990) Lupron depot (leuprolide acetate for depot suspension) in the treatment of endometriosis: a randomized, placebo-controlled, double-blind study. *Fertil Steril* 54, 419–26.

Donadio J.V. Jr., Holley K.E., Ferguson R.H. and Ilstrup D.M. (1978) Treatment of diffuse proliferative lupus nephritis with prednisone and combined prednisone and cyclophosphamide. *N Engl J Med* 299, 1151–55.

Donadio, J.V. Jr., Holley, K.E. Wagoner, R.D., Ferguson, R.H. and McDuffie, F.C. (1972) Treatment of lupus nephritis with prednisone and combined prednisone and azathioprine. *Ann Intern Med* 77, 829–35.

Donadio J.V. Jr., Holley K.E., Wagoner R.D., Ferguson R.H. and McDuffie F.C. Further observations on the treatment of lupus nephritis with prednisone and combined prednisone and azathioprine. *Arthritis Rheum* 1974, 17: 573–82.

Dooley M.A., Cosio F.G., Nachman P.H., Falkenhain M.E., Hogan S.L., Falk R.J. and Herbert L.A. Mycophenolate mofetil therapy in lupus nephritis: clinical observation. *J Am Soc Nephrol* 1999, 10: 833–9.

Dooley M.A., Hogan, S., Jennette, C, and Falk, R. (1997) Cyclophosphamide therapy of lupus nephritis: poor renal survival in black Americans. Glomerular Disease Collaborative Network. *Kidney Int* 51, 1188–95.

Droller M.J., Saral R. and Santos G. (1982) Prevention of cyclophosphamide-induced hemorrhagic cystitis. *Urology* 20, 256–8.

Dubois E.L. (1954) Nitrogen mustard in treatment of systemic lupus erythematosus. *Arch Intern Med* 93, 667–72.

Eiser A.R., Grishman E. and Dreznin S. (1993) Intravenous pulse cyclophosphamide in the treatment of type IV lupus nephritis. *Clin Nephrol* 40, 155–9.

Elliott R.W., Essenhigh D.M. and Morley A.R. (1982) Cyclophosphamide treatment for systemic lupus erythematosus. *Br Med J* 284, 1160–61.

Euler H.H., Schroeder, J.O., Harten, P., Zeuner, R.A. and Gutschmidt, H.J. (1994) Treatment-free remission in severe systemic lupus erythematosus following synchronization of plasmapheresis with subsequent pulse cyclophosphamide. *Arthritis Rheum* 37, 1784–94.

Euler H.H., Schroeder J.O., Harten P., Zeuner R.A. and Gutschmidt H.J. (1994) Treatment-free remission in severe systemic lupus erythematosus following synchronization of plasmapheresis with subsequent pulse cyclophosphamide. *Arthritis Rheum* 37, 1784–94.

Feng P.H., Jayarantnam F.J. and Tock E.P.C. (1973) Cyclophosphamide in treatment of systemic lupus erythematosus: 7 years' experience. *Br Med J* 2, 450–2.

Fogelman I. (1992) Gonadotropin-releasing hormone agonists and the skeleton. *Fertil Steril* 57, 715–24.

Fogelman I. *et al.* (1994) Goserelin (Zoladex) an the skeleton. *Br J Obstet Gynaecol* 101, S19–S23.

Fox D.A. and McCune W.J. (1994) Immunosuppressive drug therapy of systemic lupus erythematosus. *Rheum Dis Clin North Am* 20(1), 265–99.

Glicklich D. and Acharya A. (1998) Mycophenolate mofetil therapy for lupus nephritis refractory to intravenous cyclophosphamide. *Am J Kidney Dis* 32, 318–22.

Gmelig-Meyling F., Dawisha S. and Steinberg A.D. (1992) Assessment of in vivo frequency of mutated T cells in patients with systemic lupus erythematosus. *J Exp Med* 175, 297–300.

Gordon M.Y., Goldman J.M. and Gordon-Smith E.C. (1985) 4-Hydroperoxycyclophosphamide inhibits proliferation by human granulocyte-macrophage colony-forming cells (GM-CFC) but spares more primitive progenitor cells. *Leuk Res* 9, 1017–21.

Gourley M.F., Austin H.A., Scott D., Yarboro C.H., Vaughan E.M., Muir J., Boumpas D.T., Klippel J.H., Balow J.E. and Steinberg A.D. (1996) Methylprednisolone and cyclophosphamide, alone or in combination, in patients with lupus nephritis. *Ann Intern Med* 125(7), 549–57.

Hadidi T. (1970) Cyclophosphamide in systemic lupus erythematosus. *Ann Rheum Dis* 29, 673–6.

Hows J.M., Mehta A., Ward L., Woods K., Perez R. and Gordon M.Y. (1984) Comparison of mesna with forced diuresis to prevent cyclophosphamide induced haemorrhagic cystitis in marrow transplantation: a prospective randomised study. *Br J Cancer* 50, 753–6.

Illei G.G., Crane M., Austin H.A., Collins L., Gourley M.F., Yarboro C.H. *et al.* (2000) Combining pulse cyclophosphamide with pulse methylprednisolone improves long-term renal outcome in patients with lupus nephritis without added toxicity. *Unpublished work*

Ioannidis J.P.A., Boki K.A., Katsorida M.E., Drosos A.A., Skopouli F.N., Boletis J.N. *et al* (2000) Remission, relapse and re-remission of proliferative lupus nephritis treated with cyclophosphamide. *Kidney Int* 57, 258–64.

Johansen J.S. *et al.* (1988) The effect of a gonadotropin-releasing hormone agonist analog (nafarelin) on bone metabolism. *J Clin Endocrinol Metab* 67, 701–6.

Jones R.J., Collector M.I., Barber J.P., Vala M.S., Fackler M.J., May W.S. *et al.* (1996) Characterization of mouse lymphohematopoietic stem cells lacking spleen colony-forming activity. *Blood* 88, 487–91.

Kagan L.J. and Christian C.L. (1966) Clinicopathologic studies of SLE nephritis. *Arthritis Rheum* 9, 516.

Karussis D.M., Slavin S., Lehmann D. *et al.* (1992) Prevention of experimental autoimmune encephalomyelitis and induction of tolerance with acute immunosuppression followed by syngeneic bone marrow transplantation. *J Immunol* 148, 1693–8.

Karussis D.M., Vourka-Karussis U., Lehmann D., Abransky O., Ben-Nur A. and Slavin S. (1995) Immunomodulation of autoimmunity in MRL/1pr mice with syngeneic bone marrow transplantation. *Clin Exp Immunol* 100, 111–7.

Klein F.A. and Smith M.J.V. (1983) Urinary complications of cyclophosphamide therapy: etiology, prevention, and management. *South Med J* 76, 1413–6.

Knaan-Shanzer S., Houben P., Kinwel-Bohre E.P. and van Bekkum D.W. (1991) Remission induction of adjuvant arthritis in rats by total body irradiation and autologous bone marrow transplantation. *Bone Marrow Transplant* 8, 333–8.

Koyama H. *et al.* (1977) Cyclophosphamide-induced ovarian failure and its therapeutic significance in patients with breast cancer. *Cancer* 39, 1403–9.

Langevitz P., Klein L., Pras M. and Many A. (1992) The effect of cyclophosphamide pulses on fertility in patients with lupus nephritis. *Am J Reprod Immunol* 28: 157–8.

Lehman T.J., Sherry D.D., Wagner-Weiner L., McCurdy D.K., Emery H.M., Magilavy D.B., *et al.* (1989) Intermittent intravenous cyclophosphamide therapy for lupus nephritis. *J Pediatr* 114, 1055–60.

Lewis E.J., Hunsicker L.G., Lan S.P., Rohde R.D. and Lachin J.M. (1992) A controlled trial of plasmapheresis therapy in severe lupus nephritis. The Lupus Nephritis Collaborative Study Group. *N Eng J Med* 326, 1373–9.

Martin-Suarez I., D'Cruz D., Mansoor M., Ferbabdes A.P., Khamashta M.A. and Hughes G.R. (1997) Immunosuppressive treatment in severe connective tissue diseases: effects of low dose intravenous cyclophosphamide. *Ann Rheum Dis* 56, 481–7.

Martinelli R., Pereira L.J., Santos E.S. and Rocha H. (1996) Clinical effects of intermittent, intravenous cyclophosphamide in severe systemic lupus erythematosus. *Nephron* 74, 313–17.

Masala A., Faedda R., Alagna S., Satta A., Chiarelli G., Rovasio P.P., Ivaldi R., Taras M.S., Lai E. and Bartoli E. (1997) Use of testosterone to prevent cyclophosphamide-induced azoospermia. *Ann Intern Med* 126 (4), 292–5.

Miller M.L. and Steinberg A.D. (1983) Systemic lupus erythematosus–immunoregulatory therapies. *Clin Rheum Dis* 9, 617–28.

Muehrccke R.C., Kark R.M., Pirani C.L. and Pollak V.E. (1957) A clinical and pathologic study based on renal biopsies. *Medicine (Baltimore)* 36, 1.

O'Brien S., Kantarjian H. and Beran M. (1994) Fludarabine (FAMP) and cyclophosphamide therapy in chronic lymphocytic leukemia (CLL). *Ann Oncol*, 7(Suppl.3): 34 (abstract).

Plunkett W. and Gandhi V. (1997) Nucleoside analogs: Cellular pharmacology, mechanisms of action and strategies for combination therapy. In B. Cheson, M. Keating and W. Plunkett (eds) *Nucleoside Analogs in Cancer Therapy*, pp. 1–35. New York, NY: Marcel Dekker.

Pollak V.E., Pirani C.L. and Kark R.M. (1961) Effect of large doses of prednisone on the renal lesions and life span of patients with lupus glomerulonephritis. *J Lab Clin Med* 57, 495.

Puri H.C. and Campbell R.A. (1977) Cyclophosphamide and malignancy. *Lancet* 1, 1306.

Radis C.D., Kahl L.E., Baker G.L., Wasko M.C.M., Cash J.M., Gallatin A., Stolzer B.L., Agarwal A.K., Medsger, T.A. Jr. and Kwoh C.K. (1995) Effects of cyclophosphamide on the development of malignancy and on long-term survival of patients with rheumatoid arthritis. *Arthritis Rheum* 38, 1120–27.

Rivkees S.A. and Crawford J.D. (1988) The relationship of gonadal activity and chemotherapy-induced gonadal damage. *JAMA* 259, 2123–5.

Russell P.J. and Hicks J.D. (1968) Cyclophosphamide treatment of renal disease in (NZB × NZW) F$_1$ hybrid mice. *Lancet* 1, 440–46.

Schroeder J.O., Schwab U.M., Zeuner R.A., Fastenrath S. and Euler H.H. (1997) Plasmapheresis and subsequent pulse cyclophosphamide in severe systemic lupus erythematosus. Preliminary results of the LPSG-trial. *Arthritis Rheum*, 40: S325 (abstract).

Scialli A.R., Jestila K.J. and Simon J.A. (1993) Leuprolide acetate and bone mineral density measured by quantitive radiography. *Fertil Steril* 59, 674–6.

Sesso R., Monteiro M., Sato E., Kirsztajn G., Silva L. and Ajzen H. (1994) A controlled trial of pulse cyclophosphamide versus pulse methylprednisolone in severe lupus nephritis. *Lupus* 3, 107–12.

Shepherd J.D., Pringle L.E., Barnett M.J., Klingermann H.G., Reece D.E. and Phillips G.L. (1991) Mesna versus hyperhydration for the prevention of cyclophosphamide-induced hemorrhagic cystitis in bone marrow transplantation. *J Clin Oncol* 9, 2016–20.

Slater C.A., Liang M.H., McCune J.W., Christman G.M. and Laufer M.R. (1999) Preserving ovarian function in patients receiving cyclophosphamide. *Lupus* 8, 3–10.

Steinberg A.D. (1986) The treatment of lupus nephritis. *Kidney Int*, 30(5): 769–87.

Steinberg A.D. and Decker J.L. (1974) A double-blind controlled trial comparing cyclophosphamide, azathioprine and placebo in the treatment of lupus glomerulonephritis. *Arthritis Rheum* 17(6), 923–37.

Steinberg A.D., Gelfand M.G., Hardin J.A. and Lowenthal D.T. (1975) Therapeutic studies in NZB/W mice. III. Relationship between renal status and efficacy of immunosuppressive drug therapy. *Arthritis Rheum* 18, 10–14.

Steinberg A.D., Plotz P.H., Wolff S.M., Wong W.G., Agus S.G. and Decker J.L. (1972) Cytotoxic drugs in treatment of non-malignant diseases. *Ann Intern Med* 76, 619–42.

Steinberg E.B., Smith H.R. and Steinberg A.D. (1983) Studies of cyclophosphamide therapy in murine lupus–Effect of combining multiple subsets into a single randomized study. *Arthritis Rheum* 26, 1293–4.

Sztejnbok M., Stewart A. and Diamond H. (1971) Azathioprine in the treatment of systemic lupus erythematosus. A controlled study. *Arthritis Rheum* 14, 639–45.

Talar-Williams C., Hijazi Y.M., Walther M.M., Linehan W.M., Hallahan C.W., Lubensky I., Kerr G.S., Hoffman G.S., Fauci A.S. and Sneller M.C. (1996) Cyclophosphamide-induced cystitis and bladder cancer in patients with Wegener granulomatosus. *Ann Intern Med* 124, 477–84.

Varkila K. and Hurme M. (1983) The effect of cyclophosphamide on cytotoxic T-lymphocyte responses: Inhibition of helper T-cell induction in vitro. *Immunology* 48, 433–8.

Vose J.M., Reed E.C., Pippert G.C., Anderson J.R., Bierman P.J., Kessinger A., Spinolo J. and Armitage J.O. (1993) Mesna compared with continuous bladder irrigation as uroprotection during high-dose chemotherapy and transplantation: a randomized trial. *J Clin Oncol* 11(7), 1306–10.

Wallace D.J., Goldfinger D., Pepkowitz S.H., Fichman M., Metzger A.L., Schroeder J.O., *et al.* (1998) Randomized controlled trial of pulse/synchronization cyclophosphamide/apheresis for proliferative lupus nephritis. *J Clin Apheresis* 13, 163–66.

Wang C.L., Wang F. and Bosco J.J. (1995) Ovarian failure in oral cyclophosphamide treatment for systemic lupus erythematosus. *Lupus* 4, 11–14.

Yan D.C., Chou C.C., Tsai M.J., Chiang B.L., Tsau Y.K. and Hsieh K.H. (1995) Intravenous cyclophosphamide pulse therapy on children with severe active lupus nephritis. *Chung Hua Min Kuo Hsiao Erh Ko I Hsueh Hui Tsa Chih* 36, 203–9.

Yarboro C.H., Wesley R., Amantea M.A., Klippel J.H. and Pucino F. (1996) Modified oral ondansetron regimen for cyclophosphamide-induced emesis in lupus nephritis patients. *Ann Pharmacother* 30, 752–55.

7

Lupus nephritis: Treatment with continuous therapies

Gabriella Moroni and Claudio Ponticelli

The involvement of the kidney in systemic lupus erythematosus (SLE) may show a large intra and inter-individual variability. Some patients run an indolent course, some have a rapid progression to renal failure, others have an alternance of quiescience and exacerbations. Thus, it is difficult to plan a rigid therapeutical protocol. Rather, we feel that the treatment of lupus nephritis should be based on a careful evaluation of the histological picture at renal biopsy and on the monitoring of renal signs, such as plasma creatinine, proteinuria and urinary sediment.

Mild forms of lupus nephritis (pure mesangial lesions and scattered proliferative lesions)

Pure mesangial lesions or scattered focal proliferative lesions are usually associated with minor urinary abnormalities (proteinuria <1 g/day, inactive urine sediment), normal renal function and blood pressure. No controlled trial has evaluated the usefulness of treatment in these patients. Adler (Adler *et al.* 1996) proposed the use of low-dose corticosteroids, but other investigators (Ponticelli 1990; Appel and Valeri 1994) feel that no specific treatment is required, as these patients usually have an excellent renal prognosis even in the long term. Nevertheless, a continuous clinical surveillance is recommended, as in about 30% of cases the histological pattern can transform into a diffuse proliferative or a membranous glomerulonephritis (D'Agati 1998). This transformation is generally heralded either by an increase in plasma creatinine with a 'nephritic' urinary sediment (erythrocyturia, pyuria, cylindruria) or by an increase in proteinuria.

However, at presentation a minority of patients with pure mesangial lesions may show a nephrotic syndrome or even an impairment of renal function (Stankeviciute *et al.* 1997). A short course with prednisone, 1 mg/kg/day for 1 month then gradually tapered, may reverse these clinical abnormalities. The few patients who do not respond and those with significant impairment of renal function should be treated as patients with diffuse proliferative lupus nephritis.

Membranous lupus nephritis

Patients with membranous nephritis (MN), non-nephrotic proteinuria, and normal renal function have generally a benign course. These patients do not require any specific treatment but should be followed regularly in view of the possible development of nephrotic syndrome or transformation into more severe histological class. Such a transformation in MN may occur in about 40% of cases submitted to repeated renal biopsy (D'Agati 1998). More rarely, overimposed interstitial nephritis or vasculitis may occur. Thus, in patients showing a rapid increase in plasma creatinine and active urine sediment, a new renal biopsy may be helpful to detect the cause of renal function deterioration.

The prognosis of patients with MN and nephrotic syndrome is good up to 5 years (Appel *et al.* 1978). This led many investigators to discourage steroid and immunosuppressive therapy in MN. However, when the follow-up is extended to 10 years or more the renal survival in MN is even worse than that observed in diffuse proliferative glomerulonephritis (Appel *et al.* 1987). On the other hand, the 10-year renal and patient survival rates were excellent in a series in which patients were given an aggressive and prolonged treatment (Pasquali *et al.* 1993).

In a retrospective analysis (Moroni *et al.* 1998) we compared the effect of two different treatments in 19 patients with membranous lupus nephritis, all with normal renal function and nephrotic syndrome at presentation: (a) 8 patients had proteinuria less than 5 g/day and received corticosteroids alone as first treatment; (b) 11 other patients with proteinuria more than 5 g/day were treated with a 6-month regimen alternating corticosteroids and chlorambucil every other month according to a schedule we are using in idiophatic membranous glomerulonephritis (Ponticelli *et al.* 1984; Ponticelli *et al.* 1989). After a mean follow-up of 96 months, 4 of 8 patients given steroids alone were without nephrotic syndrome, compared with 10 of the 11 patients treated with corticosteroids and chlorambucil, 7 of them being without proteinuria at all. Seven of the 8 patients of group (a) had one or more relapses of the nephrotic syndrome that required new courses of therapy while the 10 responders in group (b) did not have renal flares. Three of the 8 patients given steroids alone developed renal insufficiency. One patient given corticosteroids and chlorambucil had a sudden transformation to extracapillary glomerulonephritis 26 years after treatment and eventually progressed to end stage renal disease. These results, although derived from a retrospective analysis of a small group of patients suggest that in lupus MN a combination of steroids and cytotoxic agents may be more effective than corticosteroids alone in inducing a stable remission of nephrotic syndrome and in protecting from flares and renal function deterioration.

Another therapeutic approach may consist in cyclosporine. Radhakrishnan (Radhakrishnan *et al.* 1994) gave cyclosporine plus small doses of prednisone to 10 patients with MN. Proteinuria fell to less than 1 g/day in 6 patients. In 2 patients proteinuria decreased to 1–2 g/day and the remaining 2 patients continued to excrete over 2 g/day of protein. Serum creatinine remained unchanged. Control renal biopsies showed a decrease in SLE activity but an increase in chronicity index.

Severe forms of lupus nephritis (WHO Class IV and severe Class III nephritis)

Patients with Class IV or with Class III nephritis involving many glomeruli should be treated vigorously particularly when renal biopsy shows a high activity index. Although the gold standard therapy for these forms is far to be determined (Table 7.1) corticosteroids, azathioprine and cyclophosphamide still remain the agents more frequently used for treating the severe forms of lupus nephritis.

Corticosteroids

Corticosteroids may exert several effects on inflammation and on immunologic mechanisms. When given intravenously at very high doses corticosteroids can exert some effects on inflammation and on immunologic mechanisms that are not obtained with standard doses (Kimberly *et al.* 1981; Ponticelli and Fogazzi 1989). Although corticosteroids have improved the survival of patients with lupus nephritis, there is not an absolute guide for the dosage, duration and route of administration of these agents. This uncertainty is largely caused by the fact that only few studies (Tanaka *et al.* 1992), have tried to identify an adequate biological index of the individual corticosteroid sensitivity. Thus, from a practical point of view, the indications to corticosteroid treatment are based on clinical experience, rather than on a scientific approach.

In 1964 Pollak and coworkers (Pollak *et al.* 1964) showed that low-dose prednisone was ineffective in diffuse proliferative lupus nephritis, while high-dose

Table 7.1   Therapeutic strategies for severe form of lupus nephritis

Therapy	Use
Corticosteroids (oral and intravenous)	First line therapeutic approach
Immunosuppressive agents	
Cyclophosphamide (oral and intravenous)	Frequently used with corticosteroids in severe cases
Azathioprine (oral)	Frequently used with corticosteroids in severe cases for long-term therapy
Chlorambucil oral	Insufficient experience up to now
Methotrexate (intramuscular)	Insufficient experience up to now
Mycophenolate Mofetil (oral)	Insufficient experience up to now
Cyclosporine A	Corticosteroid sparing agent, probably effective as maintenance therapy
Ancrod	Insufficient experience up to now, rescue treatment
Immunoglobulins	Insufficient experience, probably effective as maintenance therapy
Plasmapheresis	Not effective in controlled trials. Rescue treatment
Total lymphoid irradiation	Insufficient experience up to now

prednisone could improve the prognosis. After this observation, most physicians treated diffuse lupus nephritis with prednisone at doses of 1–2 mg/kg/day until the activity of the disease was quenched, which often took several months. In spite of this therapy many patients showed progressive renal disease and others developed devastating steroid-related side effects (such as hypertension, infections, accelerated atherosclerosis, obesity, diabetes, aseptic bone necrosis, cataracts and myopathy). In 1976 Cathcart (Cathcart *et al.* 1976) reported the beneficial effects of a short course of intravenous high-dose methylprednisolone pulses. Other non-controlled studies and one controlled trial in a few patients (reviewed in Ponticelli 1990) confirmed that intravenous methylprednisolone pulses (generally 1 g given every day for 3 consecutive days) could dramatically reverse the extrarenal symptoms of SLE and obtain a rapid improvement of renal function, particularly in patients with a recent increase in serum creatinine. Proteinuria tended to improve more slowly, taking as long as 6 months (Ponticelli *et al.* 1987). Once remission was achieved it could be maintained by low-dose oral prednisone, so reducing the iatrogenic risks of an intensive and prolonged corticosteroid therapy. Side effects of methylprednisolone pulses are infrequent and include flushing, tremor, nausea and altered taste. More severe but rare complications include seizures, anaphylaxis, psycosis and cardiac arrhythmia (Schuman *et al.* 1983; Freedman *et al.* 1981; Moses *et al.* 1982).

Immunosuppressive agents

The two immunosuppressive agents most widely used in SLE are cyclophosphamide and azathioprine. Cyclophosphamide is an alkylating agent which disturbs the fundamental mechanisms concerned with cell growth, mitotic activity, differentiation, and function. Azathioprine blocks purine synthesis so halting the proliferation of lymphocytes which require purines during their proliferative phase. Uncontrolled and controlled studies evaluated the efficacy of immunosuppressive agents in lupus nephritis (Donadio *et al.* 1972; Sztejnbok *et al.* 1971; Hahn *et al.* 1975; Donadio *et al.* 1976; Cade *et al.* 1973; Steinberg *et al.* 1971; Steinberg and Decker 1974; Dinant *et al.* 1982). The results of controlled trials comparing steroids with steroids plus immunosuppressive agents have been conflicting, both because the therapeutical schedules were different and because of the small number of patients enrolled in single studies. In order to achieve statistical power, Felson and Anderson (Felson and Anderson 1984) pooled together the data of eight controlled trials and showed that the risk of deterioration of renal function and renal death was significantly lower in patients assigned to receive immunosuppressive therapy than in patients given corticosteroids alone. Instead the cumulative mortality for non-renal causes was similar in the two groups. Two years later, Austin (Austin *et al.* 1986) reported the long-term results of a trial in which patients with SLE nephritis were randomly assigned to receive prednisone alone or prednisone with monthly pulses of intravenous cyclophosphamide, or with oral cyclophosphamide, or with azathioprine or with a combination of azathioprine and oral cyclophosphamide. There were no differences in renal survival among the different groups until the fifth year. At 10 years, patients given prednisone alone had a significantly worse renal survival than patients given intravenous cyclophosphamide. There was no significant difference between the groups given other immunosuppressive regimens and the group given intravenous cyclophosphamide. Analysis of serial renal biopsies showed a greater progression of sclerotic lesions in patients given prednisone alone than in patients given immunosuppressive drugs (Balow *et al.* 1984). Further trials at the NIH (Boumpas *et al.* 1992; Gourley *et al.* 1996) confirmed the validity of intravenous cyclophosphamide in lupus nephritis (see also Chapter 6).

A recent meta-analysis (Bansal and Beto 1997) of 19 prospective controlled trials showed that patient and renal survivals were significantly better in patients assigned to receive intravenous cyclophosphamide or the combination of azathioprine and oral cyclophosphamide when compared with patients given prednisone alone. Once again no difference in patient and renal survival was seen among the various immunosuppressive schedules.

These results underline the effectiveness of regimens based on an association of corticosteroids and immunosuppressive agents in lupus nephritis and their superiority over corticosteroids alone. Moreover, the use of these immunosuppressive agents may allow a reduction of the corticosteroid dose. It is still unclear which immunosuppressive drug has the best therapeutic index. The clinical impression is that cyclophosphamide is more effective in the acute phases of lupus nephritis. As a matter of fact, cyclophosphamide is a more powerful inihibitor of B cells than azathioprine and can rapidly reduce the resynthesis of autoantibodies (Cameron 1999). Experimental studies also showed a strong efficacy of cyclophosphamide in the active murine models of SLE (Steinberg 1986). However, in view of the potential risk of oncogenicity, gonadal toxicity and bladder toxicity, a high cumulative dose of cyclophosphamide may be dangerous. In this regard, it must be pointed out that the use of intravenous pulses of cyclophosphamide may allow a reduction of the cumulative dosage of this drug. A single dose of 1000 mg every month reduces by a half to a third the monthly dose when compared with an oral administration of 1–2 mg/kg/day. Azathioprine seems to be better tolerated in the long-term. This agent probably leads to a lower risk of neoplasia, to less bladder, gonadal and bone marrow toxicity than cyclophosphamide. For these reasons azathioprine is now preferred by some groups, for long–term treatments (Ponticelli 1990; Cameron 1999).

A possible alternative is represented by mycophenolate mofetil which blocks the de–novo pathway of purine synthesis, the only pathway used by lymphocytes (Eugui *et al.* 1991). The use of mycophenolate mofetil may be rational in SLE. Preliminary data of a very small sized non-controlled study suggested benefit (Dooley *et al.* 1999).[1]

Table 7.2 Suggested induction therapeutical schedule for patients with Class IV and severe Class III lupus nephritis

Drugs	Suggested dosage	Duration of therapy	Indication	Results: advantages, drawbacks
(A)				
Intravenous methylprednisolone pulse therapy	0.5–1 g/day according to the body weight	for 3 days	Moderate disease: moderate activity index and low chronicity index normal renal function with nephrotic syndrome and active urinary sediment	Satisfactory results (few controlled trials) rapid improvement of extrarenal symptoms slow decrease in proteinuria (6–12 months) saving oral steroid with reduction of side effects
+				
oral prednisone	prednisone 0.5–1 mg/kg/day	for 1 month then gradually tapered accordingly to the activity of the disease		
(B)				
Intravenous methylprednisolone pulse therapy	0.5–1 g/day according to the body weight	for 3 days	Severe disease: high activity index, with low or moderate chronicity index fibrinoid necrosis and cellular crescents recent impairment of renal function with moderate or nephrotic proteinuria and active urinary sediment	Good results: (no controlled trials) the same advantages of schedule (A) in short and long term rapid decrease in plasma creatinine infrequent severe side effects
+				
oral prednisone	prednisone 0.5–1 mg/kg/day	for 1 month then gradually tapered accordingly to the activity of the disease +		
+				
immunosuppressive agents	cyclophosphamide 1.5–2 mg/kg/day	for 2–4 months than substituted with azathioprine 1.5–2 mg/kg/day for 6–12months or more at progressively reduced dosage.		

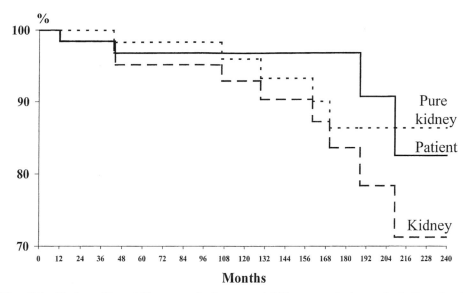

Fig. 7.1 Patient, Pure kidney survival rate and kidney survival rate including death (Kidney) in 66 patients with proliferative lupus nephritis.

86% at 20 years and the kidney survival rate including death was 93% at 10 years and 72% at 20 years (Fig. 7.1). One of the most difficult decisions concerns the treatment of patients with chronic irreversible lesions at renal biopsy. The general trend is not to increase the maintenance therapy. However, although treatment is often ineffective, a few patients with the simultaneous presence of active and chronic lesions at renal biopsy and with recent increase in plasma creatinine, may benefit from an aggressive treatment with some improvement of renal function which may remain stable even for years (Moroni *et al.* 1999). Thus, if the clinical conditions of the patient are good, a short course of intravenous high-dose methylprednisolone followed by oral prednisone and oral cyclophosphamide at doses not exceeding 1–1.5 mg/kg day may be tried.

Maintenance therapy

After obtaining the control of renal disease with induction therapy, we try to reduce progressively the dosage of prednisone up to a maintenance of 10 mg/day or to 20 mg every other day. Low-dose azathioprine is given in patients with persistent proteinuria, active sediment and/or stable renal dysfunctions. In patients with normal renal function, proteinuria less than 1 g/day and inactive urinary sediment for at least 3 years, we try to taper off treatment very gradually, over 1 year at least (Ponticelli *et al.* 1988). During this period patients are closely monitored in order to catch early any sign of reactivation of the renal disease. We could completely stop therapy in 27 patients after a median period of therapy of 29 months. At presentation, 14 patients had diffuse proliferative nephritis, 4 focal proliferative nephrits and 9 had membranous nephritis.

At stopping therapy 20 patients were in complete remission and 7 patients had normal renal function but mild-moderate proteinuria (median 1.0 g/day). Twelve of these patients never had new renal or extra-renal flares (median follow-up 139 months) and remained without therapy. The other 15 patients developed renal or extrarenal exacerbations of SLE in median 32 months after stopping treatment and were treated as flares. Four patients continued therapy while in the others a further attempt of stopping therapy was made. At the last follow-up (median 143 months) 10 patients were in complete and 5 in partial remission (median proteinuria 0.7 g/day). In patients who flared, the incidence of renal and extrarenal flares was not significantly different before and after stopping therapy (0.11 renal flare/patient/year before stopping therapy vs 0.10 after, 0.02 extrarenal flare/patient/year before stopping therapy vs 0.07 after).

The only difference between the 12 patients who never flared after stopping therapy and the 15 patients who flared was the duration of therapy before stopping. This was significantly longer in patients who did not have flares (median 51.1 months vs 20 months, $p=0.03$). The 15 patients who needed new courses of therapy had higher incidence of dyslipidemia (7/15 vs 0/12), osteoporosis (4/15 vs 0/12), arterial hypertension (9/15 vs 5/12) when compared with the 12 patients who definitively stopped therapy.

Supportive care

With the improving survival of patients the prevention of the long-term complications of SLE and of side-effects of therapy has become more and more important. Supportive care has a critical role in achieving this goal.

One of the most worrying complications of SLE is premature atherosclerosis (Moroni *et al.* 1992; Gladman and Urowitz 1987). Several factors may contribute to atherosclerosis in SLE patients: arterial hypertension, morbid obesity, smoking, dyslipidemia secondary to nephrotic syndrome or to steroid therapy, and probably high levels of plasma homocysteine. The control of arterial hypertension is critical not only for preventing cardiovascular disease but also for protecting renal function. The optimal blood pressure for patients with renal disease remains a subject of investigation. Recent data, however, pointed out that in patients with renal disease a mean blood pressure of 92 mmHg or less can protect against the risk of progressive renal failure (Klahr *et al.* 1994). Moreover the lower the blood pressure values the lower the risk of cardiovascular disease (Hansson *et al.* 1988). Sodium restriction in the diet is the first measure to obtain an adequate control of hypertension but is often insufficient. In choosing the antihypertensive agents, it must be reminded that the first goal is represented by a good control of hypertension, independently of the type of antihypertensive agents. Drugs such as β adrenergic blockers, central or peripherally acting adrenergic inhibitors, alfa 1 receptor blockers, dihydropyridinic calcium channel antagonists and direct-acting vasodilators may be quite effective in lowering blood pressure. Agents such as ACE-inhibitors, angiotensin 2 receptor antagonists, and non-dihydropyridinic calcium-channel blockers are also effective in lowering blood pressure and might theoretically offer some further advantages, as they can help in reducing urinary protein excretion (Hutchinson *et al.* 1995) and may show renoprotective properties independent of lowering blood pressure (Meyer *et al.* 1995; Maschio *et al.* 1996).

Appropriate dietetic indications to maintain ideal body weight, physical exercise and avoiding smoking should also be recommended in order to prevent atherosclerotic vascular disease. The abnormal plasma lipid concentration may accelerate atherogenesis and perhaps may contribute to progressive glomerular injury (Keane 1994). Reduced dietetic intake of cholesterol and satured fats may be effective for reducing hyperlipidemia in patients with absent or low proteinuria while it is relatively ineffective in patients with nephrotic syndrome. Hydroxymethylglutaryl co-enzyme A reductase (HMG co-A reductase) inhibitors are the agents of choice for reducing hypercholesterolemia. In patients with nephrotic syndrome these drugs can lower total cholesterol by only 35–45% while better results can be obtained in patients without proteinuria (Glassock 1997). Independently from the effects on plasma lipids, HMG co-reductase inhibitors might directly affect the progressive nature of renal disease (Massy *et al.* 1996). In fact these drugs may influence important intracellular pathways that are involved in the inflammatory and fibrogenic responses which contribute to progressive renal injury (Oda and Keane 1999). Infrequently these agents may cause myonecrosis.

In a prospective study on 337 SLE patients, elevated plasma levels of homocysteine were found to be an independent risk factor for stroke and arterial thromboses (Petri *et al.* 1996). Low levels of plasma folate, vitamin B12 and pyridoxal 5′-phosphate were frequently associated with high concentrations of plasma homocysteine. Although not supported by controlled trials, the possibility that the administration of folic acid and vitamin B12 could prevent thrombotic events in SLE patients deserves attention.

Osteoporosis is a critical problem for patients treated with corticosteroids for a long term. The risk of fractures can be reduced following the guidelines suggested by the American College of Rheumatology (American College of Rheumatology 1996). Given that bone is lost most rapidly during the first 6 months of steroid use (Aroldi *et al.* 1997) the primary prevention should begin as soon as steroids are prescribed. Patients should be submitted to evaluation of bone mineral density (BMD) of the spine and hip as baseline measurement for monitoring changes in bone mass. Patients with normal BMD should be given calcium and vitamin D supplementation. In patients who have an abnormal basal BMD (Tscore >−1) a bisphosphonate or calcitonin should be added to calcium and vitamin D supplementation. The use of hormone replacement therapy in SLE is still debated as this treatment may potentially reactivate the disease. Patients should also be informed about the toxic effects of corticosteroids on muscle, and physical exercises to maintain muscle strength should be recommended.

Note

[1] A small sized randomized controlled trial showed beneficial results with mycophenolate mofetil in lupus nephritis (Chan *et al.* 2000)

References

Adler S., Choen A.H., Glassock R.J. (1996). Secondary glomerular disease. In *The kidney* (ed. B.M. Brenner), pp. 1498–513. W.B. Saunders, Philadelphia.

American College of Rheumathology (1996). Guidelines for the prevention and treatment of glucorticoid induced osteoporosis. *Arthritis and Rheumatism*, 39(11): 1791–801.

Appel G.B., Cohen D.J., Pirani C.L., Meltzer J.I., Estes D. (1987). Long-term follow-up of patients with lupus nephritis: a study based on the classification of the World Health Organization. *American Journal of Medicine*, 83: 877–85.

Appel G.B., Valeri A. (1994). The course and treatment of lupus nephritis. *Annual Review of Medicine*, 45: 525–37.

Appel G.B., Silva F.G., Pirani C.L., Meltzer J.I., Estes D. (1978). Renal involvement in systemic lupus erythematosus (SLE): a study of fifty-six patients emphasizing histological classification. *Medicine*, 57: 371–410.

Aroldi A., Tarantino A., Montagnino G., Cesana B., Cocucci C., Ponticelli C. (1997). Effects of three immunosuppressive regimens on vertebral bone density in renal transplant recipients. *Transplantation*, 63: 380–6.

Austin H.A., III. Boumpas D.T., Vaughan E.M., Balow J.E. (1994). Predicting renal outcomes in severe lupus nephritis: contributions of clinical and histologic data. *Kidney International*, 45: 544–50.

Austin H.A., III. Klippel J.H., Balow J.E., le Riche N.G., Steinberg A.D., Plotz P.H., Decker J.L. (1986). Therapy of lupus nephritis. Controlled trial of prednisone and cytotoxic drugs. *New England Journal of Medicine*, 314: 614–9.

Balletta M., Sabella D., Magri P., Sepe V., Stanziale P., Di Luccio R., Colucci G., Fuiano G. (1992). Cyclosporin plus steriods versus steroid alone in the treatment of lupus nephritis. Contribution in *Nephrology*, 99: 129–30.

Balow J.E., Austin H.A., III. Muenz L.R., Joyce K.M., Antonovych T.T., Klippel J.H., Steinberg A.D., Plotz P.H., Decker J.L. (1984). Effect of treatment on the evolution of renal abnormalities in lupus nephritis. *New England Journal of Medicine*, 311: 491–5.

Bansal V.K., and Beto J.A. (1997). Treatment of lupus nephritis: a meta-analysis of clinical trials. *American Journal of Kidney Disease*, 29: 193–9.

Bergijk C.E., Baelde H.J., de Herr E., Bruijn J.A. (1994). Prevention of glomerulosclerosis by early cyclosporine treatment of experimental lupus nephritis. *Kidney International*, 46: 1663–6.

Boumpas D.T., Austin H.A., III. Vaughan E.M., Klippel J.H., Steinberg A.D., Yarboro C.H., Balow J.E. (1992). Controlled trial of pulse methylprednisolone versus two regimens or pulse cyclophosphamide in severe lupus nephritis. *Lancet*, 340: 741–5.

Cade R., Spooner G., Schlein E., Pickering M., De Quesada A., Holcomb A., Juncos L., Richard G., Shires D., Levin D., Hackett R., Free J., Hunt R., Fregly M. (1973). Comparison of azathioprine, prednisone, and heparin alone or combined in treating lupus nephritis. *Nephron*, 10: 37–56.

Cameron J.S. Lupus nephritis. (1999). *Journal of American Society of Nephrology*, 10: 413–24.

Cathchart E.S., Idelson B.A., Scheinberg M.A., Couser W.G. (1976). Beneficial effects of methylprednisolone 'pulse'ᵃ therapy in diffuse proliferative lupus nephritis. *Lancet*, 1: 163–6.

Chan T.M., Li F.K., Tang C.S.O., Wong R.W., Fang G.X., Ji Y.L., *et al.* Efficacy of Mycophenylate mofetil in patients with diffuse proliferative lupus nephritis. *New England Journal of Medicine 2000*, 343: 1156–62.

D'Agati V.D. (1998). Renal disease in systemic lupus erythematosus, mixed connective tissue disease, Sjogren's syndrome and rheumatoid arthritis. In *Heptinstall's pathology of the kidney*, fifth edition (eds J.C. Jannette J.L., Olson M.M., Schwartz, F.G. Silva), pp. 580. Lippincott-Raven, Philadelphia-New York.

Dinant H.J., Decker J.L., Klippel J.H., Balow J.E., Plotz P.H., Steinberg A.D. (1982). Alternative modes of cyclophosphamide and azathioprine therapy in lupus nephritis. *Annals of Internal Medicine*, 96: 728–36.

Donadio J.V., Holley K.E., Ferguson. R.H. Ilstrup D.M. (1976). Progressive lupus glomerulonephritis: treatment with prednisone and combined prednisone and cyclophosphamide. *Mayo Clinical Proceeding*, 51: 484–94.

Donadio J.V., Holley K.E., Wagoner R.D., Ferguson R.H., McDuffie F.C. (1972). Treatment of lupus nephritis with prednisone and combined prednisone and azathioprine. *Annals of Internal Medicine*, 77: 829–35.

Dooley M.A., Cosio F.G., Nachman P.H., Falkenhain M.E., Hogan S.L., Falck R.J., Hebert L.A. (1999). Mycophenolate Mofetil therapy in lupus nephritis. *Journal of American Society of Nephrology*, 10: 833–9.

Dostal C., Tesai V., Rychlik I. (1997). Cyclosporine A versus cyclophosphamide in long-term treatment of lupus nephritis. A comparative pilot study. *Arthritis and Rheumatism*, 40: 9 suppl, S57.

Eugui E.M., Almquist S., Muller C.D., Allison A.C. (1991). Lymphocyte selective cytostatic and immunosuppressive effects of mycophenolic acid in vitro: role of deoxyguanosine nucleotide depletion. *Scandinavian Journal of Immunology*, 33: 161–73.

Favre H., Miescher A., Huang P., Chatelant F., Mihatsch M.J. (1989). Cyclosporine in the treatment of lupus nephritis. *American Journal of Nephrology*, 9: 57–60.

Felson D.T., Anderson J. (1984). Evidence for the superiority of immunosuppressive drugs and prednisone over prednisone alone in lupus nephritis. *New England Journal of Medicine*, 311: 1528–33.

Feutren G., Querin S., Noel L.H., Chatenoud L., Beuraim G., Tron F., Lesavre P., Bach J.F. (1987). Effects of cyclosporine in severe systemic lupus erythematosus. *Journal of Pediatrics*, 111: 1063–8.

Freedman M.D., Schocket A.L., Chaperl N., Gerber J.G. (1981). Anaphylaxis after intravenous methylprednisolone administration. *Journal of American Medical Association*, 245: 607–8.

Fu L.W., Yang L.Y., Chen W.P., Lin C.Y. (1998). Clinical efficacy of cyclosporine A Neoral in the treatment of pediatric lupus nephritis with heavy proteinuria. *British Journal of Rheumatology*, 37: 217–21.

Gladman D.D., Urowitz M.B. (1987). Morbidity in systemic lupus erythematosus. *Journal of Rheumatology*, 14 (Suppl), 223–6.

Glassock R.J. (1997). Symptomatic therapy. In *Treatment of primary glomerulonephritis* (eds C. Ponticelli R.J., Glassock), pp. 1–24. Oxford Medical Publications, Oxford, New York, Tokyo.

8

SLE in pregnancy

Lisa R. Sammaritano and Michael D. Lockshin

General principles

Pregnancy, a common event in patients with systemic lupus erythematosus (SLE), raises issues of infertility, hypertension and preeclampsia, fetal death, measurements of disease indicators, and acceptable drug therapy. This chapter reviews these and other relevant issues.

Fertility

In the absence of premature ovarian failure associated with cyclophosphamide therapy, fertility rates are reported to be normal in SLE patients (Fraga *et al.* 1974). Renal disease, whether due to lupus or other causes, markedly affects fertility, especially in patients with severe renal dysfunction or on dialysis (Jones and Hayslett 1996; Lindheimer *et al.* 1995).

Physiologic adaptations in normal pregnancy

Normal pregnancy is an altered physiologic state. Adaptations relevant to lupus pregnancy are those in volume and blood pressure, both critically dependent on renal and cardiac function. The kidney in the pregnant patient must handle a plasma volume that is up to 50% increased over pre-pregnancy values; lupus patients with renal, vascular, or cardiac compromise may not tolerate an increase of this magnitude.

Renal and volume changes

Functional changes during pregnancy include alterations in renal hemodynamics, tubular function, osmoregulation, and volume regulation. The overall effect of these adaptations leads to a 35–50% increase both in glomerular filtration rate (GFR) and in plasma volume (40–50%). Normal mean values in creatinine (Cr) decrease, and creatinine clearance rises to 30% above that for nonpregnant women. Physiologic urinary protein excretion may double, to 300 mg/24 hours. Serum uric acid levels drop to 2.5–4.0 mg/dL. Plasma osmolality decreases, accounting, in combination with increased volume, for the physiologic edema of pregnancy (Lindheimer *et al.* 1995; Branch 1992).

Other pregnancy-induced physiologic changes

Changes in coagulation control mechanisms lead to an overall increase in hypercoagulability. Although platelet production usually increases, dilutional thrombocytopenia (Burrows and Kelton 1988) and activation of intravascular coagulation systems in normal pregnancy (Vazifi *et al.* 1986) sometimes occur.

Immunologic and hormonal changes may influence pregnancy outcome (Branch, 1992). Typical changes include depression of both cell-mediated immunity and humoral immune responses (Lockshin 1993). Estrogen, prolactin, and other hormones have immunomodulatory effects (Lahita 1992). In general, estrogens upregulate and androgens downregulate T-cell responses and immunoglobulin synthesis (Sthoeger *et al.* 1988). Pregnancy-specific proteins such as alpha-fetoprotein may also suppress lymphocyte function. Interleukins (IL-1, IL-3) and other cytokines, important in sustaining normal pregnancy, may be regulated by sex hormones as well (Hill 1992; Chaouat *et al.* 1990). Complement levels are normal or elevated, likely reflecting an increase in complement synthesis rather than a decrease in activation. Low-grade classical pathway activation, i.e., increased degradation, occurs in normal pregnancy (Lockshin 1993).

Abnormal pregnancy

Hypertensive disorders

The impact of hypertension in pregnancy ranges from negligible to severe. *Pregnancy-induced hypertension (PIH)* is defined by blood pressure of 140/90 which develops as a consequence of pregnancy and which resolves after pregnancy. *Transient hypertension* develops after the second trimester and is characterized by mild elevations of blood pressure that do not compromise the pregnancy and regress *post partum*. *Coincidental hypertension* refers to chronic hypertension that antedates pregnancy or persists *post partum*. Risks associated with coincidental hypertension include preeclampsia, eclampsia and *abruptio placentae* (Barron 1995) (Table 8.1).

Table 8.1 Common renal pregnancy complications unrelated to SLE

Complication	Clinical manifestations
Preeclampsia, eclampsia	Proteinuria, hypertension, edema, hyperuricemia, thrombocytopenia, renal insufficiency, abdominal pain, encephalopathy, convulsion
Pregnancy-induced hypertension	Hypertension, proteinuria, edema, renal insufficiency
HELLP syndrome	Hemolysis, elevated liver enzymes, thrombocytopenia (low platelets), abdominal pain, hepatic failure

Preeclampsia, also known as toxemia, usually develops late in pregnancy with hypertension, proteinuria, edema, and hyperuricemia. *Eclampsia* is severe preeclampsia that progresses to seizures. Patients with advanced preeclampsia may develop hepatic infarction or congestive heart failure. Thrombocytopenia, often severe, is common. Complement levels may be low. In its eclamptic phase, preeclampsia may be lethal. Preeclampsia is more common in patients with SLE, antiphospholipid antibody (aPL), or underlying renal disease, and in these settings tends to be early and severe. The clinical presentation of preeclampsia is easily confused with that of active SLE (Saftlas *et al.* 1990; Barron 1995).

The acronym *HELLP syndrome* refers to *h*emolysis, *e*levated *l*iver enzymes, and *l*ow *p*latelets. Patients suffer prominent hepatic transaminase abnormalities, fever, hepatic pain, and encephalopathy; thrombocytopenia can be life threatening. As in preeclampsia, fetal and/or maternal death may occur. HELLP syndrome may worsen *post partum* (Magann *et al.* 1994). Risk of severe HELLP syndrome is probably increased in patients with lupus and antiphospholipid syndrome (Ornstein and Rand 1994). Corticosteroids, used in the management of early mild HELLP, can stabilize platelet counts and prolong gestation (Magann *et al.* 1994). Short of ending the pregnancy, there is no definitive treatment. Cases of HELLP syndrome that continued after delivery have resolved with plasmapheresis (Ornstein and Rand 1994).

Hematologic complications

Thrombocytopenia occurs regularly in late normal pregnancy; it self-corrects upon delivery and usually needs no specific treatment. An increase in factors I (fibrinogen), II (prothrombin), VII, VIII, IX, and X; a decrease in protein S levels; and an inhibition of the fibrinolytic system have an overall procoagulant effect. As a result of this and of anatomic factors (e.g. venous compression by the gravid uterus), the risk of venous thromboembolism is five times higher in the pregnant than in the nonpregnant woman. Pelvic thrombophlebitis and pulmonary embolization are severe peripartum complications (Greer 1999; Toglia and Weg 1996).

APL increases risk of maternal thrombosis in untreated pregnancy. The presence of the factor V Leiden mutation and clinically silent deficiencies in antithrombin III, protein C, and protein S clearly add to risk of thrombosis in pregnancy (Bokarewa *et al.* 1996; Lee 1996; Greer 1999). The increased hypercoagulability state associated with nephrotic syndrome, common in SLE patients and often exacerbated during pregnancy, may present additional risk.

Placental complications

Abnormalities in development or function of the placenta occur in the context of many pregnancy complications, including preeclampsia and aPL. Placental abnormalities may be life threatening for the mother as well as the fetus. *Abruptio placentae* is premature separation of the normally implanted placenta, usually presenting as vaginal hemorrhage. Frequency of placental abruption is estimated at 1 in 150, with a perinatal mortality rate of 20%. Abruption is associated with pregnancy-induced or chronic hypertension. Shock, consumption coagulopathy, and renal failure may accompany severe abruption (Barron 1995; Karegard and Gennser 1986).

Other pregnancy complications

The spectrum of cardiac disease in lupus pregnancy includes valvular heart disease, pulmonary hypertension, and peripartum cardiomyopathy (O'Connell *et al.* 1986). Ischemic heart disease is a rare complication, even in patients with SLE (Thorp *et al.* 1994). Severe diabetes mellitus (DM) with nephropathy may have a significant impact on pregnancy outcome (American College of Obstetricians and Gynecologists 1994), especially if in conjunction with lupus nephritis. *Acute fatty liver of pregnancy* may lead to hepatic coma in up to 60% of cases, coagulopathy in 55% and renal failure in 55% (Pertuiset and Grunfeld 1994). Fetal death is common and maternal outcome variable.

Both pregnancy and lactation impact bone metabolism. Calcium metabolism is altered. Parathyroid hormone generally remains stable or decreases during normal pregnancy. Osteocalcin remains in the normal to low range, varying with trimester (Sowers 1996). Free 1, 25-dihydroxyvitamin D, vitamin D binding proteins and bound dihydroxyvitamin D levels all increase (Gertner *et al.* 1986). Most recent studies suggest a decrease of 5–10% in mean bone density during normal pregnancy (Koltoff *et al.* 1998; Honda *et al.* 1998). Fall in bone mass does not usually reverse until after resumption of menstruation. Even in the nonlactating woman, this may take up to 18 months (Koltoff *et al.* 1998). Lactation delays the resumption of menses and may cause a further decrease in bone density. The risk of osteoporosis is significantly increased by several factors: patients with renal dysfunction or those treated with long-term steroids may begin a pregnancy with low bone mass; corticosteroid and/or heparin therapy during pregnancy may cause frank osteoporosis, with spinal fracture rates of up to 2% (Dahlman 1993). Patients with risk factors for osteoporosis may be counselled to avoid breastfeeding.

Lupus pregnancy

Flare

Definition of flare in the nonpregnant patient is still controversial because of multiple instruments used to quantify lupus activity (Buyon *et al.* 1999). Common pregnancy complications may cause signs and symptoms commonly associated with lupus activity. There have been a number of attempts to answer the specific question, 'Does pregnancy cause SLE to flare?' but no agreement as yet (Table 8.2) (Lockshin *et al.* 1984; Petri *et al.* 1991; Urowitz *et al.* 1993; Ruiz-Irastorza *et al.* 1996). Different populations and entry criteria among clinics are likely responsible for the different conclusions (Lockshin 1992). Despite lack of consensus, it is clear both that many patients do well during pregnancy and that vigilance for flare on the part of the treating physician is always necessary.

Table 8.2 Flare rates in pregnant patients and controls, in various series

Author	Flare rate, pregnant	Flare rate, control	Author's conclusion
Lockshin 1984	25%/pregnancy (measure A) [*] 11%/pregnancy (measure B)	25% (measure A) 11% (measure B)	Pregnancy does not cause flare
Petri 1991	59%/pregnancy 1.63/person–year	53%/pregnancy 0.64/person–year	Pregnancy does cause flare
Urowitz 1993	47%/pregnancy (measure A) [†] 70%/pregnancy (measure B)	– 80% (measure B)	Pregnancy does not cause flare
Ruiz–Irastorza 1996	8.2%/month	3.9%	Pregnancy does cause flare

[*] Measure A assigns all thrombocytopenia and proteinuria to SLE; measure B attributes some of these abnormalities to toxemia.
[†] During pregnancy (measure A) and pregnancy plus 3 months (measure B).

Severe multisystemic SLE will seriously complicate pregnancy, primarily through its manifestations of high fever, hypertension, renal failure, and on occasion cardiac and respiratory failure, as well as through the treatments administered.

Thrombocytopenia is common in SLE pregnancy, especially in those patients with antiphospholipid antibody. Thrombocytopenia during gestation in patients with SLE occurs in five patterns: (1) early and mild, often in association with aPL, (2) late and tending to worsen as pregnancy progresses, usually associated with worsening fetal health and manifestations of preeclampsia or the HELLP syndrome, (3) severe, of the idiopathic thrombocytopenic purpura type, (4) moderate, accompanied by other manifestations of active SLE, responding to prednisone, and (5) the common benign thrombocytopenia of late pregnancy, unrelated to SLE. No specific test clearly differentiates one type of thrombocytopenia from another in pregnant patients with SLE. In our experience approximately one-fourth of all SLE patients experience thrombocytopenia during pregnancy (Lockshin *et al.* 1984; Lockshin 1989). Antiphospholipid antibody syndrome, active SLE, and preeclampsia are equally distributed causes. SLE-induced *anemia* amplifies the normal dilutional anemia of pregnancy and may indicate a need to use corticosteroid for protection of the fetus.

Renal manifestations

It is not clear whether patients with SLE renal disease do less well than those with other forms of glomerulonephritis. Renal prognosis in pregnancy in general depends on preexisting level of renal function and presence or absence of hypertension (Jones and Hayslett 1996; Lindheimer *et al.* 1995). Because the ability to maintain a pregnancy in patients with lupus and other types of nephritis declines with decreasing renal function, GFR but not histologic type affects risk of deterioration in renal function (Devoe *et al.* 1983; Jungers *et al.* 1982; Bobrie *et al.* 1987). Quiescent lupus for at least six months pre-conception lessens the chance of recurrent nephritis.

Most normotensive patients with mildly decreased and stable renal function do well: pregnancy success rates are over 90%, with little risk of irreversible adverse effect on renal function. Prognosis is poorer if renal function is moderately impaired (serum creatinine 1.4–3.0 mg/dL). While fetal outcome is generally good, one-third of these patients will have functional renal deterioration that persists *post partum* (Jones and Hayslett 1996; Lindheimer *et al.* 1995). Patients with severe renal function are at high risk of poor outcome. When conception does occur, the pregnancy success rate in patients receiving dialysis is less than 50%; potential complications include intraperitoneal hemorrhage and malignant hypertension (Gafter *et al.* 1990).

Although proteinuria may increase during pregnancy, the increments being 'physiologic' and unrelated to disease activity, it is always prudent to assume that a marked increase in proteinuria, especially in the presence of hypertension, indicates a problem. Rapid worsening over days is more common in preeclampsia than in SLE. In the evaluation of increasing urinary protein, clinical signs of active SLE, rising anti-dsDNA antibody and the appearance of erythrocyte casts favour the diagnosis of lupus glomerulonephritis. Normal serum complement favours preeclampsia (Table 8.3) (Lockshin *et al.* 1986; Buyon *et al.* 1986; Packham *et al.* 1992).

Pregnancy-induced thrombocytopenia may mimic SLE disease activity and so may not be helpful in distinguishing between the two conditions. New or increasing rash, lymphadenopathy, arthritis, fever, or anti-dsDNA antibody are the strongest reasons to attribute urinary or hematologic abnormalities to SLE rather than to preeclampsia.

Hypertension, thrombocytopenia, hyperuricemia, and, in some cases, hypocomplementemia occur in both lupus nephritis and preeclampsia. The interpretation of hypocomplementemic proteinuria in lupus pregnancy may be difficult. Although not common, low-grade activation of the classical pathway may be attributable to pregnancy alone (Lockshin *et al.*, 1986). Measures of alternative pathway complement activation (Ba and Bb) are abnormal in active lupus nephritis and normal in lupus pregnancies with proteinuria not due to active SLE. Evaluation of the alternative complement pathway may be the clearest way to determine whether new proteinuria in the pregnant patient is due to active SLE or to preeclampsia (Buyon *et al.* 1986). In the absence of a single definitive test, distinctions between lupus nephritis and superimposed preeclampsia must be made on clinical criteria. Renal biopsy may distinguish between lupus nephritis and preeclampsia, but is usually not feasible.

Placental pathology does not aid in differentiating SLE and antiphospholipid syndrome (APS) from preeclampsia–eclampsia. Often small in size, lupus and preeclamptic placentae demonstrate evidence of ischemia and vasculopathy. Antiphospholipid antibody placentae additionally demonstrate extensive infarction. It is usually impossible to define an underlying diagnosis on the basis of placental histologic changes alone (Salafia and Cowchock 1997; de Wolf *et al.* 1982; Sammaritano *et al.*, 1996; Hanly *et al.* 1988).

APS may cause renal insufficiency on the basis of *in situ* glomerular thrombosis, either alone or in conjunction with multisystem disease termed catastrophic APS (Neuwelt *et al.* 1997). A subset of patients with idiopathic *post partum* renal failure develops renal failure with a hemolytic-uremic syndrome-like picture related to antiphospholipid antibody (Kincaid-Smith and Nicholls 1990; Kon *et al.* 1995). Renal biopsy in aPL-related *post partum* renal failure is consistent with thrombotic microangiopathy. Thrombotic microangiopathy and classic lupus nephritis are clinically very similar; renal biopsy is often necessary. Impaired renal function, microangiopathic anemia, thrombocytopenia, and raised fibrin degradation products suggest this diagnosis. Hepatic infarction has also been closely associated with APS, especially in the presence of preeclampsia. Plasmapheresis may be life saving (Amant *et al.* 1997; Millan-Mon *et al.* 1993).

Managing pregnancy

Initial assessment

When is pregnancy best undertaken? The longer the patient is in remission, the better her chances for completing a pregnancy without exacerbation. Pregnancy

Table 8.3 Comparison between preeclampsia and lupus nephritis

Clinical measure	Preeclampsia	Lupus nephritis
C3, C4, CH$_{50}$	May be low	Almost always low
Urinalysis	Red blood cell (RBC) casts rare	RBC casts frequent
Onset of proteinuria	Commonly abrupt	Gradual or abrupt
Hepatic aminotransferases	May be increased	Rarely abnormal
Quantity of proteinuria	Will not differentiate	
Thrombocytopenia	Will not differentiate	
Hyperuricemia	Will not differentiate	
Hypertension	Will not differentiate	

is inadvisable when there is high probability of maternal or fetal death or disability and very little likelihood of a healthy child. Circumstances of this type, in addition to severe hypertension and progressive renal failure, include current use of teratogenic drugs, severe central nervous system disease, severe thrombocytopenia, and moderate-to-severe cardiopulmonary disease.

Initial pre-pregnancy evaluation of the lupus patient should include assessment of disease activity and screening for pertinent autoantibodies including anti-Ro/SSA and anti-La/SSB (predictors of neonatal lupus syndrome) and antiphospholipid antibody and lupus anticoagulant (predictors of pregnancy loss). Evaluation should also include assessment of dysfunction of renal and other relevant organ systems, and review of current medications. Table 8.4 indicates recommended initial and subsequent laboratory investigations.

Discontinuation of patient's current drugs is often necessary. Because the effect of hydroxychloroquine on the developing fetus remains unresolved, a conservative approach is to discontinue the drug for six months in advance of pregnancy. A patient taking warfarin might consider switching to heparin while she is attempting to conceive, especially if no fertility problems are anticipated. There

Table 8.4 Monitoring of the pregnant SLE patient. Note: The erythrocyte sedimentation rate is often abnormal in uncomplicated pregnancy and is not useful to follow

Recommended frequency	Monitoring test
First visit	Complete blood count, including platelets
	Urinalysis
	Creatinine clearance
	24-hour urine protein
	Anticardiolipin antibody
	Lupus anticoagulant
	Anti-SSA/Ro and anti-SSB/La antibodies
	Anti-dsDNA antibody
	Complement (C3 and C4 or CH_{50})
Monthly	Platelet count
Each trimester	Creatinine clearance[†]
	24-hour urine protein if screening urinalysis abnormal[†]
	Anticardiolipin antibody
	Complement[†]
	Anti-dsDNA antibody[†]
Weekly (3rd trimester, mothers with antiphospholipid antibody)	Antenatal fetal heart rate testing ('nonstress test'), periodic biophysical profile
At 18 and 25 weeks (mothers with anti-SSA/Ro and anti-SSB/La antibodies)	Fetal echocardiogram, ?fetal electrocardiogram

[†] More frequently if abnormal.

Table 8.5 Advice regarding discontinuation of commonly used drugs before and during pregnancy

Drug	Prior to pregnancy	During pregnancy
Prednisone	Continue at lowest effective dose	Continue at lowest effective dose
Aspirin (anti-inflammatory dose)	Continue at lowest effective dose	Discontinue or use low dose prednisone
NSAIDs	Continue at lowest effective dose	Discontinue or use low dose prednisone
Azathioprine	Consider withdrawing	Consider withdrawing
Cyclophosphamide	Discontinue	Discontinue
Methotrexate	Discontinue	Discontinue
Hydroxychloroquine	Consider discontinuing 6 months before	Consider discontinuing
Warfarin	Switch to heparin when pregnancy attempted	Switch to heparin

* NSAIDs, non-steroidal anti-inflammatory drugs.

is no documented evidence that increasing corticosteroid therapy solely because of pregnancy improves maternal or fetal prognosis. The authors do not employ such prophylactic treatment. General advice regarding commonly used drugs is displayed in Table 8.5.

Management of pregnancy: mother

Table 8.4 indicates suggested frequency of monitoring for a patient with an uncomplicated pregnancy. Clinical activity of disease, and any pregnancy abnormality, mandates more frequent observations.

General management. With qualifications, criteria for treatment of the pregnant patient do not differ from criteria for the nonpregnant patient. The choice to use antimalarial, nonsteroidal, and immunosuppressive drugs, however, is restricted by weighing potential fetal injury against control of maternal disease. Anemia (hemoglobin less than 8.0 g/dL), fever (sustained fever greater than 38.5 degrees Celsius) and hypoalbuminemia (albumin less than 3.0 g/dL) merit more aggressive treatment in the pregnant patient than they might in the nonpregnant patient because these abnormalities threaten the growing fetus. Worsening fetal health, *in the absence of clinical exacerbation of SLE*, does not justify treatment for SLE.

Thrombocytopenia, independent of antiphospholipid antibodies or preeclampsia, is not an independent predictor of fetal death. Treatment of thrombocytopenia in a pregnant lupus patient depends on clear definition of the underlying etiology. There is no documented evidence that treatment of modest thrombocytopenia ($70–150 \times 10^9$/L) improves either maternal or fetal prognosis, but many physicians interpret modest thrombocytopenia as evidence of disease activity and do treat. When thrombocytopenia is life threatening ($<30 \times 10^9$/L) or if delivery is imminent, treatment is indicated. Temporary remission of thrombocytopenia may be obtained by infusing platelets or intravenous aggregate-free immunoglobulin G (IVIG) (Yu and Lennon 1999; Newland *et al.* 1984). Intravenous immunoglobulin adds to the volume load in patients with renal dysfunction, however.

Case reports of fatalities due to pulmonary hypertension developing or worsening during pregnancy suggest that patients with lung involvement should avoid conceiving (Ray and Sermer 1996; Rubin *et al.* 1995). Anti-inflammatory doses of aspirin or nonsteroidal anti-inflammatory drugs are not recommended in pregnancy. For treatment of arthralgia or arthritis, low-dose prednisone is preferred. Corticosteroid therapy is the primary treatment for the SLE-caused anemia. Recently, safety and efficacy of human recombinant erythropoietin in pregnancy have been shown, including at least one case of SLE pregnancy with nephritis (Braga *et al.* 1996; Kontessis *et al.* 1995). Rashes may be treated with topical or systemic corticosteroid.

Management of renal disease. In our experience with 125 completed SLE pregnancies, only 15% of SLE patients entered pregnancy with preexisting renal disease. Of this 15%, two-thirds (10% of the total) developed preeclampsia, a complication that also developed in 14% of the 107 women without preexisting kidney disease. Our experience is similar to that of Nossent and Swaak (1990) but differs from the prognoses reported by Petri *et al.* (1991), who reported that more than half of their SLE patients entered pregnancy with preexisting lupus nephritis and had a high frequency of renal flare.

High-dose (60 mg/day) oral corticosteroid therapy is the initial treatment of SLE glomerulonephritis. In the pregnant patient, the risk of hypertension may be greater than in the nonpregnant patient. Obstetricians frequently use low-dose aspirin, (60–100 mg/day) to prevent preeclampsia in women identified as being at high risk (usually those with preexisting hypertension or renal disease) (Beaufils *et al.* 1985; Dekker and Sibai 1993; Schiff and Mashiach 1992). Aspirin does not reduce incidence of preeclampsia in women at low risk for this complication (Schoenfeld *et al.* 1992). No systematic study justifies the use of aspirin to prevent preeclampsia in SLE patients. Nonetheless, some physicians, including us, do prescribe this drug.

Patients with severe hypertension, on hemodialysis, or with renal transplants may achieve successful pregnancies. Peritoneal dialysis is preferred over hemodialysis, because it allows more gradual changes in volume, less risk of hypotension, and decreased risk of uterine contractions. Hemodialysis patients should be dialyzed daily to minimize high flux states and to maintain the BUN less than 40–50, since urea and other toxins do cross the placenta (Lindheimer *et al.* 1995).

Transplantation usually reverses infertility. Pregnancy prognosis of transplanted patients is good, and parallels that for women with a similar degree of renal insufficiency. It is not clear whether pregnancy affects the long-term function of the transplanted kidney (Lindheimer *et al.* 1995).

Fetus. Fetal growth and development in SLE patients may be threatened by disease activity, by abnormality of maternal renal function, by antiphospholipid antibody, and by anti-SSA/Ro and anti-SSB/La antibody. SLE activity by itself does not alter the outcome of pregnancy (Devoe *et al.* 1983). Unexplained elevation of maternal alpha-fetoprotein occurs in patients with systemic lupus erythematosus. The elevation correlates with preterm delivery, high prednisone dose, and presence of antiphospholipid antibody (Silver *et al.* 1994). It usually does not imply fetal malformation.

Maternal IgG-mediated thrombocytopenia may be transmitted to the fetus, but most infants born of thrombocytopenic mothers with SLE have normal platelet counts. Antiphospholipid antibody, while associated with placental insufficiency and intrauterine growth retardation, does not cause other abnormalities in the infant. In women with anti-SSA/Ro or anti-SSB/La antibodies, neonatal lupus (NLE) is a risk. (NLE includes transient rash, thrombocytopenia or liver function abnormalities, and permanent congenital complete heart block.) Fetal growth rate and placental function may be monitored by sonography and by weekly antepartum fetal heart rate testing (non-stress testing) beginning as early as 25 weeks (Druzin *et al.* 1987; Weiner *et al.* 1992; Adams *et al.* 1992; Kerslake *et al.* 1992).

Active lupus, of itself, does not mandate ending a pregnancy. Maternal complications that call for urgent termination of a pregnancy, regardless of fetal maturity, are more often pregnancy- than lupus-related: progressive preeclampsia, in any of its manifestations, progressive hepatic failure from fatty liver or HELLP syndrome, uncontrollable heart failure, and, sometimes, severe thrombocytopenia. Pregnancies may continue in the face of severe renal failure (including dialysis and transplant), advanced nephrosis, thrombocytopenia, and maternal neurologic disease.

Fetal death, intrauterine growth restriction, and prematurity are common in SLE pregnancies. They result from severe maternal disease, antiphospholipid antibody, or both. Prematurity most commonly results from a decision to deliver because of fetal distress. Centres differ in the frequency of premature delivery, but rates of 50% are usual. Premature rupture of membranes, often associated with corticosteroid therapy, is common (Cowchock *et al.* 1992). Other than neonatal lupus, there are no congenital, genetic, or developmental abnormalities associated with SLE. Brain and other damage may result from prematurity, placental insufficiency, or toxemia.

Antiphospholipid antibody syndrome

Risk for current pregnancy loss due to antiphospholipid antibody is a function both of prior maternal pregnancy history and of titre of anticardiolipin antibody and/or lupus anticoagulant. Table 8.6 summarizes published studies that describe risk imparted by antiphospholipid antibody in SLE patients (Out *et al.* 1991; Ramsey-Goldman *et al.* 1992; Julkunen *et al.* 1993). Some authors believe that the likelihood and severity of preeclampsia is increased in women who have antiphospholipid antibody. Hepatic infarction and renal thrombotic microan-

Table 8.6 Effect of antiphospholipid antibody on pregnancy in patients with SLE. Abbreviations: aCL, anticardiolipin antibody; lupus anticoagulant; aPL, antiphospholipid antibody (aCL and/or LAC)

Reference	Study group	Result
Out 1991	59 pregnant SLE with aPL vs.	LAC, prior loss predict new loss; aPL, prior loss predict IUGR
	54 pregnant SLE without aPL	
Ramsey-Goldman 1992	81 pregnant SLE with aPL vs.	51% adverse outcome vs. 43%; IgG aPL, prior loss predict adverse outcome
	174 pregnant SLE without aPL	
Julkunen 1993	242 SLE pregnancies vs.	LAC odds ratio 3.4; aCL and LAC predict fetal loss
	417 pregnancies	

Table 8.7 Treatment recommendations for pregnant women with antiphospholipid antibody

Patient characteristic	Recommendation
Moderate-high titre IgG or IgM aPL antibody	
Primipara or multipara, most recent pregnancy liveborn	Consider aspirin, 81 mg/d, or no therapy initially; if modest (>50 × 10^9/L) thrombocytopenia occurs, aspirin
Multipara, most recent pregnancy failure < 10 weeks (1 or 2 losses)	Aspirin
Multipara, most recent pregnancy failure ≥ 10 weeks without other explanation, or > 2 (early) loss or preeclampsia with preterm birth < 34 wks.	Aspirin while trying to conceive; add heparin, 5000 units BID at confirmation of fetal heartbeat, continue for duration of pregnancy
Low-titre IgG or IgM aPL antibody	
Primipara or multipara, no prior fetal loss	No therapy
Multipara, most recent pregnancy failure < 10 weeks (1 or 2 losses)	Aspirin
Multipara, most recent pregnancy failure ≥ 10 weeks without other explanation, or > 2 (early) loss, or preeclampsia with preterm birth < 34 wks.	Aspirin while trying to conceive; add heparin, 5000 units BID at confirmation of pregnancy, continue for duration of pregnancy
Multipara, hypertension or renal disease	Aspirin, beginning after first trimester
Negative aPL antibody	
Multipara, prior pre-eclampsia, IUGR, hypertension, or renal disease	Aspirin, beginning after first trimester

* For thrombocytopenia < 50 × 10^9/L, consider intravenous immunoglobulin and/or prednisone.

giopathy in association with early preeclampsia have occurred in several antiphospholipid antibody patients (Amant *et al.* 1997). Fetal survival, although complicated by prematurity and intrauterine growth restriction, may approach rates of up to 80%.

Our treatment recommendations are presented in Table 8.7. In women with the secondary antiphospholipid syndrome, SLE disease activity may mandate use of prednisone. The comments below apply to women with primary antiphospholipid syndrome or in those with the secondary syndrome in whom SLE is in remission. Recent studies suggest that sub-anticoagulant doses of heparin (5000 to 7000 units BID) are effective (Table 8.8) (Kutteh 1996; Rai *et al.* 1997). Low-molecular-weight heparin has been used safely and successfully (Kutteh and Ermal 1996). It is usual practice to use one 'baby' aspirin per day in conjunction with heparin. Warfarin is teratogenic and so is not used in pregnancy; subcutaneous heparin or low molecular weight heparin in full therapeutic doses is the anticoagulant of choice in women with prior thrombosis.

Drug treatment in lupus pregnancy

Physiology of drug metabolism during pregnancy

Physiologic changes during pregnancy alter maternal pharmacokinetics that in turn may affect the amount of drug reaching the mother, the placenta and the fetus (Ward 1993). In SLE, hypertension, and diabetes mellitus, disordered maternal and fetal physiology may produce placental changes that impact drug transfer from mother to fetus. Drug distribution changes with expansion of maternal blood volume (Ward 1993). In most cases there are no detailed guidelines for adjusting dose in pregnancy, or in pregnancy of patients with renal disease.

Drugs used for treating lupus

Nonsteroidal anti-inflammatory drugs (NSAIDs). Salicylates do not cause fetal anomalies (Streissguth *et al.* 1987). Aspirin in therapeutic dose, but not at 80–150 mg/day, has been associated with oligohydramnios, premature closure of the ductus arteriosus, and pulmonary hypertension. In many cases of minor arthritis or serositis during SLE pregnancy, low dose prednisone is preferable to either aspirin or NSAIDs because of its known safety and minimal placental transfer.

Antimalarials. Evidence regarding the teratogenicity of hydroxychloquine is sparse (Roubenoff *et al.* 1988), and drug safety is not established. Concerns, based on laboratory animal data, include eye and ear toxicity, which have not been reported in humans to date. While it seems prudent to avoid use of these agents during pregnancy if possible, lupus flare after discontinuation of hydroxychloroquine is a real concern.

Corticosteroids. Prednisone and methylprednisolone have minimal placental transfer and are the drugs of choice for patients requiring corticosteroid therapy (Anderson *et al.* 1981; Rayburn 1992). In conventional doses, they are safe for the fetus. Fluorinated corticosteroids (dexamethasone and betamethasone) should not

Table 8.8 Randomized controlled trials of treatment for recurrent fetal loss in women with antiphospholipid antibody

Author	No. A/B	Regimen A	Regimen B	Fetal survival A	Fetal survival B
Cowchock 1992	12/8	heparin 12000u BID + ASA 81 mg	Prednisone 40 mg + ASA 81 mg	80	75*
Kutteh 1996	25/25	heparin 13300u BID+ ASA 81 mg	ASA 81 mg	80	44
Rai 1997	45/45	heparin 5000u BID + ASA 81 mg	ASA 81 mg	70	40
Kutteh and Ermel 1996	25/25	heparin 8100u BID + ASA 81 mg	Heparin 13300u BID + ASA 81 mg	76	80

*Marked increase in fetal and maternal morbidity compared to regimen A.

Table 8.9 Lupus-specific issues which may force operative delivery

---

• Severe hypertension
• Severe thrombocytopenia
• Severe renal disease
• Immediate need to institute life-saving treatment to the mother which will be harmful
    to the fetus
• Severe maternal cardiac disease
• Severe pulmonary disease
• Deteriorating heart function in a fetus with congenital heart block
• Orthopedic indication (i.e. restricted hip range of motion)

---

therapy it is advisable to give 'stress' steroid doses beginning with the onset of labour and continuing for twenty-four hours after delivery concludes. The authors recommend against routine increases in corticosteroid dose to prevent *post-partum* flare. Anticoagulation, including aspirin, must cease with the onset of labour, to resume once risk of hemorrhage is over; reinstitution of anticoagulation one to two days after delivery is usual. Given the risk of peripartum thrombosis in APS patients, anticoagulation should continue for three months *post partum* in women with no history of thrombosis, and indefinitely in women who have suffered thromboses.

It is important to alert the neonatalogy staff about the mother's anti-Ro/SSA and anti-La/SSB status so that they may be aware of risk of rash, thrombocytopenia, and congenital heart block of neonatal lupus. The pregnancy complications of preeclampsia, HELLP syndrome, and fatty liver of pregnancy may continue to progress for several days to weeks *post partum* before they eventually regress. Treatment decisions should therefore consider the possibility of insufficient hepatic or renal clearance of drugs and presence of serious confounding illness in immediate *post partum* patients.

Breast feeding

Compounds with high molecular weights are unable to pass through cell membranes into breast milk. Since milk is mildly acidic, weak bases pass most readily into breast milk, creating a higher concentration in milk than in plasma (Gardner 1992). Aspirin and NSAIDs are highly protein-bound weak acids that do not pass easily into breast milk. The most reasonable NSAID to use is ibuprofen, 400 mg every six hours, since this has not been detected in breast milk (Townsend *et al.* 1984). The major anticoagulants are safe during breast-feeding. Heparin is too large to pass into breast milk, and warfarin (highly bound to plasma proteins and itself weakly acidic) is not detectable. For patients with SLE, the major concern is safety of corticosteroid therapy during lactation. Overall, especially with low doses and appropriate corticosteroid choice (prednisone or prednisolone), very little steroid is transmitted to breast milk. The neonatal effect (plasma level) in a woman taking a maternal dose of prednisolone of 20 mg/day or less is insignificant. Feeding just prior to ingestion of the medication (Gardner 1992) further minimizes infant corticosteroid exposure.

References

Adams D. *et al.* (1992). Antepartum testing – systemic – lupus erythematosus and associated serologic abnormalities. *American Journal of Reproductive Immunolology*, 28, 159–64.

Amant F. *et al.* (1997). Hepatic necrosis and haemorrhage in pregnant patients with antiphospholipid antibodies. *Lupus*, 6, 552–555.

American College of Obstetricians and Gynecologists (1994). Diabetes and pregnancy. Technical Bulletin 200, December 1994.

Anderson G.G. *et al.* (1981). Placental transfer of methylprednisolone following maternal intravenous administration. *American Journal of Obstetrics and Gynecology*, 140, 699–701.

Barron W.M. (1995). Hypertension. In: W.M. Barron and M.D. Lindheimer (eds) *Medical disorders during pregnancy*, pp. 1–36. Mosby, St. Louis.

Beaufils M. *et al.* (1985). Prevention of pre-eclampsia by early antiplatelet therapy. *Lancet*, 1, 840–42.

Bermas B.L and Hill J.A. (1995). Effects of immunosuppressive drugs during pregnancy. *Arthritis and Rheumatism*, 38, 722–32.

Bobrie G. *et al.* (1987). Pregnancy in lupus nephritis and related disorders. *American Journal of Kidney Disease*, IX, 339–43.

Bokarewa M.E. *et al.* (1996). Arg506 – Gln mutation in factor V and risk of thrombosis during pregnancy. *British Journal of Haematology*, 92, 473–8.

Braga J. *et al.* (1996). Maternal and perinatal implications of the use of human recombinant erythropoietin. *Acta Obstetrica et Gynecologica Scandinavica*, 75, 449–53.

Branch D.W. (1992). Physiologic adaptations of pregnancy. *American Journal of Reproductive Immunology*, 28, 120–2.

Branch D.W. *et al.* (2000). A multicenter, placebo-controlled pilot study of intravenous immune globulin treatment of antiphospholipid syndrome during pregnancy. The Pregnancy Loss Study Group. *American Journal of Obstetrics and Gynecology*, 182, 122–7.

Burrows R.F. and Kelton J.G. (1988). Incidentally detected thrombocytopenia in healthy mothers and their infants. *New England Journal of Medicine*, 319, 142–5.

Buyon J.P. *et al.* (1986). Serum complement values (C3 and C4) to differentiate between systemic lupus activity and pre-eclampsia. *American Journal of Medicine*, 81, 194–200.

Buyon J.P. *et al.* (1999). Assessing disease activity in SLE patients during pregnancy. *Lupus*, 8, 677–84.

Chaouat G. *et al.* (1990). Control of fetal survival in CBA × DBA/2 mice by lymphokine therapy. *Journal of Reproduction and Fertility*, 89, 447–58.

Cowchock F.S. *et al.* (1992). Repeated fetal losses associated with antiphospholipid antibodies, a collaborative randomized trial comparing prednisone with low dose heparin treatment. *American Journal of Obstetrics and Gynecology*, 166, 1318–23.

Dahlman T.C. (1993). Osteoporotic fractures and the recurrence of thromboembolism during pregnancy and the puerperium in 184 women undergoing thromboprophylaxis with heparin. *American Journal of Obstetrics and Gynecology*, 168, 1265–70.

de Wolf F. *et al.* (1982). Decidual vasculopathy and extensive placental infarction in a patient with repeated thromboembolic accidents, recurrent fetal loss and a lupus anticoagulant. *American Journal of Obstetrics and Gynecology*, 142, 829–34.

Dekker G.A. and Sibai B.M. (1993). Low – dose aspirin in the prevention of preeclampsia and fetal growth retardation. Rationale, mechanisms, and clinical trials. *American Journal of Obstetrics and Gynecology*, 168, 214–27.

Devoe L.D. *et al.* (1983). Renal histology and pregnancy performance in systemic lupus erythematosus. *Clinical and Experimental Hypertension*, B2(2), 325–40.

Druzin M.L. *et al.* (1987). Second – trimester fetal monitoring and preterm delivery in pregnancies with systemic lupus erythematosus and/or circulating anticoagulant. *American Journal of Obstetrics and Gynecology*, 157, 1503–10.

Fraga A. *et al.* (1974). Sterility and fertility rates, fetal wastage and maternal morbidity in systemic lupus erythematosus. *Journal of Rheumatology*, 1, 293–8.

Gafter V. *et al.* (1990). Successful pregnancies in women on regular hemodialysis treatment. *Israel Journal of Medical Science*, 26, 266–70.

Gardner D.K. (1992). Drugs in breast milk. In: W.F. Rayburn and F.P. Zuspan (eds) *Drug Therapy in Obstetrics and Gynecology*, pp. 312–25. Mosby Yearbook Company, St. Louis.

Gertner J. *et al.* (1986). Pregnancy as a state of physiologic absorptive hypercalciuria. *American Journal of Medicine*, 81, 451–6.

Greer I.A. (1999). Thrombosis in pregnancy, maternal and fetal issues. *Lancet*, 353, 1258–65.

Hanley J.G. *et al.* (1988). Lupus pregnancy. A prospective study of placental changes. *Arthritis and Rheumatism*, 31, 358–66.

Hill J.A. (1992). Cytokines considered critical in pregnancy. *American Journal of Reproductive Immunology*, 28, 123–6.

Honda A. *et al.* (1998). Lumbar bone mineral density changes during pregnancy and lactation. *International Journal of Obstetrics and Gynecology*, 63, 253–8.

Jones D.C. and Hayslett J.P. (1996). Outcome of pregnancy in women with moderate or severe renal insufficiency. *New England Journal of Medicine*, 335, 226–32.

Julkunen H. *et al.* (1993). Fetal outcome in lupus pregnancy, a retrospective case – control study of 242 pregnancies in 112 patients. *Lupus*, 2, 125–31.

Jungers P. *et al.* (1982). Lupus nephropathy and pregnancy. *Archives of Internal Medicine*, 142, 771–6.

Karegard M. and Gennser G. (1986). Incidence and recurrence rate of abruptio placentae in Sweden. *Obstetrics and Gynecology*, 67, 523–5.

Kerslake S. *et al.* (1992). Early Doppler studies in lupus pregnancy. *American Journal of Reproductive Immunology*, 28, 172–5.

Kincaid-Smith P. and Nicholls K. (1990). Renal thrombotic microvascular disease associated with lupus anticoagulant. *Nephron*, 54, 285–8.

Koltoff N. *et al.* (1998). Bone mineral changes during pregnancy and lactation, a longitudinal cohort study. *Clinical Sciences*, 94, 405–12.

Kon S.P. *et al.* (1995). Reversible renal failure due to the antiphospholipid antibody syndrome, pre-eclampsia and renal thrombotic microangiopathy. *Clinical Nephrology*, 44, 271–3.

Kontessis P.S. *et al.* (1995). Successful use of recombinant human erythropoietin in a pregnant woman with lupus nephritis. *American Journal of Kidney Disease*, 26, 781–4.

Kutteh W.H. (1996). Antiphospholipid antibody-associated recurrent pregnancy loss, treatment with heparin and low-dose aspirin is superior to low-dose aspirin alone. *American Journal of Obstetrics and Gynecology*, 174, 1584–9.

Kutteh W.H. and Ermel L.D. (1996). A clinical trial for the treatment of antiphospholipid antibody-associated recurrent pregnancy loss with lower dose heparin and aspirin. *American Journal of Reproductive Immunology*, 35, 402–7.

Lahita R.G. (1992). The effects of sex hormones on the immune system in pregnancy. *American Journal of Reproductive Immunology*, 28, 136–7.

Langevitz P. *et al.* (1992). The effect of cyclophosphamide pulses on fertility in patients with lupus nephritis. *American Journal of Reproductive Immunology*, 28, 157–8.

Lee R.V. (1996). Thromboembolic disease and pregnancy, are all women created equal? *Annals of Internal Medicine*, 125, 1001–2.

Lindheimer M.D. *et al.* (1995). Renal Disorders. In: W.M. Barron and M.D. Lindheimer (eds) *Medical Disorders During Pregnancy*, pp. 37–62. Mosby, St. Louis.

Lockshin M.D. (1989). Pregnancy does not cause systemic lupus erythematosus to worsen. *Arthritis and Rheumatism*, 32, 665–70.

Lockshin M.D. (1992). Treatment of lupus pregnancy, Can we reach consensus? (editorial). *Clinical and Experimental Rheumatology*, 10, 429–31.

Lockshin M.D. (1993). Pregnancy and systemic autoimmune disease. *Seminars in Clinical Immunology*, 5, 5–11.

Lockshin M.D. *et al.* (1984). Lupus pregnancy. Case-control prospective study demonstrating absence of lupus exacerbation during or after pregnancy. *American Journal of Medicine*, 77, 893–8.

Lockshin M.D. *et al.* (1986). Hypocomplementemia with low C1s-C1 inhibitor complex in systemic lupus erythematosus. *Arthritis and Rheumatism*, 29, 1467–72.

Magann E.F. *et al.* (1994). Antepartum corticosteroids, diseases stabilization in patients with the syndrome of hemolysis, elevated liver enzymes, and low platelets (HELLP). *American Journal of Obstetrics and Gynecology*, 171, 1148–53.

Meehan R.T. and Dorsey K.T. (1987). Pregnancy among patients with systemic lupus erythematosus receiving immunosuppressive therapy. *Journal of Rheumatology*, 14, 252–8.

Millan-Mon A. *et al.* (1993). Hepatic infarction in a pregnant patient with the 'primary' antiphospholipid syndrome. *Lupus*, 2, 275–9.

Neuwelt C.M. *et al.* (1997). Catastrophic antiphospholipid syndrome. Response to repeated plasmapheresis over three years. *Arthritis and Rheumatism*, 40, 1534–9.

Newland A.C. *et al.* (1984). Intravenous IgG for autoimmune thrombocytopenia in pregnancy. *New England Journal of Medicine*, 310, 261–2.

Nossent H.C. and Swaak T.J.G. (1990). Systemic lupus erythematosus. VI. Analysis of the interrelationship with pregnancy. *Journal of Rheumatology*, 17, 771–6.

O'Connell J.B. *et al.* (1986). Peripartum cardiomyopathy, clinical, hemodynamic, histologic and prognostic characteristics. *Journal of the American College of Cardiology*, 8, 52–8.

Ornstein M. and Rand J.H. (1994). An association between refractory HELLP syndrome and antiphospholipid syndrome during pregnancy, a report of 2 cases. *Journal of Rheumatology*, 21, 1360–4.

Out H.J. *et al.* (1991). Prevalence of antiphospholipid antibodies in patients with fetal loss. *Annals of Rheumatic Diseases*, 50, 533–7.

Packham D.K. *et al.* (1992). Lupus nephritis and pregnancy. *Quarterly Journal of Medicine*, 83, 315–24.

Table 9.3 Renal manifestations of anti-phospholipid syndrome

Renal event	Frequency	Primary APS	Secondary APS	Comments
Renal arterial lesions				
Renal artery stenosis	≤10%	60, 81–89, 91a	90, 91	May be accompanied by HTN (~100%), ischemic ARF, and renal infarction; HTN and ARF both potentially reversible with release of occlusion
Renal infarction	~1%	60, 83, 85, 88, 91a, 93, 95, 98	91, 94, 96, 97	Usually clinically silent, but may be accompanied by HTN, hematuria, flank pain, or reversible ARF
Renal vein lesions				
Renal vein thrombosis	<1% (1° APS) ~10% (2° APS)	88, 99, 100	101–103	aPL significantly increases risk in association with other risk factors; clinical features include loin pain, hematuria, pulmonary embolism, enlarged kidneys
Microvasculature				
TMA	>50% (1° APS with renal findings) ~10% (2° APS)	54, 86, 89, 95, 98, 104, 105, 111–114, 117–119, 124–125, 128–142	54, 73, 96, 105, 108–110, 112a, 114–116, 120–125, 143–145	Presentation may range from ARF with widespread intrarenal thrombosis to chronic mild renal insufficiency and bland urinary sediment; accompanied by HTN (~80%), proteinuria (~90%), and hematuria (~50%)

Selected references

Table 9.3 Renal manifestations of anti-phospholipid syndrome *continued*

Renal event	Frequency	Selected references		Comments
		Primary APS	Secondary APS	
TMA (chronic) and mild CRF		96, 124, 131–133	96	
TMA (acute) and reversible ARF		86, 105, 111, 114, 119, 130, 135, 136, 140	105, 114, 125, 138, 143, 144	
TMA (acute) and ARF requiring dialysis		89, 104, 113, 117, 128, 129, 131, 134, 141, 142	73, 105, 139, 145	
TMA and nephrotic proteinuria		89, 104, 124, 125, 128, 134, 137	144	
Glomerular lesions Non-ischemic, non–TMA glomerular disease		80, 124, 146, 147		
Adrenal failure		88, 89, 95, 98, 136, 139		

tension (often severe), ischemic loss of renal function, hemorrhage, cortical necrosis, or renal infarction. The severity of presentation usually relates to the acuteness of thrombosis and the extent of occlusion. Thus, renal insufficiency occurring in association with APS can present anywhere along a spectrum from explosive and rapidly progressive to clinically silent and indolent. Depending on the size of vessels affected, renal failure has two predominant etiologies, thrombotic microangiopathy and ischemia.

Renal artery lesions

Renal artery stenosis has been well documented in patients with APS (60, 81–91, 91a). While the coexistence of APS and renal artery stenosis in no way establishes causality, the absence of significant risk factors for vascular disease in many of these patients makes such a link highly likely. Angiography revealed both unilateral (60, 83–89, 91, 91a) and bilateral (81–83, 90) renal artery stenoses, often with nearly complete occlusion (81–83, 86, 87). In several cases, the kidney represented only one of several organ systems affected by arterial thrombosis (83, 88, 89, 91a). Thrombosis of the suprarenal (92) and infrarenal (93) aorta, with hypertension and/or renal infarction, has also been described. The prevalence of renal artery stenosis among APS patients is difficult to assess. In a series of 70 unselected patients with primary APS, 2 (3%) had evidence of renal artery stenosis (60). In two other series of patients with primary APS, both selected, renal artery stenosis was found in 2 of 16 (13%) patients selected for renal involvement of any sort (89), and in 1 of 14 (7%) patients who underwent abdominal computerized tomography (CT) for non-renal reasons (88).

Hypertension, usually severe or malignant, was present in virtually every case of renal artery stenosis (79–91). Several cases were accompanied by ARF (81–83, 85, 87), in one instance leading to end-stage renal disease and maintenance hemodialysis (82). Renal biopsies in two cases revealed glomerular ischemia, without evidence of glomerular thrombotic microangiopathy (82, 87). A causal relationship between the stenoses and hypertension was demonstrated in two patients whose hypertension was successfully treated by angioplasty (81) or ipsilateral nephrectomy (80). Angioplasty also led to resolution of ARF (80). In two additional cases, treatment with urokinase and anticoagulation resulted in stabilization and improvement of renal function (83, 87).

Important unresolved issues relate to the histologic nature of the renal artery stenoses and the mechanism behind their generation. The occurrence of renal artery stenoses in several children suggests that APS can lead to thrombosis in otherwise healthy arteries (87, 90). Alternatively, thrombosis may occur as a secondary phenomenon in arteries whose walls have already been damaged by atherosclerosis or vasculitis. A final possibility, suggested by the occurrence of renal artery stenoses in two patients with fibromuscular dysplasia (83), is that endothelial damage from post-stenotic turbulence may provide a nidus for aPL-induced thrombosis.

Renal infarction

Renal infarction in association with APS can have several etiologies: *in situ* thrombosis of a renal artery or its branches; embolism from a pre-existing renal artery stenosis or thrombus; or bland embolism from a cardiac valve lesion (79, 80). Most infarctions were incidentally detected after the event, appearing as single or multiple wedge-shaped scars on abdominal CT (83, 85, 88, 93, 94) and autopsy (95) or as areas of hypoperfusion on intravenous pyelogram (96), scintigraphy (97), and renal arteriography (83, 85, 91, 97). In one case of acute renal infarction, abdominal CT with contrast showed bilaterally enlarged kidneys with areas of decreased contrast enhancement, consistent with infarction (98). When performed, renal arteriography frequently revealed an area of diminished or absent perfusion, with retraction of the renal cortex, but no evidence of renal artery stenosis, consistent with either an embolic etiology or recanalization of an arterial thrombus (91, 97). Signs and symptoms, when present, included flank or loin pain, hematuria, hypertension, and reversible loss of renal function (83, 91, 91a). The prevalence of renal infarction appears to be less than that for renal artery stenosis, occurring in 1 of 70 (1%) unselected patients with primary APS (60), in 2 of 130 (2%) unselected patients with secondary APS (91), and in 1 of 14 (7%) patients who underwent abdominal CT for non-renal reasons (88).

Renal vein thrombosis

While an association exists between APS and renal vein thrombosis (79, 80, 88, 99–103), the relative contributions of aPL vs. other established risk factors, in particular the nephrotic syndrome, remain unresolved. The development of renal vein thrombosis in patients with primary APS (88, 99, 100) would tend to suggest that aPL can act as a sole etiologic agent, but, in each of these cases, additional risk factors, such as prior eclampsia and post-partum proteinuria (2 g/day) (99), could be identified, or the case history lacked sufficient detail to fully assess the role of aPL (88, 100). In fact, in several large series of patients with primary APS, no cases of renal vein thrombosis were described (56, 58, 60, 62, 63, 89, 104–106). The situation with secondary APS in association with SLE is somewhat clearer. While aPL may not constitute so great a risk factor as the presence of nephrotic syndrome (107), APS does appear to substantially increase the risk for renal vein thrombosis among SLE patients. Thus, renal vein thrombosis occurred in 3 of 18 (17%) SLE patients with LA and in none of 59 SLE patients without LA (102). Adding to the significance of this result is the fact that the mean follow-up time of the group without LA was almost twice that of the group with LA (7.9 and 4.7 years, respectively) (102).

Like renal artery stenosis, renal vein thrombosis may be bilateral (101) and may occur in association with other large vein thromboses (88, 102). The clinical presentation of renal vein thrombosis in patients with APS did not differ from that in patients with other predisposing conditions. Clinical features included loin pain, hematuria, renal enlargement, and, in one case of bilateral renal vein

Table 9.4 Histopathologic manifestations of anti-phospholipid syndrome

Pathophysiologic process	Renal parenchymal element		
	Glomeruli	Vasculature	Interstitium
Acute TMA	Light: Intracapillary fibrin thrombi Glomerular congestion Endothelial cell swelling and degeneration Focal mesangiolysis and mesangial hypercellularity IF: Glomerular capillary wall staining for fibrin-related antigens Virtual absence of staining for complement or immunoglobulins EM: Separation of endothelium from glomerular basement membrane by fluffy electrolucent material Absence of electron dense deposits	Light: Arterial and arteriolar fibrin thrombi Degeneration and loss of endothelial lining Medial accumulation of fibrinous or cellular material Fibrinoid necrosis	Light: Mild interstitial edema Mild interstitial cellular infiltrate (lymphocytes and plasma cells) Acute tubular necrosis
Chronic TMA	Light: Global glomerulosclerosis Occasional focal segmental glomerulosclerosis Glomerular hypoperfusion Double contour or 'tram-tracking' of capillary walls Mesangial sclerosis EM: Glomerular basement membrane widening with mesangial interposition	Light: Thrombotic organization with recanalization Fibrous intimal hyperplasia Intimal accumulation of connective tissue components (collagen and elastin) Arterio- and arteriolosclerosis	Light: Interstitial fibrosis Tubular atrophy Focal cortical atrophy

Table 9.4 Histopathologic manifestations of anti-phospholipid syndrome *continued*

Pathophysiologic process	Renal parenchymal element		
	Glomeruli	Vasculature	Interstitium
Ischemia due to large vessel thrombosis	Light: Global glomerulosclerosis (late) Retraction or shrinkage of glomerular tuft Capillary collapse Wrinkling of capillary walls Hyperplasia of juxtaglomerular apparatus Cystic enlargement of Bowman's space	Light: Arterio- and arteriolosclerosis	Light: Interstitial fibrosis Tubular atrophy Focal cortical atrophy

Renal histopathologic features of APS

The renal histopathologic features of APS reflect two pathophysiologic processes, TMA and ischemia secondary to upstream renal arterial thromboses (65, 89, 127, 155). The changes of TMA are not at all specific to APS and can be seen in a variety of acute and chronic diseases and syndromes, including HUS/TTP, malignant hypertension, scleroderma, radiation nephritis, post-partum or pregnancy-associated renal failure, HELLP syndrome, nephropathy associated with bone marrow transplantation, HIV infection, transplant glomerulopathy, and various drug-induced thrombotic angiopathies (cyclosporine, FK506, and chemotherapeutic agents, such as mitomycin C). While the acute changes of TMA are usually fairly prominent, the chronic changes can be quite subtle and are easily overlooked unless one approaches the biopsy findings with a high index of suspicion. In the following discussion, we will contrast acute with chronic changes at the level of the glomerulus, interstitium, and vasculature (Table 9.4).

Acute glomerular changes attributable to TMA include glomerular congestion and the presence of intracapillary fibrin thrombi (64, 86, 89, 96, 102, 104, 105, 112a, 124, 125, 128, 130, 133, 134, 153). In general, there is an absence of inflammation (65, 89, 105). Clumps of red blood cells, platelets, and fibrin thrombi narrow or obliterate the lumens of glomerular capillaries (89). Glomerular endothelial cells, at times swollen and degenerative, can appear separated from the underlying capillary wall (89, 124, 155). The mesangium may be widened, with focal areas of mesangiolysis and occasional hypercellularity (86, 87, 96, 104, 124, 125, 128). Immunofluorescence reveals a predominance of fibrin-related antigens, lying along the glomerular capillary walls (86, 89, 105, 124, 125, 128). Staining for complement or immunoglobulins is at most focal and sparse, and markedly decreased in comparison with fibrin (86, 87, 89, 97, 105, 124, 125, 128). On electron microscopy, the endothelium is separated from the glomerular basement membrane by an accumulation of fluffy electron lucent material (86, 104, 105, 124, 125). The same electron lucent material may also be seen in mesangial areas. No electron dense deposits are seen (124).

Chronic glomerular changes from TMA reflect healing and scarring of these acute changes. As opposed to acute TMA, fibrin thrombi are only rarely seen (64, 87, 89, 96, 105, 114, 125, 132). Glomeruli may be obsolescent due to global sclerosis (64, 89, 104, 124, 125, 128, 133). Though rarer, lesions of focal segmental glomerulosclerosis can also be seen (89). Glomeruli may show evidence of ischemic hypoperfusion, with combinations of any of the following: shrunken retracted tufts, capillary collapse, wrinkled capillary walls, hyperplasia of the juxtaglomerular apparatus, or cystic enlargement of Bowman's space (87, 89, 96, 104, 105, 114, 124, 128, 130, 132). The capillary walls are often thickened, with a double contour or 'tram-track' appearance (89, 104, 105, 114, 124, 125, 130). The mesangium may have areas of sclerosis. Fibrin is still the predominant antigen detected by immunofluorescence, but its staining is much less intense than that seen in acute TMA. Electron microscopy shows widening of the glomerular basement membrane, with areas of mesangial interposition accounting for the double contours on light microscopy (104, 105, 124, 125). Effacement of the visceral epithelial cells from the glomerular basement membrane may also be seen, especially in those patients with significant proteinuria (124). Significantly less electron lucent material is seen, and there are again no electron dense deposits.

Acute interstitial changes include edema and a mild cellular infiltrate, consisting predominantly of lymphocytes and plasma cells (86, 124, 125, 128, 130). Acute tubular necrosis may also be seen. These changes may progress to tubular atrophy and interstitial fibrosis (87, 89, 96, 97, 105, 114, 124, 128, 132, 133). So-called focal cortical atrophy occurs within the superficial cortex, just beneath the renal capsule, and appears as well-demarcated foci or triangles of scarring and atrophy (89, 96, 114). The sharp borders of focal cortical atrophy suggest previous infarction. Focal cortical atrophy results in alterations of all elements of the renal parenchyma in a pattern that has been said to be highly suggestive of APS (89). The lesions of focal cortical atrophy include dense interstitial fibrosis, tubular atrophy and thyroidization, global sclerosis of glomeruli with occasional cystic dilatation, and fibrous intimal hyperplasia of arteries and arterioles with positive intimal staining for fibrin (89). Areas of focal cortical atrophy were found in 10 of 16 (62%) primary APS patients who underwent renal biopsy for renal insufficiency, abnormal urinalysis, and/or systemic hypertension (89).

Vascular involvement by TMA extends from the preglomerular arterioles up to the small interlobular arteries. During the acute phase, fibrin thrombi containing fragmented erythrocytes, leukocytes, and platelets narrow or occlude the vascular lumen (86, 89, 104, 105, 112a, 124, 125, 128, 133). Accumulations of fibrinous and cellular material may also be seen in the subendothelial space, leading to degeneration and loss of the endothelial lining (89, 124, 128), or they may be seen within the media of larger vessels (89). Thrombi eventually organize into fibrocellular and fibrous vascular occlusions, which in later stages can be recanulated by endothelialized channels (89, 114, 124, 144). Organization of thrombi within the interlobular arteries and their branches is usually accompanied by fibrous intimal hyperplasia, characterized by intimal thickening in association with an intense myofibroblastic intimal cellular proliferation (64, 87, 89, 96, 97, 104, 105, 114, 125, 130, 132, 134, 144). Intimal thickening in some cases may also be attributable to accumulation of connective tissue components, such as collagen and elastin (89). Fibrous intimal projections often bulge into the vascular lumen and reduce luminal size (89, 96, 105, 114, 132). An onion-skin arrangement of intimal fibrosis is a frequent end result. The lesions of arterio- and arteriolosclerosis should be distinguished from those of fibrous intimal hyperplasia, which are usually much more cellular in nature (89).

True vasculitis is rarely, if ever, seen in primary APS (65, 89, 155). While there is enormous confusion and controversy regarding the terminology for vascular lesions associated with SLE, vaso-occlusive disease in association with APS, irrespective of the size of the vessel involved, is universally due to thrombosis (65). When seen in secondary APS, vasculitis is attributable to SLE or other accompanying rheumatologic disorders.

Risk factors

An important issue in deciding whom to treat is the identification of those patients at increased risk for a thrombotic episode in association with aPL. It should be recalled that many patients have laboratory evidence of aPL without clinical consequence. While the exact percentage of such patients among the normal population cannot be determined in the absence of systematic screening studies, as many as 30% of SLE patients with positive aCL lacked any clinical evidence of APS (62). The two most important risk factors predictive of future thrombosis appear to be a previous history of thrombosis (156) and an elevated titre of aCL IgG (≥35 standardized phospholipid units) (59, 156, 157), both of which increased the risk for thrombosis up to 5-fold, though not all studies agree (37). The following factors did not significantly impact the risk of thrombosis among patients with APS: category of APS (primary vs. secondary); age; gender; co-existence of thrombocytopenia; hypertension; or concurrent use of corticosteroids, azathioprine, or cyclophosphamide (37, 59, 156, 157).

Treatment

Outside of case reports, the issue of treatment of the renal manifestations of APS has not been addressed. Nonetheless, certain conclusions can be drawn from the literature, based upon the assumption that the pathophysiology of APS within the kidney does not differ substantively from that within other vascular beds or organ systems. Treatment decisions fall into three main areas: prophylaxis, prevention of further large vessel thromboses, and treatment of acute TMA.

Prophylaxis

A nested case-control study within the Physician's Health Study examined the role of aspirin (325 milligrams per day) as a prophylactic agent (157). While male physicians with aCL titres above the 95th percentile had an increased risk for deep venous thrombosis and pulmonary embolus, aspirin offered no protection (157). Among secondary APS patients with SLE, the use of hydroxychloroquine may be protective against the development of thrombosis (66). In lieu of data to the contrary, modification of risk factors for vascular disease would seem prudent. We base this recommendation on the putative role of vascular injury in promoting aPL-associated thrombosis (32, 33) plus the growing association of aPL with Ox-LDL (38–42).

Treatment after a thrombotic event

A beneficial role for anticoagulation in decreasing the rate of recurrence of thromboses has been shown in three retrospective studies (37, 158, 159). In a small series of 19 APS patients examined solely with respect to thromboembolic events, the recurrence rate at 8 years was 0% for those patients receiving oral anticoagulation (159). Among patients whose anticoagulation was stopped, the recurrence rate was 50% at 2 years, and 78% at 8 years (159). In the two larger series, protection (venous and arterial) was directly correlated with the level of anti-coagulation (37, 158). Among 70 APS patients, intermediate- (INR [International Normalized Ratio], 2.0–2.9) and high- (INR ⩾3.0) intensity treatment with warfarin significantly reduced the rate of thrombotic recurrence, whereas low-intensity treatment (INR ⩽ 1.9) did not confer significant protection (158). Similar results were found in a series of 147 APS patients, for whom high-intensity warfarin (INR ⩾3.0) was significantly more effective than low-intensity warfarin (INR <3.0) in preventing further thrombotic events (37). Aspirin alone has been shown in two studies to be ineffective in reducing the rate of thrombotic recurrence (37, 158).

Several additional points warrant mention. First, discontinuation of warfarin is associated with an increased risk of thrombosis, especially in the first 6 months after stopping anticoagulation (37, 159). As the rate of recurrence among patients who are not optimally anticoagulated can be as high as 70% (37, 158, 159), treatment with warfarin should probably be long-term, if not life-long. Second, the lack of a standardized thromboplastin for determination of the INR plus the potential interference of aPL with measurement of the INR can create problems in monitoring the level of anticoagulation in APS patents (160). Finally, several case reports have documented the effectiveness of intravenous urokinase in the treatment of renal artery stenosis (83, 87, 91a).

Acute TMA

Recommendations for treatment of the renal manifestations of acute TMA are based entirely on case reports. As acute TMA is present in the vast majority of patients with catastrophic APS (139), the efficacy of various treatment protocols can be best assessed with respect to this patient population. Recovery from catastrophic APS occurred in 13 of 20 (65%) patients who underwent plasmapheresis, in 22 of 35 (63%) patients who received anticoagulation (heparin or coumadin), in 19 of 35 (54%) patients given corticosteroids, in 4 of 8 (50%) patients who received intravenous gammaglobulin, and in 7 of 41 (41%) patients who received cyclophosphamide (139). Most patients received combinations of these therapies. The most effective combination was anticoagulation, steroids, and plasmapheresis or intravenous gammaglobulin, for which recovery occurred in 14 of 20 (70%) patients (139). The rationale for plasmapheresis in treatment of acute TMA is based on the documented effectiveness of plasmapheresis in treating HUS/TTP. In addition to its effectiveness in patients with catastrophic APS, plasmapheresis has also proven effective in numerous (105, 111, 117, 125, 139, 144, 145), but not all (113), case reports of TMA. The fibrinolytic agents streptokinase and urokinase have also been used to treat acute TMA with varying success (91a, 139). As emphasized in our discussion of catastrophic APS, thrombosis tends to be a self-perpetuating process (91a), so that an aggressive therapeutic approach is warranted in these patients. At present, our best

30. Viard J.P., Amoura Z., and Bach J.F. (1992). Association of anti-beta 2 glycoprotein I antibodies with lupus-type circulating anticoagulant and thrombosis in systemic lupus erythematosus. *American Journal of Medicine*, 93, 181–186.

31. Belmont H.M., Abramson S.B., and Lie J.T. (1996). Pathology and pathogenesis of vascular injury in systemic lupus erythematosus. Interactions of inflammatory cells and activated endothelium. *Arthritis and Rheumatism*, 39, 9–22.

32. Arnout J. (1996). The pathogenesis of the antiphospholipid syndrome: a hypothesis based on parallelisms with heparin-induced thrombocytopenia. *Thrombosis and Haemostasis*, 75, 536–541.

33. Ames P.R.J. (1994). Antiphospholipid antibodies, thrombosis and atherosclerosis in systemic lupus erythematosus: a unifying 'membrane stress syndrome' hypothesis. *Lupus*, 3, 371–377.

34. Belmont H.M., Buyon J., Giorno R., and Abramson S. (1994). Up-regulation of endothelial cell adhesion molecules characterizes disease activity in systemic lupus erythematosus. the Shwartzman phenomenon revisited. *Arthritis and Rheumatism*, 37, 376–383.

35. Boshkov L.K., Warkentin T.E., Hayward C.P., Andrew M., and Kelton J.G. (1993). Heparin-associated thrombocytopenia and thrombosis: clinical and laboratory studies. *British Journal of Haematology*, 84, 322–328.

36. Makhoul R.G., Greenberg C.S., and McCann R.L. (1986). Heparin-associated thrombocytopenia and thrombosis: a serious clinical problem and potential solution. *Journal of Vascular Surgery*, 4, 522–528.

37. Khamashta M.A., Cuadrado M.J., Mujic F., Taub N.A., Hunt B.J., and Hughes G.R.V. (1995). The management of thrombosis in the antiphospholipid-antibody syndrome. *New England Journal of Medicine*, 332, 993–997.

38. Witztum J.L., and Steinberg D. (1991). Role of oxidized low density lipoprotein in atherogenesis. *Journal of Clinical Investigation*, 88, 1785–1792.

39. Vaarala O., Alfthan G., Jauhiainen M., Leirisalo-Repo M., Aho K., and Palosuo T. (1993). Crossreaction between antibodies to oxidised low-density lipoprotein and to cardiolipin in systemic lupus erythematosus. *Lancet*, 341, 923–925.

40. Puurunen M., Manttari M., Manninen V., Tenkanen L., Alfthan, G., Ehnholm C., Vaarala, O., Aho K., and Palosuo T. (1994). Antibody against oxidized low-density lipoprotein predicting myocardial infarction. *Archives of Internal Medicine*, 154, 2605–2609.

41. Vaarala O., Manttari, M., Manninen V., Tenkanen L., Puurunen M., Aho K., and Palosuo T. (1995). Anti-cardiolipin antibodies and risk of myocardial infarction in a prospective cohort of middle-aged men. *Circulation*, 91, 23–27.

42. Hörkkö S., Miller E., Dudl E., Reaven P., Curtiss L.K., Zvaifler N.J., Terkeltaub R., Pierangeli S.S., Branch D.W., Palinski W., and Witztum J.L. (1996). Antiphospholipid antibodies are directed against epitopes of oxidized phospholipids: recognition of cardiolipin by monoclonal antibodies to epitopes of oxidized low density lipoprotein. *Journal of Clinical Investigation*, 98, 815–825.

43. Rauch J. and Janoff A. (1992). The nature of anti-phospholipid antibodies. *Journal of Rheumatology*, 19, 1782–1785.

44. Bevers E.M., Comfurius P., and Zwaal R.F.A. (1983). Changes in membrane phospholipid distribution during platelet activation. *Biochimica Biophysica Acta*, 736, 57–66.

45. Schwartz R.S., Tanaka Y., Fidler I.J., Chiu D.T., Lubin B., and Schroit A.J. (1985). Increased adherence of sickled and phosphatidylserine-enriched human ery-

throcytes to cultured human peripheral blood monocytes. *Journal of Clinical Investigation*, 75, 1965–1972.

46. Schroit A.J., Madsen J.W., and Tanaka Y. (1985). *In vivo* recognition and clearance of red blood cells containing phosphatidylserine in their plasma membranes. *Journal of Biological Chemistry*, 260, 5131–5138.

47. Fadok V.A., Voelker D.R., Campbell P.A., Cohen J.J., Bratton D.L., and Henson P.M. (1992). Exposure of phosphatidylserine on the surface of apoptotic lymphocytes triggers specific recognition and removal by macrophages. *Journal of Immunology*, 148, 2207–2216.

48. Shi W., Chong B.H., and Chesterman C.N. (1993). β2-glycoprotein I is a requirement for anticardiolipin antibodies binding to activated platelets: differences with lupus anticoagulants. *Blood*, 81, 1255–1262.

49. Vázquez-Mellado J., Llorente L., Richaud-Patin Y., and Alarcón-Segovia D. (1994). Exposure of anionic phospholipids upon platelet activation permits binding of β2 glycoprotein I and through it that of IgG antiphospholipid antibodies. Studies in platelets from patients with antiphospholipid syndrome and normal subjects. *Journal of Autoimmunity*, 7, 335–348.

50. Price B.E., Rauch J., Shia M.A., Walsh M.T., Lieberthal W., Gilligan H.M. O'Laughlin T., Koh J.S., and Levine J.S. (1996). Antiphospholipid autoantibodies bind to apoptotic, but not nonapoptotic, thymocytes in a β2-glycoprotein I-dependent manner. *Journal of Immunology*, 157, 2201–2208.

51. Manfredi A.A., Rovere P., Galati G., Heltai S., Bozzolo E., Soldini L., Davoust J., Balestrieri G., Ticani A., and Sabbadini M.G. (1998). Apoptotic cell clearance in systemic lupus erythematosus: I. Opsonization by antiphospholipid antibodies. *Arthritis and Rheumatism*, 41, 205–214.

52. Jacobson M.D. (1996). Reactive oxygen species and programmed cell death. *Trends in Biological Sciences*, 21, 83–86.

53. Hörkko S., Miller E., Branch D.W., Palinski W., and Witztum J.L. (1997). The epitopes for some antiphospholipid antibodies are adducts of oxidized phospholipid and β2 glycoprotein I (and other proteins). *Proceedings of the National Academy of Sciences, USA*, 94, 10356–10361.

54. Levine J.S., Koh J.S., Subang R., and Rauch J. (1999). Apoptotic cells as immunogen and antigen in the antiphospholipid syndrome. *Experimental and Molecular Pathology*, 66, 82–98.

55. Wilson W.A., Gharavi A.E., Koike T., Lockshin M.D., Branch D.W., Piette J.-C., Brey R., Derksen R., Harris E.N., Hughes G.R.V., Triplett D.A., and Khamashta M.A. (1999). International consensus statement on preliminary classification criteria for definite antiphospholipid syndrome. Report of an international workshop. *Arthritis and Rheumatism*, 42, 1309–1311.

56. Dührsen U., Paar D., Kölbel C., Boekstegers A., Metz-Kurschel U., Wagner R., Kirch W., Meusers P., König E., and Brittinger G. (1987). Lupus anticoagulant associated syndrome in benign and malignant systemic disease – analysis of ten observations. *Klinische Wochenschrift*, 65, 852–859.

57. McHugh N.J., Maymo J., Skinner R.P., James I., and Maddis P.J. (1988). Anticardiolipin antibodies, livedo reticularis, and major cerebrovascular and renal disease in systemic lupus erythematosus. *Annals of the Rheumatic Diseases*, 47, 110–115.

58. Alarcón-Segovia D., and Sanchez-Guerrero J. (1989). Primary antiphospholipid syndrome. *The Journal of Rheumatology*, 16, 482–488.

148. Stratta P., Canavese C., Ferrero S., Grill A., Salomone M., Schinco P.C., Fusaro E., Montaruli B., Santi S., and Piccoli G. (1999). Catastrophic antiphospholipid syndromes in systemic lupus erythematosus. *Renal Failure*, 21, 49–61.

149. Weidmann C.E., Wallace D.J., Peter J.B., Knight P.J., Bear M.E., and Klinenberg J.R. (1988). Studies of IgG, IgM, and IgA antiphospholipid antibody isotypes in systemic lupus erythematosus. *The Journal of Rheumatology*, 15, 74–79.

150. Gulko P.S., Reveille J.D., Koopman W.J., Burgard S.L., Bartolucci A.A., and Alarcón G.S. (1993). Anticardiolipin antibodies in systemic lupus erythematosus: clinical correlates, HLA associations, and impact on survival. *The Journal of Rheumatology*, 20, 1684–1693.

151. Ishii Y., Nagasawa K., Mayumi T., and Niho Y. (1990). Clinical importance of persistence of anticardiolipin antibodies in systemic lupus erythematosus. *Annals of the Rheumatic Diseases*, 49, 387–390.

152. Perdiguero M., Boronat M., Marco P., and Rivera F. (1995). The role of antiphospholipid antibodies in lupus nephropathy. *Nephron*, 71, 35–39.

153. Kant K.S., Pollak V.E., Weiss M.A., Glueck H.I., Miller M.A., and Hess E.V. (1981). Glomerular thrombosis in systemic lupus erythematosus: prevalence and significance. *Medicine*, 60, 71–86.

154. Asherson R.A. (1992). The catastrophic antiphospholipid syndrome. *The Journal of Rheumatology*, 19, 508–512.

155. Appel G.B., Pirani C.L., and D'Agati V.D. (1994). Renal vascular complications of systemic lupus erythematosus. *Journal of the American Society of Nephrology*, 4, 1499–1515.

156. Finazzi G., Brancaccio V., Moia M., Ciavarella N., Mazzucconi M.G., Schinco, P.C., Ruggeri M., Polgliani E., Gamba G., Rossi E., Baudo F., Manotti C., D'Angelo A., Palareti G., De Stefano V., Berrettini M., and Barbui T. (1996). Natural history and risk factors for thrombosis in 360 patients with antiphospholipid antibodies: A four-year prospective study from the Italian registry. *American Journal of Medicine*, 100, 530–536.

157. Ginsburg K.S., Liang M.H., Newcomer L., Goldhaber S.Z., Schur P.H., Hennekens C.H., and Stampfer M.J. (1992). Anticardiolipin antibodies and the risk for ischemic stroke and venous thrombosis. *Annals of Internal Medicine*, 117, 997–1002.

158. Rosove M.H., and Brewer P.M.C. (1992). Antiphospholipid thrombosis: Clinical course after the first thrombotic event in 70 patients. *Annals of Internal Medicine*, 117, 303–308.

159. Derksen R.H., de Groot P.G., Kater L., and Nieuwenhuis H.K. (1993). Patients with antiphospholipid antibodies and venous thrombosis should receive long term anticoagulant treatment. *Annals of the Rheumatic Diseases*, 52, 689–692.

160. Moll S., and Ortel T.L. (1997). Monitoring warfarin therapy in patients with lupus anticoagulants. *Annals of Internal Medicine*, 127, 177–185.

PART II

10

Vasculitis classification

J. Charles Jennette, Ronald J. Falk and David B. Thomas

Introduction

The hallmark of vasculitis is inflammation of vessel walls. Thus, the diagnosis of vasculitis requires recognition of signs and symptoms of vascular inflammation. However, there are numerous complexities to the diagnosis of vasculitis. First, there are numerous variants of vasculitis defined by different causes, different pathogenic mechanisms, different distributions of vessel involvement, different types of inflammatory vascular injury, and different disease associations (see Tables 10.1 and 10.2, and Fig. 10.1). Second, the pathologic lesions of vasculitis are rather nonspecific and evolve over time from acute to chronic inflammatory lesions to sclerosing lesions. Third, many different organs can be affected and different patients with the same vasculitis may have very different distributions of organ involvement. Fourth, many of the signs and symptoms of vasculitis are nonspecific and mimic and can be mimicked by other types of inflammatory or ischemic single organ or multi-system disease. Fifth, the etiology of most forms of vasculitis is poorly understood or unknown thus requiring categorization of vasculitides on the basis of clinicopathologic or syndromatic definitions. And finally, in part because of the aforementioned difficulties, there is no complete agreement about how to name, categorize, or diagnose most forms of vasculitis.

The lack of a unified system for diagnostic categorization has caused many problems. Distinct types of vasculitis have been given multiple names and different names have been used for the same type of vasculitis. This chapter will emphasize the Chapel Hill Nomenclature System (Table 10.2), which was developed through a collaboration of physicians from diverse fields, including rheumatology, immunology, nephrology, pulmonology, nephrology, and pathology (1). This system does not include all forms of vasculitis, but rather focuses on some of the most distinctive categories of so-called primary vasculitides. For example, lupus vasculitis and rheumatoid vasculitis are not included and will not be discussed in this chapter.

The Chapel Hill Nomenclature System divides vasculitides into three groups: large vessel vasculitis; medium-sized vessel vasculitis; and small vessel vasculitis (Table 10.2). Although these names imply that the size of the vessels affected by inflammation is the primary criterion for categorizing vasculitides, this is not the case. Figure 10.1 shows that there is substantial overlap among categories with

Table 10.1 Major categories of vasculitis

Large vessel vasculitis
  Giant cell arteritis
  Takayasu arteritis

Medium-sized vessel vasculitis
  Polyarteritis nodosa
  Kawasaki disease

Small vessel vasculitis
  Anca small vessel vasculitis
    Microscopic polyangiitis
    Wegener's granulomatosis
    Churg-Strauss syndrome
    Drug-induced ANCA vasculitis
  Immune complex small vessel vasculitis
    Henoch-Schönlein purpura
    Cryoglobulinemic vasculitis
    Lupus vasculitis
    Rheumatoid vasculitis
    Goodpasture's syndrome
    Serum sickness vasculitis
    Drug-induced immune complex vasculitis
    Infection-induced immune complex vasculitis
    Sjögren's syndrome vasculitis
    Hypocomplementemic urticarial vasculitis
    Behçet's disease
  Paraneoplastic small vessel vasculitis
    Carcinoma induced vasculitis
    Lymphoproliferative neoplasm induced vasculitis
    Myeloproliferative neoplasm induced vasculitis
  Inflammatory bowel disease vasculitis

---

respect to the size and type of vessel involved. In fact, adequate diagnostic categorization requires a complex integration not only of clinical data but also historical data, demographic data, serologic data, and pathologic data to reach the proper diagnosis. The reference to vessel size is also misleading because, from a pathologic perspective, the type of vessel and the type of inflammation are more specific for the major categories of vasculitis than is vessel size alone. In essence, during the active acute phase, the large vessel vasculitides manifest as granulomatous arteritis, the medium-sized vessel vasculitides as necrotizing arteritis, and the small vessel vasculitides as necrotizing polyangiitis.

This chapter will briefly review the distinctive features of a number of relatively common systemic vasculitides with an emphasis on those features that

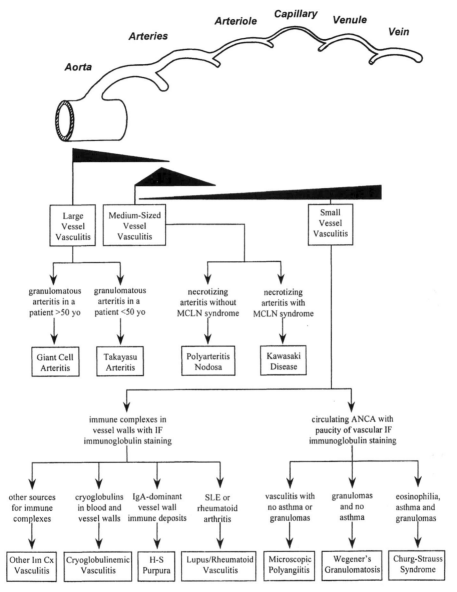

Fig. 10.1 Predominant vascular involvement by large vessel vasculitides, medium–sized vessel vasculitides, and small vessel vasculitides as indicated by the positions and heights of the solid triangles. The algorithm suggests clinical and pathologic features that discriminate among different diagnostic categories of vasculitis. (Abbreviations: yo = years old, MCLN = mucocutaneous lymph node syndrome, IF = immunofluorescence microscopy, ANCA = anti-neutrophil cytoplasmic autoantibodies, Im Cx = immune complex, SLE = systemic lupus erythematosus, and H-S = Henoch-Schönlein.

Table 10.2 Names and definitions of vasculitis adopted by the Chapel Hill Consensus Conference on the nomenclature of systemic vasculitis. Modified from Reference 1 with permission.

Large vessel vasculitis[1]

Giant cell (temporal) arteritis	Granulomatous arteritis of the aorta and its major branches, with a predilection for the extracranial branches of the carotid artery. *Often involves the temporal artery. Usually occurs in patients older than 40 and often is associated with polymyalgia rheumatica.*
Takayasu arteritis	Granulomatous inflammation of the aorta and its major branches. *Usually occurs in patients younger than 40.*

Medium-sized vessel vasculitis[1]

Polyarteritis nodosa (classic polyarteritis nodosa)	Necrotizing inflammation of medium-sized or small arteries without glomerulonephritis or vasculitis in arterioles, capillaries or venules.
Kawasaki disease	Arteritis involving large, medium-sized and small arteries, and associated with mucocutaneous lymph node syndrome. *Coronary arteries are often involved. Aorta and veins may be involved. Usually occurs in children.*

Small vessel vasculitis[1]

Wegener's granulomatosis[2]	Granulomatous inflammation involving the respiratory tract, and necrotizing vasculitis affecting small to medium-sized vessels, e.g. capillaries, venules, arterioles, and arteries. *Necrotizing glomerulonephritis is common.*
Churg–Strauss syndrome[2]	Eosinophil-rich and granulomatous inflammation involving the respiratory tract and necrotizing vasculitis affecting small to medium-sized vessels, and associated with asthma and blood eosinophilia
Microscopic polyangiitis (microscopic polyarteritis)[2]	Necrotizing vasculitis with few or no immune deposits affecting small vessels, i.e. capillaries, venules, or arterioles. *Necrotizing arteritis involving small and medium-sized arteries may be present. Necrotizing glomerulonephritis is very common. Pulmonary capillaritis often occurs.*
Henoch–Schönlein purpura	Vasculitis with IgA-dominant immune deposits affecting small vessels, i.e. capillaries, venules, or arterioles. *Typically involves skin, gut and glomeruli, and is associated with arthralgias or arthritis.*

Table 10.2 Names and definitions of vasculitis adopted by the Chapel Hill Consensus Conference on the nomenclature of systemic vasculitis. Modified from Reference 1 with permission.   *continued*

Essential cryoglobulinemic vasculitis	Vasculitis with cryoglobulin immune deposits affecting small vessels, i.e. capillaries, venules, or arterioles, and associated with cryoglobulins in serum. *Skin and glomeruli are often involved.*
Cutaneous leukocytoclastic angiitis	Isolated cutaneous leukocytoclastic angiitis without systemic vasculitis or glomerulonephritis.

[1] Large artery refers to the aorta and the largest branches directed toward major body regions (e.g. to the extremities and the head and neck); medium-sized artery refers to the main visceral arteries (e.g. renal, hepatic, coronary and mesenteric arteries), and small artery refers to the distal arterial radicals that connect with arterioles. Note large and medium-sized vessel vasculitides do not involve vessels smaller than arteries.
[2] Strongly associated with antineutrophil cytoplasmic autoantibodies (ANCA).

allow diagnostic differentiation. Most of these vasculitides and their clinical management are discussed in more detail elsewhere in this book.

Large vessel vasculitides (granulomatous aortitis and arteritis)

The large vessel vasculitides affect the aorta and its major branches, such as those to the head and neck, and to the extremities. Takayasu arteritis and giant cell arteritis (less appropriately called temporal arteritis) are the two major categories of large vessel vasculitis. In both, the acute phase of injury is characterized by transmural infiltration by mononuclear leukocytes (lymphocytes, monocytes, and macrophages) with varying amounts of granulomatous inflammation including multinucleated giant cells. Chronic disease has predominantly sclerosis with scant inflammation. This less specific pathologic appearance may complicate pathologic diagnosis, for example leading to confusion with hypertensive arteriosclerosis or atherosclerosis. The inflammation or scarring or both cause narrowing of arteries and causes ischemic symptoms, for example pulselessness and claudication.

Takayasu arteritis

William Savory in 1856 (2) probably made the first detailed clinical description of Takayasu arteritis; however, patients with pulseless disease who probably had Takayasu arteritis were described as early as the mid-eighteenth century (3). Mikito Takayasu, for whom the disease is named, was a Japanese ophthalmologist who identified the ocular complications of this disease in 1908 (4).

Takayasu arteritis is characterized pathologically by granulomatous inflammation that most often affects the aorta and its major branches, but also can affect the pulmonary arteries (5–7). Synonyms include 'aortic arch syndrome' and 'pulseless disease' because the arteries arising from the aorta often are narrowed causing diminished or absent pulses, especially in the upper extremities. Frequent signs and symptoms of Takayasu arteritis include fever, arthralgias, weight loss, reduced pulses, vascular bruits, claudication and renovascular hypertension (5, 8). Takayasu arteritis has been reported most often in Asia, has a strong female predilection, usually is diagnosed in individuals who are between 10 and 20 years old, and only rarely occurs after the 50 years stage. Patient age is very useful for distinguishing between Takayasu arteritis and giant cell arteritis because giant cell arteritis rarely occurs before 50 years of age (5).

Giant cell arteritis

Hutchinson gave a detailed account of giant cell arteritis in 1890, in which he emphasized the involvement of the temporal arteries (9). This resulted in the widespread use of the term 'temporal arteritis' for this category of vasculitis. However, the systemic distribution of this disease is now well recognized. Thus, the term giant cell arteritis is more appropriate than temporal arteritis. In addition, not all patients with giant cell arteritis have temporal artery involvement and vasculitides other than giant cell arteritis (e.g. polyarteritis nodosa, Wegener's granulomatosis, and microscopic polyangiitis) can cause temporal artery inflammation (1). Polymyalgia rheumatica is associated with giant cell arteritis (10, 11), and thus is a useful aid for diagnosis. Once again, however, not all patients with giant cell arteritis have polymyalgia rheumatica, and not all patients with polymyalgia rheumatica have giant cell arteritis.

Giant cell arteritis affects the aorta and its major branches, and has a predilection for the extracranial branches of the carotid artery. However, giant cell arteritis can affect arteries in almost any organ as long as they have elastic laminae. Giant cell arteritis usually affects multiple body regions, but may be isolated to a single organ, such as uterus, ovary, breast, and brain.

Giant cell arteritis is most common in people of northern European ancestry and over 95% of patients are more than 50 years old (12, 13). The most common symptom is headache. Other common manifestations are blindness, deafness, jaw claudication, tongue dysfunction, extremity claudication, and reduced pulses. Over 50% of patients with giant cell arteritis have polymyalgia rheumatica, which is characterized by stiffness and aching in the neck and the proximal muscles of the shoulders and hips. Older age, polymyalgia rheumatica, and preferential involvement of branches of the carotid artery are useful in differentiating giant cell arteritis from Takayasu arteritis. However, none of these features are pathognomonic.

Medium-sized vessel vasculitis (necrotizing arteritis)

Necrotizing arteritis was first recognized because of the nodular and aneurysmal lesions in arteries that are caused by the necrotizing acute inflammation. Adolf Kussmaul and Rudolf Maier reported the first definitive description of a patient with necrotizing arteritis in 1866 (14). Their patient had typical features of systemic vasculitis, including fever, anorexia, muscle weakness, myalgias, paresthesias, abdominal pain and oliguria. Postmortem examination demonstrated nodular inflammatory lesions in medium-sized and small arteries throughout the body. Kussmaul and Maier named the disease 'periarteritis nodosa'. In 1903, Ferrari introduced the more appropriate term 'polyarteritis nodosa', which refers to the involvement of multiple different arteries by transmural inflammation (15). Polyarteritis nodosa is now the most widely used term, and is advocated by the Chapel Hill Nomenclature System (1).

Until additional distinctive categories of vasculitis with necrotizing arteritis were recognized, all patients with necrotizing arteritis were diagnosed as having polyarteritis nodosa (16–20). Over the years, however, numerous observations have confirmed that necrotizing arteritis identical to that seen in polyarteritis nodosa can occur as a component of many other clinically and pathologically distinct forms of vasculitis (1, 19, 20). For example, necrotizing arteritis that can be confused with polyarteritis nodosa also occurs in Kawasaki disease, microscopic polyangiitis, Wegener's granulomatosis, and Churg-Strauss syndrome. These different variants of vasculitis each have distinctive manifestations, natural histories, and treatment requirements. Thus, it is very important to properly categorize a patient who has necrotizing arteritis rather than making a reflex diagnosis of polyarteritis nodosa.

Polyarteritis nodosa

Because of the historical use of the category polyarteritis nodosa as a wastebasket for all forms of vasculitis with necrotizing arteritis, most of the literature on polyarteritis nodosa prior to the 1990s includes conclusion based on populations of patients with various combinations of both polyarteritis nodosa and microscopic polyangiitis. Using the Chapel Hill Nomenclature System definitions (Table 10.2), polyarteritis nodosa can be separated from microscopic polyangiitis by the absence of signs and symptoms of involvement of vessels other than arteries in polyarteritis nodosa (e.g. absence of glomerulonephritis, alveolar capillaritis, dermal venulitis) and the presence of such involvement in microscopic polyangiitis (1).

Pathologically, polyarteritis nodosa is characterized in the acute phase by necrotizing arteritis, often with arterial aneurysm, which actually are pseudoaneurysm formed by erosion of the necrotizing process through the arterial walls and into adjacent tissues. Thrombosis, infarction, and hemorrhage often accompany the arterial inflammation and necrosis. Any calibre artery can be affected by polyarteritis nodosa, from the main visceral artery to the smallest of arteries, such as epineural arteries. Histologically, the lesions begin with acute inflammation and fibrinoid necrosis, evolve through chronic inflammation, and culminate in arterial sclerosis.

Polyarteritis nodosa often involves the gastrointestinal tract, heart, kidneys, skin and peripheral nerves. The major clinical manifestations include fever, peripheral neuropathy, myalgias, abdominal pain, and signs and symptoms of renal disease (21, 22). When reading the literature about polyarteritis nodosa, one must determine whether data are derived from patients with polyarteritis nodosa alone (as defined in this chapter), or from patients with a mixture of polyarteritis nodosa and microscopic polyangiitis. Table 10.3 shows an attempt by Guillevin and Lhote to distinguish between the clinical manifestations of polyarteritis nodosa and microscopic polyangiitis (22, 23). A major distinction between polyarteritis nodosa and microscopic polyangiitis is the high frequency of glomerulonephritis and pulmonary involvement in microscopic polyangiitis but not polyarteritis nodosa (22, 24–27). Anti-neutrophil cytoplasmic autoantibodies (ANCA) are frequent in patients with microscopic polyangiitis, as will be discussed in more detail later; however, ANCA are not frequent in patients who have arteritis that is not accompanied by inflammatory involvement of capillaries or venules. ANCA are not frequent in polyarteritis nodosa (22, 28).

Table 10.3 Clinical differences between polyarteritis nodosa and microscopic polyangiitis. Modified from Reference 22

Clinical feature	Polyarteritis nodosa	Microscopic polyangiitis
Microaneurysms by angiography	Yes	No (?rare)
Rapidly progressive nephritis	No	Yes (very common)
Pulmonary hemorrhage	No	Yes
Renovascular hypertension	Yes (10%–33%)	No
Peripheral neuropathy	Yes (50%–80%)	Yes (10%–20%)
Positive hepatitis B serology	Uncommon	No
Positive ANCA serology	Rare	Frequent
Relapses	Rare	Frequent

Kawasaki disease

Kawasaki disease is an acute febrile illness that usually occurs in young children (29–32). The *sine qua non* of Kawasaki disease is the mucocutaneous lymph node syndrome, which is characterized by polymorphous erythematous rash, erythema of the palms and soles, erythema of the oropharyngeal mucosa, conjunctivitis, indurative edema and desquamation of the extremities, and nonsuppurative lymphadenopathy. The mucocutaneous lymph node syndrome was first described by Tomisaku Kawasaki in 1967 (33). Necrotizing arteritis involving medium-sized and small arteries is an important complication of Kawasaki disease that was first reported by Tanaka, Naoe and Kawasaki (34, 35). The necrotizing arteritis of Kawasaki disease should not be mistakenly diagnosed as polyarteritis nodosa because corticosteroid treatment may increase the risk of coronary artery aneurysms in Kawasaki disease. Kawasaki disease usually is treated with aspirin and intravenous gamma globulin therapy rather than high dose corticosteroids and cyclophosphamide as would be used for polyarteritis nodosa (35–38).

The acute arteritis of Kawasaki disease is a necrotizing process that usually has less conspicuous fibrinoid necrosis than polyarteritis nodosa (31). Early inflammatory changes are most extensive in the media and are characterized by edema and disassociation of smooth muscle cells. Transmural involvement eventually occurs, and there may be extensive intimal thickening or thrombosis, or both, that can cause ischemia and infarction.

The arteritis of Kawasaki disease affects small and medium-sized arteries, and frequently involves the coronary arteries (30, 31, 39, 40). This may result in coronary artery aneurysms, thrombosis, and myocardial infarction. Although rare, Kawasaki disease is the most common cause of childhood myocardial infarction.

The diagnostic differentiation between polyarteritis nodosa and Kawasaki disease should not be a problem because the presence or absence of the mucocutaneous lymph node syndrome is an absolute discriminator between these two diagnoses.

Small vessel vasculitis (necrotizing polyangiitis)

Small vessel vasculitis is characterized by the involvement of vessels smaller than arteries, that is, involvement of capillaries, venules, or arterioles. Arteries also may be involved, but all forms of small vessel vasculitis affect predominantly vessels other than arteries, and in many instances arteries are not involved at all. The frequency of arterial involvement varies among different vasculitides. For example, arterial involvement is extremely rare in Henoch-Schönlein purpura or cryoglobulinemic vasculitis, whereas it is relatively frequent in Wegener's granulomatosis and microscopic polyangiitis. Of the many variants of small vessel vasculitis, some of which are listed in Table 10.1, this chapter will focus on the diagnostic categorization of Wegener's granulomatosis, microscopic polyangiitis, Churg-Strauss syndrome, Henoch-Schönlein purpura, and cryoglobulinemic vasculitis. More details about these and other vasculitides can be found in other chapters of this book.

Wegener's granulomatosis, microscopic polyangiitis and Churg-Strauss syndrome

Wegener's granulomatosis, microscopic polyangiitis, and Churg-Strauss syndrome once were included in the same diagnostic category with polyarteritis nodosa because they often have necrotizing arteritis as a component of the vasculitic process. However, careful evaluation of pathologic and clinical features resulted in the recognition of distinctive clinicopathologic variants of vasculitis that warrant separate categorization. Heinz Klinger (41) and Friedrich Wegener (42) recognized what they considered to be a variant of polyarteritis nodosa that had destructive necrotizing inflammation that often affected the upper and lower respiratory tract. In 1954, Gabriel Godman and Jacob Churg described in more detail the full spectrum of pathologic and clinical features of what is now called 'Wegener's granulomatosis' (19). These features include necrotizing 'angiitis', necrotizing granulomatous inflammation of the respiratory tract, and necrotizing glomerulonephritis. Patients with limited expressions of Wegener's granulomatosis also occur; for example, patients with disease confined to the respiratory tract (43).

Jacob Churg and Lotte Strauss described another variant of necrotizing vasculitis in 1951 characterized by asthma, eosinophilia, granulomatous inflammation, necrotizing vasculitis (including necrotizing arteritis) and focal necrotizing glomerulonephritis (17). This variant of necrotizing vasculitis is now called Churg-Strauss (1).

In their classic 1954 article that definitively described Wegener's granulomatosis, Godman and Churg also concluded that Wegener's granulomatosis and Churg-Strauss syndrome are closely related to each other, and both also are closely related to what they called 'microscopic periarteritis' (19). They further concluded that Wegener's granulomatosis, Churg-Strauss syndrome and microscopic periarteritis (which is now usually called microscopic polyangiitis) are

distinct from polyarteritis nodosa. These conclusions are supported by recent observations that anti-neutrophil cytoplasmic autoantibodies (ANCA) are frequent
in patients with Wegener's granulomatosis, microscopic polyangiitis, and Churg-
Strauss syndrome, but are infrequent in patients with polyarteritis nodosa (as
defined by the Chapel Hill Nomenclature System) (20, 22, 44–46).

Thus, ANCA are a useful diagnostic serologic marker for microscopic
polyangiitis, Wegener's granulomatosis and Churg-Strauss syndrome. However, a
positive ANCA result is not absolutely specific or sensitive, and thus must be interpreted in light of the other data (47, 48). Approximately 80% to 90% of
active untreated Wegener's granulomatosis or microscopic polyangiitis patients,
and approximately 60% of Churg-Strauss syndrome patients are ANCA-positive.

ANCA in patients with vasculitis or glomerulonephritis are specific for proteins in the cytoplasmic granules of neutrophils and the lysosomes of monocytes
(44, 45). The two major types of ANCA cause two staining patterns, cytoplasmic
(C-ANCA) and perinuclear (P-ANCA), when they are detected using indirect
immunofluorescence microscopy. The P-ANCA pattern is an artefact of substrate preparation that results in redistribution of the antigen from cytoplasm to
nucleus during substrate preparation (49). Enzyme immunoassay (EIA) reveals
that most C-ANCA have specificity for proteinase 3 (PR3-ANCA) (50–53) and
most P-ANCA have specificity for myeloperoxidase (MPO-ANCA) (54).

Patients with Wegener's granulomatosis usually have C-ANCA (PR3-ANCA),
patients with microscopic polyangiitis have slightly more P-ANCA (MPO-
ANCA) than C-ANCA (PR3-ANCA), and patients with Churg-Strauss syndrome have predominantly P-ANCA (MPO-ANCA).

Henoch-Schönlein purpura

In the 1800s Johann Schönlein and Eduard Henoch reported the association of
purpura with arthralgias, arthritis, abdominal pain, and nephritis (55, 56). In the
early 1900s this syndrome was called 'Henoch's purpura', and more recently
'Schönlein-Henoch purpura' or 'Henoch-Schönlein purpura'. The former is his-
torically more correct but the latter correctly emphasizes the more extensive contributions that Henoch made to the recognition of this syndrome of vasculitic
manifestations.

Many variants of small vessel vasculitis can produce the syndrome described
by Henoch and Schönlein (20). For example, cryoglobulinemic vasculitis, microscopic polyangiitis, Wegener's granulomatosis, Churg-Strauss syndrome, lupus
vasculitis, rheumatoid vasculitis, and serum sickness vasculitis all can manifest
purpura, abdominal pain, arthralgias, and nephritis. Thus, the term Henoch-
Schönlein purpura has little specific value in patient management unless it is
confined to a more restricted group of patients who have similar and predictable
natural histories and appropriate therapy. Fortunately, advances in immunopathology and serology have provided a number of tools for differentiating
among clinically and histologically indistinguishable categories of small vessel
vasculitis. This has resulted in refining the definitions of a number of diagnostic

terms, including Henoch-Schönlein purpura, Goodpasture's syndrome, microscopic polyangiitis, and polyarteritis nodosa (20).

The advent of immunofluorescence microscopy allowed the identification of granular deposits of immunoglobulins and complement within vessel walls of patients with certain types of vasculitis. Examination of patients with Henoch-Schönlein purpura revealed a distinct group, often children, who had IgA-dominant immune deposits in the walls of cutaneous vessels (57). This distinguished these patients from patients with other types of vascular immune deposits, such as patients with cryoglobulinemic vasculitis who have granular vascular deposits of IgM and IgG (58), and from patients with little or no vascular immunoglobulin localization, such as patients with Wegener's granulomatosis, microscopic polyangiitis, and Churg-Strauss syndrome (20, 22, 44–46). As mentioned earlier, these latter patients with so-called pauci-immune small vessel vasculitis also have a relatively specific serologic marker, i.e. ANCA.

By current approaches to diagnostic categorization, a patient with signs and symptoms of small vessel vasculitis who has IgA-dominant vascular immune deposits should be diagnosed as Henoch-Schönlein purpura, while a patient with the same clinical presentation who has circulating cryoglobulins and vascular cryoglobulin deposits should be diagnosed as cryoglobulinemic vasculitis, and a patient with the same clinical presentation who has no vascular immune deposits but has circulating ANCA should be diagnosed as microscopic polyangiitis (1, 20). A caveat to this last diagnosis is whether or not there is evidence for granulomatous inflammation or asthma. If there is granulomatous inflammation and no asthma, the proper diagnosis is Wegener's granulomatosis. If there is asthma and eosinophilia, the proper diagnosis is Churg-Strauss syndrome.

Cryoglobulinemic vasculitis

Cryoglobulinemic vasculitis is caused by cryoglobulins that localize in small vessel walls and incite inflammation (58). Purpura, arthralgias and nephritis are the most common manifestations (59). Cryoglobulinemic vasculitis must be differentiated from other small vessel vasculitides that cause the same signs and symptoms of small vessel disease. For example, Henoch-Schönlein purpura and microscopic polyangiitis also frequently cause purpura, arthralgias and nephritis. Useful although not completely specific diagnostic markers for cryoglobulinemic vasculitis include mixed (type II) cryoglobulinemia, rheumatoid factor activity, and laboratory evidence for hepatitis C virus infection (59–62). Very low serum C4 with normal or slightly low C3 is a characteristic abnormality (61, 62). IgA-dominant immune deposits in vessels, for example in skin or kidney biopsy specimens, indicate Henoch-Schönlein purpura rather than cryoglobulinemic vasculitis. Positive serologic testing for ANCA suggests a pauci-immune small vessel vasculitis, such as Wegener's granulomatosis or microscopic polyangiitis, rather than cryoglobulinemic vasculitis.

Conclusion

Diagnostic categorization of vasculitis is a complex process that requires knowledgeable integration of clinical, laboratory, and pathologic data. One should be cautious not to rush to conclusions based on the first bits of evidence. Carefully consider what features should be present, and, equally important, what features should be absent to confirm the diagnosis.

References

1. Jennette J.C., Falk R.J., Andrassy K. *et al.* Nomenclature of systemic vasculitides. Proposal of an international consensus conference. *Arthritis Rheum* 1994, 37: 187–192.
2. Savory W.S. Case of a young woman in whom the main arteries of both upper extremities and of the left side of the neck were throughout completely obliterated. *Med Chir Trans Lond* 1856, 39: 205–219.
3. DiGiacomo V. A case of Takayasu's disease occurred over two hundred years ago. *Angiology* 1984, 35: 750–754.
4. Takayasu M. Case with unusual changes of the central vessels in the retina. *Acta Soc Opthamology* 1908, 12: 554.
5. Arend W.P., Michel B.A., Bloch D.A. *et al.* The American College of Rheumatology 1990 criteria for the classification of Takayasu arteritis. *Arthritis Rheum* 1990, 33: 1129–1134.
6. Lie J.T. Takayasu arteritis. In: A. Churg and J. Churg (eds) *Systemic Vasculitides*. New York: Igaku-Shoin, 1991: 159–179.
7. Churg J. Large vessel vasculitis. Clin *Exp Immunol* 1993, 93 Suppl. 1: 11–12.
8. Lupi-Herrera E., Sanchez-Torres G., Marcushamer J., Mispireta J., Horwitz S. and Vela J.E. Takayasu's arteritis. Clinical study of 107 cases. *Am Heart J* 1977, 93: 94–103.
9. Hutchinson J. Diseases of the arteries. On a peculiar form of thrombotic arteries of the aged which is sometimes productive of gangrene. *Arch Surg* 1890, 1: 323–329.
10. Paulley J.W. Anathritic rheumatoid diseases. *Lancet* 1956, 2: 946.
11. Hamrin B. Polymyalgia arteritica. *Acta Med Scand* [Suppl.] 1972, 533: 1–131.
12. Hamilton C.R. Jr, Shelley W.M. and Tumulty P.A. Giant cell arteritis: including temporal arteritis and polymyalgia rheumatica. *Medicine* 1971, 50: 1–27.
13. Hunder G.G., Bloch D.A., Michel B.A. *et al.* The American College of Rheumatology 1990 criteria for the classification of giant cell arteritis. *Arthritis Rheum* 1990, 33: 1122–1128.
14. Kussmaul A. and Maier R. Uber eine bisher nicht beschreibene eigenthumliche Arterienerkrankung (Periarteritis nodosa), die mit Morbus Brightii und rapid fortschreitender allgemeiner Muskellahmung einhergeht. *Dtsch Arch Klin Med* 1866, 1: 484–518.
15. Ferrari E. Ueber Polyarteritis actua nodosa (sogenannte Periarteriitis nodosa), und ihre Beziehungen zur Polymyositis and Polyneuritis acuta. *Beitr Pathol Anat* 1903, 34: 350–386.

16. Zeek P.M., Smith C.C. and Weeter J.C. Studies on periarteritis nodosa. III. The differentiation between the vascular lesions of periarteritis nodosa and of hypersensitivity. *Am J Pathol* 1948, 24: 889–917.

17. Churg J. and Strauss L. Allergic granulomatosis, allergic angiitis and periarteritis nodosa. *Am J Pathol* 1951, 27: 277–301.

18. Zeek P.M. Periarteritis nodosa: a critical review. *Am J Clin Pathol* 1952, 22: 777–790.

19. Godman G.C. and Churg J. Wegener's granulomatosis. Pathology and review of the literature. *Arch Pathol Lab Med* 1954, 58: 533–553.

20. Jennette J.C. and Falk R.J. Small Vessel Vasculitis. *N Engl J Med* 1997, 337: 1512–23.

21. Arkin A. A clinical and pathological study of periarteritis nodosa. A report of five cases, one histologically healed. *Am J Pathol* 1930, 6: 401–426.

22. Guillevin L., Lhote F., Amouroux J., Gherardi R., Callard P. and Casassus P. Antineutrophil cytoplasmic antibodies, abnormal angiograms and pathological findings in polyarteritis nodosa and Churg-Strauss syndrome: indications for the classification of vasculitides of the polyarteritis nodosa group. *Br J Rheumatol* 1996, 35: 958–964.

23. Lhote F. and Guillevin L. Polyarteritis nodosa, microscopic polyangiitis, and Churg-Strauss syndrome. Clinical aspects and treatment. *Rheum Dis Clin North Am* 1995, 21: 911–947.

24. Davson J., Ball J. and Platt R. The kidney in periarteritis nodosa. *Q J Med* 1948, 17: 175–202.

25. Heptinstall R.H. Polyarteritis (periarteritis) nodosa, Wegener's syndrome, and other forms of vasculitis. In: R.H. Heptinstall (ed.) *Pathology of the Kidney*, 4th edn, Boston: Little, Brown and Company, 1992: 1097–1162.

26. Rose G.A. and Spencer H. Polyarteritis nodosa. *Q J Med* 1957, 26: 43–82.

27. Dickson W.E.C. Polyarteritis acuta nodosa and periarteritis nodosa. *J Pathol Bact* 1908, 12: 31–57.

28. Kirkland G.S., Savige J., Wilson D., Heale W., Sinclair R.A. and Hope R.N. Classical polyarteritis nodosa and microscopic polyarteritis with medium vessel involvement – a comparison of the clinical and laboratory features. *Clin Nephrol* 1997, 47: 176–80.

29. Bell D.M., Brink E.W., Nitzkin J.L. *et al.* Kawasaki syndrome: description of two outbreaks in the United States. *N Engl J Med* 1981, 304: 1568–1575.

30. Gribetz D., Landing B. and Larson E. Kawasaki disease: mucocutaneous lymph node syndrome (MCLNS). In: A. Churg and J. Churg (eds) *Systemic Vasculitides*, New York: Igaku-Shoin, 1991: 257–272.

31. Naoe S., Takahashi K., Masuda H. and Tanaka N. Kawasaki disease. With particular emphasis on arterial lesions. *Acta Pathol Jpn* 1991, 41: 785–797.

32. Rauch A.M. and Hurwitz E.S. Centers for Disease Control (CDC) case definition for Kawasaki syndrome [letter]. *Pediatr Infect Dis* 1985, 4: 702–703.

33. Kawasaki T. MLNS showing particular skin desquamation from the finger and toe in infants. *Allergy* 1967, 16: 178–189.

34. Tanaka N., Naoe S. and Kawasaki T. Pathological study on autopsy cases of mucocutaneous lymph node syndrome. *J Jap Red Cross Cent Hosp* 1971, 2: 85–94.

35. Nagashima M., Matsushima M., Matsuoka H., Ogawa A. and Okumura N. High-dose gammaglobulin therapy for Kawasaki disease. *J Pediatr* 1987, 110: 710–712.

36. Furusho K., Kamiya T., Nakano H. *et al.* High-dose intravenous gammaglobulin for Kawasaki disease. *Lancet* 1984, 2: 1055–1058.
37. Newburger J.W., Takahashi M., Burns J.C. *et al.* The treatment of Kawasaki syndrome with intravenous gamma globulin. *N Engl J Med* 1986, 315: 341–347.
38. Rowley A.H., Duffy C.E. and Shulman S.T. Prevention of giant coronary artery aneurysms in Kawasaki disease by intravenous gamma globulin therapy. *J Pedriatr* 1988, 113: 290–294.
39. Fujiwara H. and Hamashima Y. Pathology of the heart in Kawasaki disease. *Pediatrics* 1978, 61: 100–107.
40. Hirose S. and Hamashima Y. Morphological observations on the vasculitis in the mucocutaneous lymph node syndrome. A skin biopsy study of 27 patients. *Eur J Pedriatr* 1978, 129: 17–27.
41. Klinger H. Grenzformen der Periarteritis nodosa. *Frankf Ztschr Pathol* 1931, 42: 455–480.
42. Wegener F. Uber eine eigenartige rhinogene Granulomatose mit besonderer Beteiligung des Arteriensystems under der Nieren. *Beitr Pathol Anat* 1939, 102: 36–68.
43. Carrington C.B. and Liebow A. Limited forms of angiitis and granulomatosis of Wegener's type. *Am J Med* 1966, 41: 497–527.
44. Kallenberg C.G., Brouwer E., Weening J.J. and Tervaert J.W. Anti-neutrophil cytoplasmic antibodies: current diagnostic and pathophysiological potential. *Kidney Int* 1994, 46: 1–15.
45. Jennette J.C. and Falk R.J. Anti-neutrophil cytoplasmic autoantibodies: Discovery, specificity, disease associations and pathogenic potential. *Adv Pathol Lab Med* 1995, 8: 363–377.
46. Savige J., Davies D., Falk R.J., Jennette J.C. and Wiik A. Antineutrophil cytoplasmic antibodies (ANCA) and associated diseases. *Kidney Int* 2000, 57: 846–862.
47. Lim L.C.L., Taylor III J.G., Schmitz J.L. *et al.* Diagnostic usefulness of antineutrophil cytoplasmic autoantibody serology: comparative evaluation of commercial indirect fluorescent antibody kits and enzyme immunoassay kits. *Am J Clin Pathol* 1999, 111: 363–369.
48. Hagen E.C., Daha M.R., Hermans J. *et al.* Diagnostic value of standardized assays for anti-neutrophil cytoplasmic antibodies in idiopathic systemic vasculitis. EC/BCR Project for ANCA Assay Standardization. *Kidney Int* 1998 53: 743–753.
49. Charles L.A., Falk R.J. and Jennette J.C. Reactivity of anti-neutrophil cytoplasmic autoantibodies with HL-60 cells. *Clin Immunol Immunopathol* 1989, 53: 243–253.
50. Goldschmeding R., van der Schoot C.E., ten Bokkel Huinink D. *et al.* Wegener's granulomatosis autoantibodies identify a novel diisopropylfluorophosphate-binding protein in the lysosomes of normal human neutrophils. *J Clin Invest* 1989, 84: 1577–1587.
51. Jennette J.C., Hoidal J.R. and Falk R.J. Specificity of anti-neutrophil cytoplasmic autoantibodies for proteinase 3 [letter, comment]. *Blood* 1990, 75: 2263–2264.
52. Ludemann J., Utecht B. and Gross W.L. Anti-neutrophil cytoplasm antibodies in Wegener's granulomatosis recognize an elastinolytic enzyme. *J Exp Med* 1990, 171: 357–362.
53. Niles J.L., McCluskey R.T., Ahmad M.F. and Arnaout M.A. Wegener's granulomatosis autoantigen is a novel neutrophil serine proteinase. *Blood* 1989, 74: 1888–1893.

54. Falk R.J. and Jennette J.C. Anti-neutrophil cytoplasmic autoantibodies with specificity for myeloperoxidase in patients with systemic vasculitis and idiopathic necrotizing and crescentic glomerulonephritis. *N Engl J Med* 1988, 318: 1651–1657.

55. Schönlein J.L. Allgemeine und spezielle Pathologie und Therapie. Vol. 2. Herisau, Germany: Literatur-Comptoir, 1837.

56. Henoch E. Uber den zusammenhang von purpura und intestinal-stoerungen. *Berl Klin Wochenschur* 1868, 5: 517–519.

57. Arkin A. A clinical and pathological study of periarteritis nodosa. A report of five cases, one histologically healed. *Am J Pathol* 1930, 6: 401–426.29.

58. Meltzer M., Franklin E.C., Elias K., McCluskey R.T. and Cooper N. Cryoglobulinemia – a clinical and laboratory study. II. Cryoglobulins with rheumatoid factor activity. *Am J Med* 1966, 40: 837–856.

59. Gorevic P.D., Kassab H.J., Levo Y. *et al.* Mixed cryoglobulinemia: clinical aspects and long-term follow-up of 40 patients. *N Engl J Med* 1980, 69: 287–308.

60. Agnello V., Chung R.T. and Kaplan L.M. A role for hepatitis C virus infection in type II cryoglobuliema. *N Engl J Med* 1992, 327: 1490–1495.

61. D'Amico G. and Fornasieri A. Cryoglobulinemic glomerulonephritis: a membranoproliferative glomerulonephritis induced by hepatitis C virus infection. *Am J Kidney Dis* 1995, 25: 361–369.

62. Agnello V. and Romain P.L. Mixed cryoglobulinemia secondary to hepatitis C virus infection. *Rhem Dis Clin N Am* 1991, 18: 164–170.

11

Immunopathogenesis of systemic vasculitis

Anne Ben-Smith and Caroline O.S. Savage

Introduction

Vasculitis is defined as inflammation of blood vessel walls, which may present as a primary disease or secondary to another disease process. Clinically, vasculitis can be subdivided according to the size and type of vessel affected and whether or not there is associated granuloma formation (1). The incidence of primary systemic vasculitis is estimated at 42 per million per year in the UK (2), with up to 50% of cases associated with the presence of ANCA (*anti-neutrophil cytoplasmic antibodies*) directed against lysosomal constituents of neutrophils and monocytes. This review will focus on such ANCA-associated vasculitides, which include Wegener's granulomatosis (WG), microscopic polyangiitis (MPA) and Churg-Strauss syndrome (CSS).

ANCA

The association of ANCA with WG, CSS and MPA has led to the hypothesis that ANCA are involved in the pathogenesis of these disorders. The antibodies are present in patient sera (3, 4) and titres may correlate with disease activity (5). ANCA are mainly directed at two target antigens, proteinase 3 (PR3) and myeloperoxidase (MPO) that are both localized within neutrophil azurophil granules and monocyte lysosomes (4, 6). PR3 is a 29 kDa serine proteinase (pI 9.2) with proteolytic activity towards several physiological substrates including elastase and extracellular matrix proteins (7). MPO is a highly cationic chloride peroxidase of 140 kDa (pI > 11) that generates hypochlorous acid from H_2O_2 and Cl^-. Its activities include the killing of ingested bacteria, activation of latent metalloproteins and generation of reactive oxygen species (8). PR3-ANCA are found in the majority of patients with WG, as well as a proportion of patients with MPA, whereas MPO-ANCA occur in about 70% of patients with MPA and 50% of patients with CSS (9). By indirect immunohistochemistry, PR3-ANCA can be shown to bind to normal, acetone-fixed neutrophils to produce a granular cytoplasmic (or cANCA) staining pattern, whereas MPO-ANCA produces a perinuclear (or pANCA) staining pattern. The different staining patterns are artefacts of ethanol fixation of the neutrophils, which may result in myeloperoxidase migrating towards the nucleus. Both MPO-ANCA and PR3-ANCA target a relatively small number of antigenic epitopes and bind to conformational rather than linear epitopes (10, 11). MPO-ANCA are generally oligoclonal in nature. The clonotypes appear stable over time and between patients suggesting a restriction of self-reactive epitopes (12).

Less commonly, ANCA may also be directed against other antigens such as elastase (13), lactoferrin (14) and bactericidal/permeability-increasing protein (BPI) (15). ANCA have also been described in association with other diseases including inflammatory bowel disease (16) autoimmune liver disease (17) and rheumatoid arthritis (18). Specificity is usually towards targets other than PR3 or MPO.

Evidence for immune involvement

There is little doubt that ANCA-associated disorders are immune-mediated. Although the vasculitic lesions contain little complement or deposited immunoglobulin (19), the initial lesions are associated with the presence of lysed neutrophils within the vessels (20). This is followed by mononuclear cell infiltration and, in WG and CSS, there may be associated granuloma formation (21). These disorders are clinically responsive to immunosuppressive therapies, which have transformed the prognosis of WG from a two-year mortality of over 90% (22) to five-year survival rates of better than 80%. Intravenous immunoglobulin has also been used for treatment of patients with ANCA-associated vasculitis, leading to clinical improvement and a general reduction in ANCA titres (23).

There is no direct evidence to support the hypothesis that these disorders are autoimmune. Although there have been attempts to develop animal models (see later), there are no satisfactory models at present and transfer of ANCA alone fails to induce disease. Also, there have been no cases of placental transfer of autoantibodies in the twenty documented cases of pregnant women with ANCA-associated vasculitis (24). However, there is considerable circumstantial evidence. Several studies have reported a strong association between ANCA titres and disease activity in WG (3, 25, 26) and rising ANCA titres can be used to predict relapses (27). Moreover, circulating autoreactive T cells, as well as B cells and autoantibodies, can be detected in such patients (28, 29). Small-scale studies undertaken to treat refractory WG with anti-thymocyte globulin or humanized anti-lymphocyte monoclonal antibodies also suggest a role for cell-mediated autoimmunity (30).

There is some evidence for genetic susceptibility to vasculitis, with occasional reports of occurrence in related individuals (31, 32). No consistent MHC associations have been found that would point firmly to a T cell dependent autoimmune response. There have been conflicting reports of positive associations with, among others, HLA B8 (33), DR2 (34) and DQw7 (35), negative associations with DR13DR6 (36), or lack of association (37). However, there is an interesting association between deficiency of α1-antitrypsin (the main inhibitor of PR3) and PR3-ANCA positive vasculitis (38), and the PiZ allele is associated with severe disease and poor prognosis (39). A number of studies have also examined polymorphisms in Fcγ receptors bound by ANCA on the surface of neutrophils and monocytes. The NA1 allele of FcγRIII was shown to be a significant risk factor for disease severity and renal involvement in WG (40). Although a later study found no association between the NA1 allele and renal disease, there was a significant increase in NA1 homozygosity in patients with MPO-ANCA positive vasculitis (41). No association has been found between ANCA-associated vasculitis and FcγRII polymorphisms (42). There have also been reports of increased frequency of the complement factor C3 allotype C3F in ANCA-associated vasculitis (43). Taken together, these data suggest that whilst an appropriate genetic background may predispose, or even be necessary for development of disease, additional factors also contribute to pathogenesis.

ANCA and disease pathogenesis

There is good evidence *in vivo* to support neutrophil activation as an important factor in early vasculitis. Initial lesions are associated with the presence of lysed neutrophils within the vessels (20, 44). Renal biopsies from patients with active WG contain activated neutrophils that co-localize with the potent neutrophil chemoattractant, IL-8, by *in situ* hybridization and immunohistochemistry (45) and show positive staining for H_2O_2 and extracellular PR3, MPO and elastase (46). In this latter study, ANCA samples from the same patients were able to activate primed normal neutrophils to undergo a respiratory burst and degranulate. Moreover, the numbers of activated neutrophils correlated with the degree of renal impairment as assessed by serum creatinine (46). There was, however, no correlation between the capacity of ANCA to stimulate normal neutrophils *in vitro* with either the numbers of activated neutrophils present in the biopsies or renal function, suggesting that ANCA alone cannot be implicated in mediating vasculitic tissue damage.

Patient neutrophils exist in a primed state with upregulation of CD66b, CD64, and CD63 (47) and high PR3 expression on the cell surface (48). *In vitro* studies have shown that priming of neutrophils with cytokines such as TNFα (49) TGFβ (50) or IL-8 (51) leads to the translocation of both MPO and PR3 to the neutrophil surface where they are then available for ANCA binding. PR3 and MPO can also translocate to the cell surface as cells become apoptotic (52). It is believed that ANCA IgG bind the surface-expressed antigens via their F(ab′)$_2$ portions and trigger neutrophil activation by ligation of constitutively expressed Fcγ receptors, FcγRIIa and FcγRIIIb (53). This results in intracellular signalling cascades that include tyrosine phosphorylation (54), PKC translocation (54) and PI 3-kinase activation (53). Signal transduction activates a respiratory burst with the release of reactive oxygen species (55) and leukotrienes (56), degranulation (55) and secretion of pro-inflammatory cytokines (57). Adhesion via β2 integrins is also required for neutrophil activation by ANCA (58, 59).

In vitro, neutrophil activation by ANCA can cause endothelial cell injury (60). Cytokine-primed neutrophils can adhere to cytokine-activated endothelium, while ANCA mediated release of cytotoxic products may cause direct injury. In addition, the anionic nature of endothelial cells can lead to charge-related binding of the cationic proteins PR3 and MPO, followed by ANCA binding to these antigens and subsequent endothelial cell cytotoxicity (61) or apoptosis (62). Such endothelial injury may precede and promote the vasculitic lesions.

Stimulation of neutrophils by ANCA and by IL-8, secreted by monocytes and neutrophils in response to ANCA, produces rapid actin cytoskeletal reorganization (63, 64). These changes in the neutrophil cytoskeleton lead to decreased deformability and frustration of neutrophil trafficking. TNFα priming of neutrophils downregulates the expression of the IL-8 receptor CXCR2 (65), reducing their ability to respond to an IL-8 chemotactic gradient and transmigrate into tissues. This results in intravascular retention of neutrophils (65). *In vivo*, this may result in trapping of neutrophils within capillary circulatory systems such as the glomerulus, preventing transmigration and thereby directing inflammation towards the glomerular endothelium (45). That the earliest vasculitic lesions are thrombotic, necrotic and contain small numbers of neutrophils is consistent with development of such mechanisms.

Following ANCA stimulation, the fate of neutrophils is unknown. ANCA can induce accelerated apoptosis in neutrophils (66). However, this ANCA-induced apoptosis is dysregulated, since the morphological changes of apoptosis develop without accelerated surface expression of phosphatidylserine, necessary for successful clearance of such apoptotic cells by scavenging phagocytes. Failure to clear these neutrophils *in vivo* may result in progression to secondary necrosis (67) and also result in the intravascular leukocytoclasis that typifies vasculitic lesions (44) and further endothelial injury. Complementary pro-inflammatory processes may also follow from the presence of ANCA antigens on the surface of apoptotic neutrophils (52), allowing opsonization of these cells by ANCA, which may increase their uptake by macrophages. Macrophage phagocytosis of opsonized apoptotic cells stimulates further inflammatory cytokine release, including TNFα, and persistence of the inflammatory reaction producing greater tissue damage (68).

Role of T lymphocytes

Histological studies have shown the presence of T cells in necrotizing small vessel vasculitis. Renal, lung and nasal biopsies contain CD3+ cells, which are predominantly activated CD4+ memory T cells (69). There are also increased numbers of CD3+ cells in the bronchial lavage of patients with WG. Within vasculitic lesions, there is enhanced expression of MCP-1, MIP-1α, MIP-1β and RANTES (70) and VCAM-1 (71), all of which promote T cell recruitment.

In addition, a role for T cells in systemic vasculitis is suggested by beneficial responses of some patients to treatment with monoclonal anti-T cell (CD4, CD52) antibodies (72). Antigen-specific T cells have been detected in the peripheral blood of patients with ANCA-positive vasculitis (28, 29) and also from the sputum of patients with WG (73). Such T cells may participate in pathogenesis of vasculitis at the initiation and effector stages of the immune response. Antigen specific T cells persist in peripheral blood of patients in remission (28), suggesting that T cells may contribute to the tendency for vasculitis patients to relapse.

A role for T cells is also consistent with T cell-dependent immunoglobulin class switching of ANCA and the presence of high affinity antibodies (74). There is some evidence that the developing T cell response is Th1-like, driven by IFNγ and IL-2 (75). Cytokine analysis of peripheral blood T cells, nasal mucosal tissue or bronchoalveolar lavage fluid from patients with WG showed enhanced IFNγ production (76). TCR V gene analysis has suggested that abnormal expansions of T cells may be present (77, 78), while isolation of BV8$^+$ CD4$^+$ T cells with a common dominating CDR3 motif from four patients with WG suggest that T cells may be responding to specific peptide antigens (79).

Role of monocytes

Like neutrophils, monocytes express MPO and PR3 on their cell surface, which are available for ANCA binding (48). ANCA stimulation of TNFα primed monocytes activates the release of the chemoattractants IL-8 (80) and MCP-1 (81). The subsequent infiltration of mononuclear cells at these sites may then lead to a sustained cellular inflammatory response.

Macrophages form a major component of the inflammatory cells in vasculitic lesions (21). These cells secrete pro-inflammatory cytokines such as TNFα and IL-1 which have multiple effects on the vascular endothelium, including increased expression of adhesion molecules for leukocytes and induced secretion of IL-1, IL-6, IL-8 and GM-CSF from the endothelial cell itself (82). Macrophage-derived IL-1 and TNFα also contribute to activation of lymphocytes and neutrophils (83).

A further role for macrophages is in the processing and presentation of autoantigens (possibly from apoptotic neutrophils) to CD4$^+$ T cells. It is likely that macrophages contribute to escalation and progression of vasculitic injury, particularly within the glomerulus (75).

Role of infection

Infectious agents have been postulated in the aetiology of WG. There are conflicting reports as to whether onset of symptoms is more common in winter (84–86). Infection often precedes a rise in antibody level and clinical disease activity (27, 87). Parvovirus B19 has been linked to WG (88), although this was not substantiated using PCR (89). Chronic nasal carriage of *Staphylococcus aureus* is a significant risk factor for disease relapse (27, 90), particularly in patients carrying superantigen-positive staphylococcal strains, suggesting a role for staphylococcal enterotoxins as superantigens in disease induction (91). In this study of active and quiescent disease in WG, there was significant expansion of superantigen reactive Vβ$^+$ subset of T cells, although this did not correlate with elevated T cell activation (91). Cotrimoxazole therapy may have beneficial effects on control of disease activity (92) and reduce relapse rates (93), but whether this is via effects on *Staphylococcus aureus* or via other immunomodulatory activities remains to be determined.

Non-infectious environmental factors

Drugs

There have been several reports of an association between use of the antithyroid drug propylthiouracil and the development of ANCA-positive vasculitis (94, 95). It has been suggested that MPO, which is involved in the formation of reactive metabolites from propylthiouracil, may bind covalently to one of the metabolites forming an immune complex with the metabolite acting as a hapten (96). These complexes could then induce ANCA formation and, in genetically susceptible individuals, lead to the development of vasculitis. Other drugs that are associated with ANCA-positive vasculitis include hydrallazine (97) and penicillamine (98). A number of cases of Churg-Strauss syndrome have followed the introduction of leukotriene receptor antagonists, but whether the vasculitis is secondary to the drug or whether the drug permits a reduction of steroid dose and the manifestation of latent Churg Strauss syndrome, is not clear (99). However, the association of any drug exposure and vasculitis has never been subjected to a case control study.

Silica and hydrocarbons

Three small hospital-based case control studies previously found an association between ANCA-associated vasculitis with renal involvement and silica exposure, with odds ratios between 6 and 12 (100). However, a more recent case control study of renal and non-renal WG did not confirm this association (86). Hydrocarbon exposure may also have a pathogenic role in renal vasculitis, as evidenced by epidemiological data and animal models (101).

Animal models

There are no satisfactory models of ANCA-associated vasculitic disorders and this has hindered both the understanding of pathogenesis and the ability to test new treatments in vasculitis. However, the main animal models currently available are summarized below (for a more detailed review, see Heeringa *et al.* 1998 (102).

Anti-MPO-associated necrotizing crescentic glomerulonephritis

Brown Norway rats develop anti-human MPO antibodies after immunization with human MPO (103). Necrotizing proliferative glomerulonephritis can then be induced by perfusing kidneys with neutrophil lysosomal enzyme extract (consisting primarily of myeloperoxidase) followed by either H_2O_2 perfusion or clamp ischaemia. Although MPO, IgG and complement factor C3 can be detected after perfusion along the glomerular basement membrane at 24 hours, immune deposits are absent at 4 and 10 days after perfusion. This model suggests that initial local immune complex formation precedes the development of ANCA-related pauci-immune glomerulonephritis and raises the possibility that in such human disorders, immune complexes are transiently deposited on the endothelium but are rapidly cleared by phagocytes. However, other attempts to reproduce this animal model have resulted in significant immune complex deposition (104). Interestingly, another study found that circulating anti-MPO antibodies aggravated subnephritogenic anti-GBM disease, suggesting that anti-MPO antibodies could have pathogenic co-factor potential (105).

Mercuric chloride (HgCl₂)-induced vasculitis

Exposure to $HgCl_2$ in Brown Norway rats induces an autoimmune syndrome mediated by Th2-dependent polyclonal B cell activation (106). This is associated with the development of several autoantibodies including anti-glomerular basement membrane and anti-MPO antibodies. There is widespread tissue injury including a necrotizing leucocytoclastic vasculitis of the gut and lung and also some evidence that bacterial infection may contribute to vascular injury (107). However, in this model, there is no associated glomerulonephritis and a lack of correlation of anti-MPO levels with the extent of the vasculitic lesions. Moreover, human ANCA-positive vasculitis has a more Th1-like profile.

Spontaneous vasculitis in mice

Autoimmune MRL/lpr mice have been used extensively to study immunopathological mechanisms in vasculitis. At an early age, pathogen-free mice spontaneously develop lymphoproliferation, proliferative glomerulonephritis and a perivascular infiltration around small and medium muscular arteries consisting of CD4⁻CD8⁻ T cells (108, 109). These gradually infiltrate the adventitia and result in selective vascular smooth muscle cell necrosis without antibody deposition. The smooth muscle cells that appear to be the target for the cell-mediated hypersensitivity response may help direct the process since they express increased levels of MHC class II antigens and can secrete IL-1 (109, 110). By 16 weeks of age, a second phase of vascular damage is evident, characterized by neutrophil infiltration and fibrinoid necrosis of vascular walls that is believed to be immune-complex mediated (108, 111). There is also evidence of polyclonal B cell stimulation with the development of numerous autoantibodies including anti-MPO IgG. However, with regard to ANCA-associated vasculitis, the polyclonal nature of the autoantibody response and discordance between development of renal vasculitis and presence of anti-MPO antibodies makes it difficult to define their precise pathophysiological role.

SCG/Kj mice develop a crescentic glomerulonephritis together with anti-MPO antibodies that can bind to murine neutrophils (112). However, transfer of MPO-specific hybridomas induces proteinuria but no vasculitis or nephritis (113), suggesting that if MPO and neutrophils are necessary for development of vasculitis, they are not sufficient.

Altogether, perhaps the most important observation from the animal models is that ANCA alone are not pathogenic. Additional factors inducing priming or activation of neutrophils and monocytes are required initially, after which the inflammatory process may be exacerbated by ANCA.

Summary

The aetiology of ANCA-associated vasculitis is unknown. However, from all the available data, a model for immune mechanisms involved in the pathogenesis of ANCA-associated vasculitis may be proposed as follows. An initiating episode, e.g. a bacterial infection, which is normally associated with the release of pro-inflammatory cytokines, neutrophil and monocyte activation and degranulation of PR3 and MPO, breaks tolerance to MPO and PR3 in genetically susceptible individuals. This results in the development of ANCA autoantibodies. Cytokines released due to local infection or inflammatory responses cause upregulation of adhesion molecules on endothelium, priming of neutrophils and allow ANCA to activate neutrophils with damage localized to the endothelium, resulting in early lesions. ANCA activation of neutrophils and release of IL-8 reduces their deformability and leads to blockage of vessels. Such neutrophils also undergo accelerated apoptosis but fail to be cleared, so proceed to secondary necrosis. These cells show accelerated and dysregulated apoptosis and release reactive oxygen intermediates and lysosomal enzymes resulting in endothelial cell damage and necrosis. ANCA-mediated LTB4, IL-1β, IL-8 and MCP-1 production amplify the inflammatory response. Damage and activation of endothelial cells produces pro-inflammatory chemokines and cytokines with influx of monocytes and T cells, intensifying the tissue damage. Antigen-specific memory T cells persist following disease remission with the potential of reactivation and disease relapse.

The immunopathogenic mechanisms involved in ANCA-associated vasculitis are a complex interaction of a variety of mechanisms acting in concert to bring about necrotizing inflammation of blood vessel walls. Further definition of these processes and the development of a better animal model will advance the ultimate goal of better treatment regimes.

References

1. Savage C., Harper L. and Adu D. Primary systemic vasculitis. *Lancet* 1997, 349: 553–558.
2. Scott D.G.I. and Watts R.A. Classification and epidemiology of systemic vasculitis. *Br J Rheumatol* 1994, 33: 879–900.
3. van der Woude F.J., Rasmussen N., Lobatto S., *et al.* Autoantibodies against neutrophils and monocytes: tool for diagnosis and marker of disease activity in Wegener's granulomatosis. *Lancet* 1985, 1: 425–429.
4. Falk R.J. and Jennette J.C. Anti-neutrophil cytoplasmic autoantibodies with specificity for myeloperoxidase in patients with systemic vasculitis and idiopathic necrotising and crescentic glomerulonephritis. *New Eng J Med* 1988, 318: 1651–1657.

5. Egner W. and Chapel H.M. Titration of antibodies against neutrophil cytoplasmic antigens is useful in monitoring disease activity in systemic vasculitis. *Clin Exp Immunol* 1990, 82: 244–249.

6. Campanelli D., Melchoir M., Fu Y., *et al.* Cloning of cDNA for proteinase 3: a serine protease, antibiotic, and autoantigen from human neutrophils. *J Exp Med* 1990, 172: 1709–1715.

7. Rao N.V., Wehner N.G., Marshall B.C., Gray W.R., Gray B.H. and Hoidal J.R. Characterization of proteinase-3 (PR-3), a neutrophil serine proteinase. *J Biol Chem* 1991, 266: 9540–9548.

8. Weiss S.J. Tissue destruction by neutrophils. *New England J Med* 1989, 320: 365–376.

9. Kallenberg C., Brouwer E., Weening J. and Cohen Tervaret J. Anti-neutrophil cytoplasmic antibodies: current diagnosis and pathophysiological potential. *Kidney Int* 1994, 46: 1–15.

10. Williams R., Staud R., Malone C., Payabyab J., Byres L. and Underwood D. Epitopes on proteinase 3 recognised by antibodies from patients with Wegener's granulomatosis. *J Immunol* 1994, 152: 4722–4737.

11. Short A.K. and Lockwood C.M. Studies of epitope restriction on myeloperoxidase (MPO), an important antigen in systemic vasculitis. *Clin Exp Immunol* 1997, 110: 270–276.

12. Nachman P., Reisner H., Yang J., Jennette J. and Falk R. Shared idiotypy among patients with myeloperoxidase-antineutrophil cytoplasmic autoantibody associated glomerulonephritis and vasculitis. *Lab Invest* 1996, 75: 519–527.

13. Goldschmeding R., van der Schoot C.E., ten Bokkel Huinink D., *et al.* Wegener's granulomatosis autoantibodies identify a novel diisopropylfluorphosphate-binding protein in the lysosomes of normal human neutrophils. *J Clin Invest* 1989, 84: 1577–1587.

14. Lesavre P. Antineutrophil cytoplasmic autoantibodies antigen specificity. *Am J Kidney Dis* 1991, 18: 159–163.

15. Zhao M.H., Jones S.J. and Lockwood C.M. Bactericidal/permeability-inducing protein (BPI) is an important antigen for anti-neutrophil cytoplasmic autoantibodies (ANCA) in vasculitis. *Clin Exp Immunol* 1995, 99: 49–56.

16. Mulder A.H., Broekroelofs J., Horst G., Limburg P.C., Nelis G.F. and Kallenberg C.G. Anti-neutrophil cytoplasmic antibodies (ANCA) in inflammatory bowel disease: characterisation and clinical correlates. *Clin Exp Immunol* 1994, 95: 490–497.

17. Hardarson S., Labrecque D.R., Mitros F.A., Neil G.A. and Goeken J.A. Antineutrophil cytoplasmic antibody in inflammatory bowel and hepatobiliary diseases. High prevalence in ulcerative colitis, primary sclerosing cholangitis and autoimmune hepatitis. *Am J Clin Path* 1993, 99: 277–281.

18. Savige J.A., Gallicchio M.C., Stockman A., Cummingham T.J. and Rowley M.J. Anti-neutrophil cytoplasm antibodies in rheumatoid arthritis. *Clin Exp Immunol* 1991, 86: 92–98.

19. Weiss M. and Crissman J. Renal biopsy findings in Wegener's granulomatosis: Segmental necrotising glomerulonephritis with glomerular thrombosis. *Hum Pathol* 1984, 15: 943–856.

20. Hooke D., Gee D. and Atkins R. Leukocyte analysis using monoclonal antibodies in glomerulonephritis. *Kidney Int* 1987, 31: 964–972.

21. Churg J. and Churg A. Idiopathic and secondary vasculitis: a review. *Mod Pathol* 1989, 2: 144–160.

22. Walton E.W. Giant-cell granuloma of the respiratory tract (Wegener's granulomatosis). *BMJ* 1958, 2: 265–270.
23. Jayne D.R.W., Davies M.J., Fox C.J.V., Black C.M. and Lockwood C.M. Treatment of systemic vasculitis with pooled intravenous immunoglobulin. *Lancet* 1990, 337: 1137–1139.
24. Kumar A., Mohan A., Gupta R., Singal V.K. and Garg O.P. Relapse of Wegener's granulomatosis in the first trimester of pregnancy: a case report. *Br J Rheumatol* 1998, 37: 331–333.
25. Nolle B., Specks U., Ludemann J., Rohrbach M.S., DeRemee R.A. and Gross W.L. Anticytoplasmic autoantibodies: their immunodiagnostic value in Wegener's granulomatosis. *Ann Intern Med* 1989, 111: 28–40.
26. Cohen Tervaert J.W., van der Woude F.J., Fauci A.S., *et al.* Association between active Wegener's granulomatosis and anticytoplasmic antibodies. *Arch Intern Med* 1989, 149: 2461–2465.
27. Cohen Tervaert J.W., Huitema M.G., Hene R.J., *et al.* Prevention of relapses in Wegener's granulomatosis by treatment based on antineutrophil cytoplasmic antibody titre. *Lancet* 1990, 336: 709–711.
28. King W., Brooks C., Holder R., Hughes P., Adu D. and Savage C. T lymphocyte responses to anti-neutrophil cytoplasmic autoantibody (ANCA) antigens are present in patients with ANCA-associated systemic vasculitis and persist during disease remission. *Clin Exp Immunol* 1998, 112: 539–546.
29. Griffith M.E., Coulthart A. and Pusey C.D. T cell responses to myeloperoxidase (MPO) and proteinase 3 (PR3) in patients with systemic vasculitis. *Clin Exp Immunol* 1996, 103: 253–258.
30. Jayne D.R.W. Immunotherapy for ANCA-associated systemic vasculitis. *Clin Exp Immunol* 1998, 112: 12.
31. Stoney P., Davies W., Ho S., Paterson I. and Griffith I. Wegener's granulomatosis in two siblings: a family study. *J Laryngol Otol* 1991, 105: 123–124.
32. Nowack R., Lehmann H., Flores-Suarez L.F., Nanhou A. and van der Woude F. Familial occurrence of systemic vasculitis and rapidly progressive glomerulonephritis. *Am J Kidney Dis* 1999, 34: 364–373.
33. Katz P, Alling DW, Haynes BF and Fauci AS. Association of Wegener's granulomatosis with HLA-B8. *Clin Immunol Immunopathol* 1979, 14: 268–270.
34. Elkon K.B., Sutherland D.C., Rees A.J., Hughes G.R.V. and Batchelor J.R. HLA frequencies in systemic vasculitis. Increase in HLA-DR2 in Wegener's granulomatosis. *Arthritis Rheum* 1983, 26: 102–105.
35. Spencer S.J.W., Burns A., Gaskin G., Pusey C.D. and Rees A.J. HLA class II specificities and the development and duration of vasculitis with antibodies to neutrophil cytoplasmic antigens. *Kidney Int* 1992, 41: 1059–1063.
36. Hagen E.C., Stegeman C.A., D'Amaro J., *et al.* Decreased frequency of HLA DR13 DR6 in Wegener's granulomatosis. *Kidney Int* 1995, 48: 801–805.
37. Zhang L., Jayne D., Zhao M.H., Lockwood C.M. and Olivera D.G.B. Distribution of MHC class II alleles in primary systemic vasculitis. *Kidney Int* 1995, 47: 294–298.
38. Esnault V.L.M., Testa A., Audrain M., *et al.* Alpha1-antitrypsin genetic polymorphism in ANCA-positive systemic vasculitis. *Kidney Int* 1993, 43: 1329–1332.
39. Segelmark M., Elzouki A.-N., Weislander J. and Eriksson S. The PiZ gene of α1-antitrypsin as a determinant of outcome in Pr3-ANCA positive vasculitis. *Kidney Int* 1995, 48: 844–50.

40. Kimberly R.P., Edberg J.C., Weinstein E., *et al.* Association of the FcγRIIIb-NA1 allele with renal disease in Wegener's granulomatosis (WG). *Clin Exp Immunol* 1998, 112: 26.

41. Tse W.Y., Abadeh S., Jefferis R., Savage C.O.S. and Adu D. Neutrophil FcγRIIIb allelic polymorphism in anti-neutrophil cytoplasmic antibody (ANCA)-positive systemic vasculitis. *Clin Exp Immunol* 2000, 119: 574–577.

42. Tse W.Y., Abadeh S., McTiernan A., Jefferis R., Savage C.O.S. and Adu D. No association between neutrophil FcγRII allelic polymorphism and ANCA-positive systemic vasculitis. *Clin Exp Immunol* 1999, 117: 198–205.

43. Persson U., Truedsson L., Westman K.W.A. and Segelmark M. C3 and C4 allotypes in anti-neutrophil cytoplasmic autoantibody (ANCA)-positive vasculitis. *Clin Exp Immunol* 1999, 116: 379–382.

44. Donald K.J., Edwards R.L. and McEvoy J.D.S. An ultrastructural study of the pathogenesis of tissue injury in limited Wegener's granulomatosis. *Pathology* 1976, 8: 161–169.

45. Cockwell P., Brooks C., Adu D. and Savage C. Interleukin 8: a pathogenetic role in antineutrophil cytplasmic autoantibody (ANCA)-associated glomerulonephritis. *Kidney Int* 1999, 55: 852–863.

46. Brouwer E., Huitema M.G., Mulder A.H.L., *et al.* Neutrophil activation *in vitro* and *in vivo* in Wegener's granulomatosis. *Kidney Int* 1994, 45: 1120–1131.

47. Muller Kobold A., Mesander G., Stegeman C., Kallenberg, C. and Cohen-Tervaert J. Are circulating neutrophils intravascularly activated in patients with anti-neutrophil cytoplasmic antibody (ANCA)-associated vasculitis? *Clin Exp Immunol* 1998, 114: 491–499.

48. Muller Kobold A., Kallenberg C. and Cohen Tervaert J. Leucocyte membrane expression of proteinase 3 correlates with disease activity in patients with Wegener's granulomatosis. *Br J Rheumatol* 1998, 37: 901–907.

49. Csernok E., Ernst M., Schmitt W., Bainton D.F. and Gross W.L. Activated neutrophils express proteinase 3 on their plasma membrane *in vitro* and *in vivo*. *Clin Exp Immunol* 1994, 95: 244–250.

50. Csernok E., Szymkowiak C.H., Mistry N., Daha M.R., Gross W.L. and Kekow J. Transforming growth factor-beta (TGF-β) expression and interaction with proteinase 3 (PR3) in anti-neutrophil cytoplasmic antibody (ANCA)-associated vasculitis. *Clin Exp Immunol* 1996, 105: 104–111.

51. Rainger G., Fischer A. and Nash G. Endothelial-borne platelet-activating factor and Interleukin 8 rapidly immobilise rolling neutrophils. *Am J Physiol* 1997, 272: H114-H122.

52. Gilligan H., Bredy B., Brady H., *et al.* Antineutrophil cytoplasmic autoantibodies interact with primary granule constituents on the surface of apoptotic neutrophils in the absence of neutrophil priming. *J Exp Med* 1996, 184: 2231–2241.

53. Ben-Smith A., Dove S.K., Martin A., Wakelam M.J.O. and Savage C.O.S. Antineutrophil cytoplasm autoantibodies from patients with systemic vasculitis activate neutrophils via distinct signalling cascades compared to conventional Fcγ receptor ligation.

54. Radford D.J., Lord J.M. and Savage C.O.S. The activation of the neutrophil respiratory burst by anti-neutrophil cytoplasm autoantibody (ANCA) from patients with systemic vasculitis requires tyrosine kinases and protein kinase C activation. *Clin Exp Immunol* 1999, 118: 171–179.

89. Nikkari S., Vainiojnpaa R., Toivanen P., Gross W., Mistry E., *et al.* Wegener's granulomatosis and parvovirus B 19 infection: comment on the concise communication by Nikkari *et al.*, reply. *Arthritis Rheum* 1995, 38: 1175.

90. Stegeman C.A., Cohen Tervaert J.W., Sluiter W.J., Manson W.L., de Jong P.E. and Kallenberg C.G.M. Association of chronic nasal carriage of Staphylococcus aureus and higher relapse rates in Wegener's granulomatosis. *Ann Intern Med* 1994, 120: 12–17.

91. Popa E., Bos N., Stegeman C., Kallenberg C. and Cohen Tervaert F. Skewed TCR Vβ usage in Wegener's granulomatosis suggests stimulation by superantigens. *J Am Soc Nephrol* 1997, 8: A2528.

92. DeRemee R.A., McDonald T.J. and Weiland L.H. Wegener's granulomatosis: observations on treatment with antimicrobial agents. *Mayo Clin Proc* 1985, 60: 27–32.

93. Stegeman C.A., Cohen Tervaert J.W., De Long P.E. and Kallenberg C.G.M. Cotrimoxazole for the prevention of relapses of Wegener's granulomatosis. *New Eng J Med* 1996, 335: 16–20.

94. Kitihara T., Hiromusa K., Maezawa A., *et al.* Case of propylthiouracil-induced vasculitis associated with anti-neutrophil cytoplasmic antibody; review of literature. *Clin Nephrol* 1997, 47: 336–340.

95. Harper L., Cockwell P. and Savage C.O.S. Case of propylthiouracil-induced ANCA associated small vessel vasculitis. *Nephrol Dial Transplant* 1998, 13: 455–458.

96. Waldhauser L. and Uetrecht J. Oxidation of propylthiouracil to reactive metabolites by activated neutrophils. Implications for agranulocytosis. *Drug Metab Dispos* 1991, 19: 354–359.

97. Short A.K. and Lockwood C.M. Antigen specificity in hydralazine associated ANCA positive systemic vasculitis. *QJM* 1995, 88: 775–783.

98. Mathieson P.W., Peat D.S., Short A. and Watts R.A. Coexistent membranous nephropathy and ANCA-positive crescentic glomerulonephritis in association with penicillamine. *Nephrol Dial Transplant* 1996, 11(5): 863–866.

99. D'Cruz D.P., Barnes N.C. and Lockwood M.C. Difficult asthma or Churg-Strauss syndrome? Steroids may be masking undiagnosed cases of Churg-Strauss syndrome. *BMJ* 1999, 318: 475–476.

100. Tervaert J.W., Stegeman C.A. and Kallenberg C.G. Silicon exposure and vasculitis. *Curr Opin Rheumatol* 1998, 10(1): 12–17.

101. Pai P., Bone J.M. and Bell G.M. Hydrocarbon exposure and glomerulonephritis due to systemic vasculitis (letter). *Nephrol Dial Transplant* 1998, 13: 1321–1323.

102. Heeringa P., Brouwer E., Cohen Tervaert J.W., Weening J.J. and Kallenberg C.G.M. Animal models of anti-neutrophil cytoplasmic antibody associated vasculitis. *Kidney Int* 1998, 53: 253–263.

103. Brouwer E., Huitema M.G., Klok P.A., *et al.* Antimyeloperoxidase-associated proliferative glomerulonephritis: an animal model. *J Exp Med* 1993, 177: 905–914.

104. Yang J.J., Jennette J.C. and Falk R.J. Immune complex glomerulonephritis is induced in rats immunised with heterologous myeloperoxidase. *Clin Exp Immunol* 1994, 97: 466–473.

105. Heeringa P., Brouwer E., Klok P.A., *et al.* Autoantibodies to myeloperoxidase aggrevate mild anti-glomerular-basement membrane mediated glomerular injury. *Am J Pathol* 1996, 149: 1695–1706.

106. Mathieson P.W., Qasim F.J. and Esnault V.L.M. Animal models of systemic vasculitis. *J Autoimmun* 1993, 6: 251–264.

107. Mathieson P.W., Thiru S. and Oliveira D.B.G. Mercuric chloride-treated Brown Norway rats develop widespread tissue injury including necrotising vasculitis. *Lab Invest* 1992, 67: 121–129.

108. Alexander E.L., Moyer C.F., Travlos G.S., Roths J.B. and Murphy E.D. Two histopathologic types of inflammatory vascular disease in MRL/MP autoimmune mice: models for human vasculitis in connective tissue disease. *Arthritis Rheum* 1985, 28: 1146–1155.

109. Moyer C.F., Strandberg J.D. and Reinisch C.L. Systemic mononuclear vasculitis in MRL/MP-lpr/lpr mice. A histologic and immunochemical analysis. *Am J Pathol* 1987, 127: 229–242.

110. Moyer C.F. and Reinisch C.L. The role of vascular smooth muscle cells in experimental autoimmune vasculitis. I. The initiation of delayed type hypersensitivity angiitis. *Am J Pathol* 1984, 117: 380–390.

111. Bereden J.H.M., Hang L., McConahey J. and Dixon F.J. Analysis of vascular lesions in murine SLE. I. Association with serologic abnormalities. *J Immunol* 1983, 130: 1699–1705.

112. Kinjoh K., Kyoguko M. and Good R.A. Genetic selection for crescent formation yields mouse strain with rapidly progressive glomerulonephritis and small vessel vasculitis. *Proc Natl Acad Sci USA* 1993, 90: 3413–3417.

113. Kinjoh K., Good R.A., Nemito K., Falk R.J. and Jennette J.C. Hybridomas from SCG/j mice produce P-ANCA with specificity for myeloperoxidase (MPO) and induce proteinuria in nude mice. *Clin Exp Immunol* 1995, 101: 37.

12

Pathology of vasculitis

Franco Ferrario and Maria Pia Rastaldi

Introduction

A pauci-immune necrotizing crescentic glomerulonephritis is the morphological hallmark of ANCA-associated microscopic vasculitis (1, 2). The lesion can vary widely as far as degree and diffusion, and characterizes fundamentally Wegener's granulomatosis, microscopic polyarteritis and its renal limited variant. Although less common, Churg-Strauss syndrome belongs to the same group of ANCA-related small vessels vasculitis, and shows a similar renal involvement, in which the presence of eosinophil infiltration can be a distinguishing feature, but its absence does not exclude the diagnosis (3).

Considering our experience with the review of 231 cases for the Italian Renal Immunopathology Group and of 117 biopsies for the EUVAS group (http://www.vasculitis.org), we have not found in renal biopsies of ANCA-associated renal vasculitis a statistical difference among the diseases as far as the quality and the diffusion of morphological lesions, as shown in Table 12.1. It follows that, for instance, the presence of periglomerular granulomas cannot be considered as diagnostic for Wegener's granulomatosis, because they are present also in cases of renal limited vasculitis. On the contrary, true interstitial granulomas are, although difficult to identify when the underlying structure is not recognizable and very rare, probably the unique morphological distinguishing finding for Wegener's granulomatosis (4, 5). For these reasons, we will describe in this chapter the four entities as a whole.

Pathology

Renal biopsy remains a fundamental instrument for both diagnosis and in particular for management of these disease entities, especially because the degree of clinical symptoms is frequently unrelated with the level and the activity of renal lesions (6). The microscopic finding of a diffuse necrotizing crescentic glomerulonephritis can in fact be present in a patient with only mild renal failure and frequently in our experience the highest levels of serum creatinine correspond best with sclerosing lesions.

In these last years, since the discovery of ANCA-tests (7, 8) and their prevalent association with these forms, diagnosis has greatly improved. In 1994, their

Table 12.1 Main histological features in ANCA-associated renal vasculitis, according to our experience on 117 case study for the EUVAS group

Diagnosis (No. cases)	Necrosis <30%	Necrosis >60%	Crescents <30%	Crescents >60%	Periglomerular infiltrates (+/++)	Periglomerular granulomas	Renal arteritis
WG* (51)	68%	9%	51%	32%	34%	10%	14%
MPA* (48)	76%	16%	31%	32%	39%	12%	8%
RLV* (18)	82%	12%	22%	45%	45%	6%	6%

Results are expressed as percentages

* WG = Wegener's granulomatosis, MPA = micropolyarteritis, RLV = renal limited vasculitis.

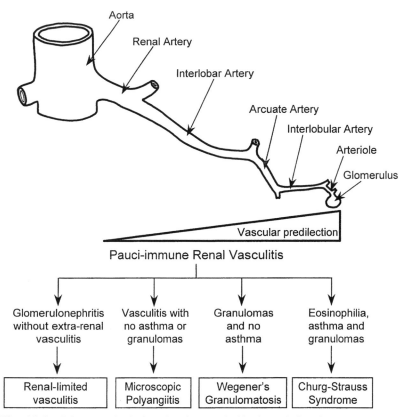

Fig. 13.1 Diagram depicting, in the top half, the relative frequency of involvement by pauci-immune renal vasculitis of different segments of the renal vasculature (as indicated by the relative height of the triangle), and, in the bottom half, an algorithm for categorizing pauci-immune renal vasculitis based on clinical and pathologic features.

Because the glomerular lesion is the same in patients with Wegener's granulomatosis, microscopic polyangiitis, Churg-Strauss syndrome, and renal-limited pauci-immune crescentic glomerulonephritis, additional findings must be used to differentiate among these different variants of pauci-immune renal vasculitis. In a patient with pauci-immune crescentic glomerulonephritis, a diagnosis of Wegener's granulomatosis is warranted if there is clinical or pathologic evidence for necrotizing granulomatous inflammation, usually in the upper or lower respiratory tract (7). A diagnosis of Churg-Strauss syndrome is appropriate if there is a history of asthma and eosinophilia along with granulomatous pulmonary disease. A diagnosis of microscopic polyangiitis is appropriate if there is systemic pauci-immune necrotizing small vessel vasculitis without evidence for granulomatous inflammation or asthma. Finally, if there is no evidence for extra-renal vasculitis, granulomatous inflammation, or asthma, a diagnosis of renal-limited vasculitis or pauci-immune crescentic glomerulonephritis alone is appropriate.

Note that nonspecific constitutional signs and symptoms, such as myalgias, arthralgias, weight loss or fever, are not adequate to conclude that there is extra-renal vasculitic disease in a patient with pauci-immune crescentic glomerulonephritis.

There is no need to delay treatment in a patient with pauci-immune crescentic glomerulonephritis until the patient is categorized as renal-limited disease, microscopic polyangiitis, Wegener's granulomatosis, or Churg-Strauss syndrome. The treatment is the same when there is major organ damage, and delay of treatment is likely to worsen the outcome. A generic term, such as ANCA-associated small vessel vasculitis, can be used as a working diagnosis until enough data are collected to categorize the patient more precisely.

Clinical manifestations

Clinical features of extra-renal pauci-immune vasculitis that are shared by patients with microscopic polyangiitis, Wegener's granulomatosis, and Churg-Strauss syndrome include purpura, erythematous cutaneous nodules, mononeuritis multiplex, imaging showing arterial aneurysms, visceral infarcts, gut perforation, melena, and pulmonary hemorrhage causing radiographic consolidation or hemoptysis. Pathologic confirmation is supplied by tissue biopsy specimens that show necrotizing arteritis, arteriolitis, venulitis or capillaritis, or chronic sclerosing changes consistent with earlier necrotizing angiitis.

Clinical evidence for upper respiratory tract or ocular involvement includes necrotizing sinusitis or rhinitis with ulceration or crusting, otitis media, conjunctivitis, scleritis, uveitis, keratitis, proptosis, orbital pseudotumor, or subglottic stenosis. Note that these features can be present in Wegener's granulomatosis, microscopic polyangiitis, or Churg-Strauss syndrome, and thus do not confirm the presence of granulomatous inflammation. In the absence of infection, strong clinical evidence for granulomatous inflammation includes pulmonary nodules or cavities, or destructive bone or cartilage lesions in the upper respiratory tract. These findings, even in the absence of pathologic confirmation of necrotizing granulomatous inflammation, justify the diagnosis of Wegener's granulomatosis in a patient with pauci-immune crescentic glomerulonephritis, especially if the patient also has ANCA.

Table 13.3 provides rough approximations of the frequency of involvement of different organs by pauci-immune small vessel vasculitis (10). Accurate determinations of organ system involvement are difficult if not impossible to obtain because all series are biased by the referral pattern to the physicians conducting the study. For example, patients referred to nephrologists will have a disproportionately high frequency of renal involvement, those referred to pulmonologists will have more pulmonary disease, those to rheumatologists more musculoskeletal disease, those to neurologists more neural disease, and so on. However, when multiple series are examined, Wegener's granulomatosis appears to have the highest frequency of respiratory tract involvement, microscopic polyangiitis the highest frequency of renal involvement, and Churg-Strauss syndrome the highest

Table 13.3 Approximate frequency of organ system involvement in pauci-immune small vessel vasculitis

	Microscopic polyangiitis (%)	Wegener's granulomatosis (%)	Churg-Strauss syndrome (%)
Cutaneous	40	40	60
Renal	90	80	45
Pulmonary	50	90	70
Ear, nose and throat	35	90	50
Musculoskeletal	60	60	50
Neurologic	30	50	70
Gastrointestinal	50	50	50

Revised from reference 10 with permission.

frequency of cutaneous and peripheral nerve involvement. Churg-Strauss syndrome has less frequent and less severe renal disease than Wegener's granulomatosis or microscopic polyangiitis. The major cause for morbidity and mortality in patients with Churg-Strauss syndrome is coronary arteritis and myocarditis (22, 23), which are rare in microscopic polyangiitis and Wegener's granulomatosis.

Wegener's granulomatosis

Approximately 90% of patients with Wegener's granulomatosis have evidence for upper or lower respiratory tract disease, or both (24–26). The most common upper respiratory tract manifestation is destructive sinusitis with hemorrhagic or purulent sinus drainage and sinus pain. Necrosis of the nasal septum can result in septal perforation or saddle nose deformity. Otitis media can be severe and may cause injury to the facial nerve resulting in facial paralysis. Tracheal inflammation and sclerosis causes airway stenosis in approximately 15% of adults and 50% of children (26).

The two major expressions of lower respiratory tract involvement are nodular, sometimes cavitary, lesions caused by necrotizing granulomatous inflammation, and pulmonary hemorrhage caused by hemorrhagic alveolar capillaritis. Patients with Churg-Strauss syndrome also develop necrotizing granulomatous inflammation, usually with conspicuous eosinophils. The presence of necrotizing granulomatous inflammation rules out microscopic polyangiitis (7). Hemorrhagic pulmonary alveolar capillaritis occurs in patients with Wegener's granulomatosis, microscopic polyangiitis or Churg-Strauss syndrome, and thus is of no value in differentiating between these variants of pauci-immune small vessel vasculitis.

Churg-Strauss syndrome

Churg-Strauss syndrome is distinguished from the other variants of pauci-immune small vessel vasculitis by the presence of asthma and eosinophilia (>10%

eosinophils in the peripheral blood). Eosinophilia without asthma is not specific, because patients with microscopic polyangiitis or Wegener's granulomatosis may have marked eosinophilia. Churg-Strauss syndrome often evolves through three phases (22, 23, 27). Patients initially have allergic rhinitis and asthma, followed by the development of eosinophilic infiltrative disease, such as eosinophilic pneumonia or gastroenteritis. Several years to decades later, evidence for small vessel vasculitis and granulomatous inflammation develops.

Microscopic polyangiitis

Microscopic polyangiitis has pauci-immune systemic small vessel vasculitis that is pathologically indistinguishable from the vasculitis in patients with Wegener's granulomatosis and Churg-Strauss syndrome (8, 10). The absence of immune deposits in vessel walls, including glomerular capillaries, distinguishes microscopic polyangiitis from immune complex mediated vasculitides, such as Henoch-Schönlein purpura and cryoglobulinemic vasculitis.

Wegener's granulomatosis and Churg-Strauss syndrome have distinctive clinicopathologic features that distinguish them from microscopic polyangiitis (7, 10, 22, 23, 27). In a patient with pauci-immune small vessel vasculitis, microscopic polyangiitis is a diagnosis by exclusion. That is, a diagnosis of microscopic polyangiitis is appropriate only when none of the specific features of Wegener's granulomatosis or Churg-Strauss syndrome are identified (7). In some patients, an initial diagnosis of microscopic polyangiitis will subsequently be changed to Wegener's granulomatosis or Churg-Strauss syndrome as additional features are identified or develop. This is not a major management problem, because all three variants of pauci-immune renal vasculitis are treated similarly when there is major organ damage. Similarly, patients who initially appear to have renal-limited pauci-immune crescentic glomerulonephritis may later develop manifestations of systemic small vessel vasculitis, such as Wegener's granulomatosis or microscopic polyangiitis, months to years later (28).

Approximately 80% to 90% of patients with microscopic polyangiitis have renal involvement that almost always includes necrotizing glomerulonephritis with crescents (8, 10, 29, 30). Most patients with microscopic polyangiitis have overt glomerulonephritis as an early manifestation of disease. In our practice, microscopic polyangiitis and renal-limited pauci-immune crescentic glomerulonephritis are the most common causes for rapidly progressive glomerulonephritis, especially in older adults. An ANCA test should be obtained in any patient with clinical evidence for aggressive nephritis.

Anti-neutrophil cytoplasmic autoantibodies (ANCA)

Anti-neutrophil cytoplasmic autoantibodies (ANCA) are a major serologic marker for pauci-immune renal vasculitis (13–17). In patients with glomerulonephritis or vasculitis, the two major antigen specificities of ANCA are for myeloperoxidase (MPO) (13) and proteinase 3 (PR3) (31–34), which are proteins in the primary granules of neutrophils and the lysosomes of monocytes. PR3-ANCA produce a cytoplasmic staining pattern (C-ANCA pattern) when ethanol-fixed neutrophils are used as substrate for an indirect immunofluorescence assay, while MPO-ANCA produce a perinuclear staining pattern (P-ANCA pattern) (13). Most patients with renal-limited pauci-immune crescentic glomerulonephritis have P-ANCA (MPO-ANCA) (16, 17). Most patients with Wegener's granulomatosis have C-ANCA (PR3-ANCA) (16, 17). Patients with microscopic polyangiitis have an approximately equal frequency of P-ANCA and C-ANCA, or more P-ANCA, depending on the study (16, 17, 29, 35). Although not as extensively studied, P-ANCA (MPO-ANCA) appears to be more frequent than C-ANCA (PR3-ANCA) in patients with Churg-Strauss syndrome (22).

ANCA are not confined to patients with pauci-immune crescentic glomerulonephritis. Approximately a quarter to a third of patients with anti-GBM disease have ANCA (36–39). This dual reactivity results from two different antibody populations rather than one crossreacting population (39, 40). The epitope specificity of anti-GBM antibodies is the same in patients with anti-GBM alone compared to those with both ANCA and anti-GBM antibodies (40). Compared to patients with anti-GBM alone, these patients with both anti-GBM and ANCA are older, often have features of systemic small vessel vasculitis, and have a better prognosis for renal survival with treatment.

Up to a quarter of patients with crescentic glomerulonephritis who have glomerular immune complex deposits are ANCA positive (16). These patients have more extensive necrosis and crescents than ANCA-negative patients with glomerular immune complexes.

Diagnostic ANCA testing should include both indirect immunofluorescence assay for C-ANCA and P-ANCA, and immunochemical assay (such as enzyme immunoassay) for PR3-ANCA and MPO-ANCA (16, 17, 41). This improves the specificity of a positive result for pauci-immune small vessel vasculitis without significantly reducing sensitivity. As illustrated in Table 13.4, the clinical signs and symptoms in a patient influence the predictive value of an ANCA test result. For example, in a patient with clinical evidence for rapidly progressive glomerulonephritis (RPGN), a positive ANCA result indicates a greater than 90% likelihood that the patient has some variant of pauci-immune renal vasculitis and a negative result reduces the likelihood to approximately 15% (16). In contrast, in a patient with weak evidence for pauci-immune renal vasculitis, such as hematuria with normal renal function and no clinical evidence for extrarenal vasculitis, a positive ANCA result predicts less than a 70% likelihood of pauci-immune renal vasculitis (16). Therefore, in a patient with good clinical evidence for pauci-immune renal vasculitis, a positive ANCA result is strong confirmation of pauci-immune renal vasculitis and might warrant institution of high dose corticosteroid treatment while awaiting tissue confirmation by renal biopsy. In a patient with weak evidence for vasculitis, however, a positive ANCA result should at least prompt an expeditious and thorough search for confirmatory evidence for pauci-immune renal vasculitis. A positive ANCA result in the absence of substantial supporting evidence for small vessel vasculitis is not sufficient cause for instituting aggressive immunosuppressive treatment.

Table 13.4 Predictive value of combined IFA and EIA ANCA testing

Adult with:	Prevalence (pre-test likelihood) (%)	PPV (post-test likelihood) (%)	NPV (post-test unlikelihood) (%)
RPGN Hematuria,	47	95	85
Proteinuria, Cr >3mg/dl Hematuria,	21	84	95
Proteinuria, Cr 1.5–3mg/dl Hematuria,	7	60	99
Proteinuria, Cr <1.5 mg/dl	2	29	100

Data derived from an analysis of 2315 patients, with ANCA assay sensitivity 81% and specificity 96%. From reference 16.

ANCA-associated pauci-immune crescentic glomerulonephritis and systemic vasculitis can be induced by drugs, including propylthiouracil (42–44), penicillamine (45–47) and hydralazine (48). This is an important possibility to consider, because removal of the drug results in disappearance of ANCA and resolution of the nephritis and vasculitis.

Treatment

Pauci-immune renal vasculitis usually is an aggressive immune-mediated disease that warrants aggressive immunosuppressive therapy. In their study of patients with renal vasculitis who were treated during the late 1970s and early 1980s, Serra, Cameron and associates observed a patient survival of only 38% at five years (2, 6). With current immunosuppressive regimens, five year renal and patient survival has improved to 60% to 80% (29, 49, 50). Although there is no doubt that immunosuppressive therapy is beneficial in patients with severe pauci-immune renal vasculitis, it is important to realize that approximately a third of patient deaths, especially in elderly patients, are directly related to complication of the treatment (6). The treatment of pauci-immune small vessel vasculitis is complicated by high recurrence rate after successful induction of remission, which requires additional immunosuppressive maintenance therapy or retreatment regimens. Complications of prolonged immunosuppressive therapy include life-threatening infections, hemorrhagic cystitis, ovarian and testicular failure, and cancer (6, 51). The daunting challenge is to give enough but not too much immunosuppression.

Prednisolone and cyclophosphamide

All variants of pauci-immune renal vasculitis are treated similarly when there is active major organ involvement, such as progressive acute glomerulonephritis. Treatment can be divided into remission induction, remission maintenance, and relapse treatment (52). Corticosteroids alone may be adequate for ameliorating indolent limited disease, but are inadequate for patients with active major organ damage (26). The currently accepted standard treatment for pauci-immune renal vasculitis is a combination of corticosteroids and cytotoxic drugs. This treatment approach results in a high frequency of remission, good patient survival, and frequent recovery of renal function (30, 51, 53–55).

For example, in a study of 70 patients with ANCA-positive pauci-immune renal vasculitis, Falk *et al.* obtained 75% renal survival at 2 years using high dose corticosteroids or corticosteroids combined with cyclophosphamide (55). Patients with renal-limited disease had the same renal and patient survival as those with systemic vasculitis. Oral cyclophosphamide and intravenous cyclophosphamide were equally effective for inducing remission. Patients treated with corticosteroids alone had a lower initial remission rate and three times greater risk for relapse compared to patients treated with corticosteroids plus cyclophosphamide (53). Patients treated with corticosteroids alone also have a higher mortality than patients treated with combination therapy (29).

The relative efficacy of oral cyclophosphamide versus intravenous cyclophosphamide is unclear. Both are similarly effective at inducing remission (50, 55). Patients on oral cyclophosphamide have less toxic effects but have a higher rate of remissions (50, 55). The administration of intravenous cyclophosphamide can be carefully regulated. More evidence is required before the relative value of oral versus intravenous cyclophosphamide can be settled.

The induction treatment regimen frequently used at UNC is intravenous methylprednisolone at 7 mg/kg/day for 3 days followed by tapering doses of oral prednisone. This is combined with oral cyclophosphamide at 2 mg/kg/day, or intravenous cyclophosphamide at 0.5 g/m2/month adjusted upward to 1 g/m2 based on the leukocyte count (53). Corticosteroids usually are discontinued after attaining remission and the cyclophosphamide is continued for 6 to 12 months.

Another potentially less toxic but equally or more effective approach is to convert from cyclophosphamide to azathioprine after remission is achieved, after as little as 3 months of cyclophosphamide treatment (56–58). This approach has resulted in equal or better relapse rates compared to conventional therapy.

Methotrexate and trimethoprim-sulfamethoxazole may have an adjunctive role in ameliorating indolent smouldering or limited disease but are not adequate for remission induction or maintenance in patients with active major organ involvement by pauci-immune small vessel vasculitis.

The optimum duration of initial immunosuppressive therapy is unknown. Early regimens used for the treatment of Wegener's granulomatosis called for a year or more of therapy with cyclophosphamide. Such prolonged treatment results in a high frequency of complications (59–60). In patients who respond well, cyclophosphamide treatment for as short as 6 months may be adequate, but this has not been proven.

Plasmapheresis

The role of plasmapheresis in the treatment of pauci-immune renal vasculitis is not clear. Several studies have demonstrated little or no value (6, 61–64). However, Pusey *et al.* found evidence that plasmapheresis was beneficial in patients who already were dialysis dependent at the time therapy was begun (64). Gianviti *et al.* also have suggested a benefit from plasmapheresis, but this was based on a retrospective uncontrolled study (65). Although there is no proof of its effectiveness, plasmapheresis often is used in patients with severe pulmonary hemorrhage because of the hope that this will be beneficial in this extremely life-threatening situation.

Intravenous gamma globulin

Intravenous gamma globulin therapy has been tried in a small number of patients with pauci-immune renal vasculitis who have been resistant to conventional therapy (66–68). The anecdotal data from these patients suggest a possible benefit but are not conclusive.

Other treatments

Additional treatments of uncertain value include mofetil mycophenolate, cyclosporine, soluble TNF receptor antagonists, dozoxyspermaglytoline, and humanized antibodies to leukocyte antigens. These or similar agents may prove to be of value, but for now the mainstay of therapy for patients with active pauci-immune renal vasculitis remains corticosteroids and cyclophosphamide.

Prognostic factors

Serum creatinine at the time of diagnosis and institution of treatment is the best predictor of outcome (29, 69), which indicates that rapid diagnosis and initiation of treatment are critically important for an optimum outcome. A number of systems have been designed to assess disease activity and damage in patients with pauci-immune renal vasculitis, including the five-factor score (FFS) (29), Birmingham Vasculitis Activity Score (BVAS) (70), and the Vasculitis Damage Index (VDI) (71). The value of these tools for predicting outcomes and directing treatment is still being evaluated. A variety of renal biopsy findings have been evaluated as potential prognostic indicators. The percentage of normal glomeruli appears to be the best indicator identified so far (72). ANCA antigen specificity is of limited prognostic value. Patients with C-ANCA (PR3-ANCA) have more rapid initial deterioration of renal function compared to patients with P-ANCA

(MPO-ANCA); however, eventual clinical outcomes are similar (73). One study has suggested that monitoring of ANCA levels during the course of pauci-immune renal vasculitis is useful for directing treatment (74). However, the value of ANCA levels for modulating treatment is unsubstantiated (75).

Relapse

Approximately a third to a half of the patients with pauci-immune renal vasculitis who attain remission have at least one relapse within 5 years (30, 51, 53, 76). Relapses usually are treated with a regimen similar to induction therapy with approximately two-thirds of patients showing a response (26, 54).

End stage renal failure

Renal replacement therapy with dialysis or transplantation has special challenges in patients with end stage renal disease (ESRD) caused by pauci-immune renal vasculitis (77–84). In particular, patients with ESRD who are on dialysis or have renal transplants may have relapse of extrarenal disease; and patients with renal transplants may have recurrence of renal disease. In spite of these problems, pauci-immune renal vasculitis patients do not have significantly worse graft or patient survival than other ESRD patients (77). An accurate rate of recurrence of vasculitis and glomerulonephritis is difficult to obtain. One attempt estimates an approximately 15% recurrence rate (84). Recurrences do not correlate with the initial variant of pauci-immune renal vasculitis, type of anti-rejection therapy, or persistent ANCA positivity (84). Transplantation should not be deferred because of persistent ANCA positivity if there is no clinical evidence for active vasculitic disease. Systemic and renal recurrences usually respond to high dose corticosteroid and cyclophosphamide treatment (77). The current recommendation is to use standard approaches to renal replacement therapy in patients who develop ESRD secondary to pauci-immune renal vasculitis, but to be vigilant for recurrent disease.

References

1. Stilmant M.M., Bolton W.K., Sturgill B.C., Schmitt G.W. and Couser W.G. Crescentic glomerulonephritis without immune deposits: clinicopathologic features. *Kidney Int* 1979, 15: 184–195.
2. Serra A., Cameron J.S., Turner D.R. *et al.* Vasculitis affecting the kidney: presentation, histopathology and long-term outcome. *Q J Med* 1984, 53: 181–207.
3. Serra A. and Cameron J.S. Clinical and pathologic aspects of renal vasculitis. *Seminars in Nephrology.* 1985, 5: 15–33.
4. Balow J.E. Renal vasculitis. *Kidney Int* 1985, 27: 954–964.
5. Croker B.P., Lee T. and Gunnells J.C. Clinical and pathologic features of polyarteritis nodosa and its renal-limited variant: primary crescentic and necrotizing glomerulonephritis. *Human Pathol* 1987, 18: 48–44.

6. Cameron J.S. Renal vasculitis: microscopic polyarteritis and Wegener's granuloma. *Contributions to Nephrology* 1991, 94: 38–46.

7. Jennette J.C., Falk R.J., Andrassy K. *et al*. Nomenclature of systemic vasculitides: The proposal of an international consensus conference. *Arthritis Rheum* 1994, 37: 187–192.

8. Jennette J.C. and Falk R.J. The pathology of vasculitis involving the kidney. *Am J Kidney Dis* 1994, 24: 130–141.

9. D'Amico G., Sinico R.A. and Ferrario F. Renal vasculitis. *Nephrol Dial Transplant* 1996, 11 [Suppl.] 9: 69–74

10. Jennette J.C. and Falk R.J. Small vessel vasculitis. *N Engl J Med* 1997, 337: 1512–1523.

11. Ronco P., Mougenot B., Bindi P., Noel L.H., Mignon F. and Lesavre P. Les glomerulonehrites extracapillaires 'idiopathiques' sans depot immune sont des vascularites: analyse clinique et serologique. *Bull Acad Natl Med* 1993, 177: 481–494.

12. Godman G.C. and Churg J. Wegener's granulomatosis: pathology and review of the literature. *Arch Pathol* 1954, 58: 533–553.

13. Falk R.J. and Jennette J.C. Anti-neutrophil cytoplasmic autoantibodies with specificity for myeloperoxidase in patients with systemic vasculitis and idiopathic necrotizing and crescentic glomerulonephritis. *N Engl J Med* 1988, 318: 1651–1657.

14. Kallenberg C.G., Brouwer E., Weening J.J. and Tervaert J.W. Anti-neutrophil cytoplasmic antibodies: current diagnostic and pathophysiological potential. [Review]. *Kidney Int* 1994, 46: 1–15.

15. Jennette J.C. and Falk R.J. Anti-neutrophil cytoplasmic autoantibodies: Discovery, specificity, disease associations and pathogenic potential. *Adv Pathol Lab Med* 1995, 8: 363–377.

16. Lim L.C.L., Taylor III J.G., Schmitz J.I., *et al*. Diagnostic usefulness of antineutrophil cytoplasmic autoantibody serology: comparative evaluation of commercial indirect fluorescent antibody kits and enzyme immunoassay kits. *Am J Clin Pathol* 1999, 111: 363–369.

17. Hagen E.C., Daha M.R., Hermans J., *et al*. Diagnostic value of standardized assays for anti-neutrophil cytoplasmic antibodies in idiopathic systemic vasculitis. EC/BCR Project for ANCA Assay Standardization. *Kidney Int* 1998, 53: 743–753.

18. Bonsib S.M. and Walker W.P. Pulmonary-renal syndrome: clinical similarity amidst etiologic diversity. *Mod Pathol* 1989, 2: 129–137.

19. Niles J.L., Bottinger E.P., Saurina G.R., *et al*. The syndrome of lung hemorrhage and nephritis is usually an ANCA-associated condition. *Arch Intern Med* 1996, 156: 440–445.

20. Schena F.P. Survey of the Italian Registry of Renal Biopsies. Frequency of the renal diseases for 7 consecutive years. *Nephrol Dial Transplant* 1997, 12: 418–426.

21. Lane S.E., Scott D.G., Heaton A. and Watts R.A. Primary renal vasculitis in Norfolk – increasing incidence or increasing recognition? *Nephrol Dial Transplant* 2000, 15: 23–27.

22. Lhote F. and Guillevin L. Polyarteritis nodosa, microscopic polyangiitis, and Churg-Strauss syndrome. *Rheum Dis Clin of N Am* 1995, 21: 911–947.

23. Masi A.T., Hunder G.G., Lie J.T. *et al*. The American College of Rheumatology 1990 criteria for the classification of Churg-Strauss syndrome (allergic granulomatosis and angiitis). *Arthritis Rheum* 1990, 33: 1094–1100.

24. Fauci A.S., Haynes B.F., Katz P. and Wolff S.M. Wegener's granulomatosis: prospective clinical and therapeutic experience with 85 patients for 21 years. *Ann Intern Med* 1983, 98: 76–85.

25. Leavitt R.Y., Fauci A.S., Bloch D.A. *et al.* The American College of Rheumatology 1990 criteria for the classification of Wegener's granulomatosis. *Arthritis Rheum* 1990, 33: 1101–1107.

26. Duna G.F., Galperin C. and Hoffman G.S. Wegener's granulomatosis. *Rheum Dis Clin North Am* 1995, 21: 949–986.

27. Lanham J.G., Elkon K.B., Pusey C.D. and Hughes G.R. Systemic vasculitis with asthma and eosinophilia: a clinical approach to the Churg-Strauss syndrome. *Medicine* 1984, 63: 65–81.

28. Woodworth T.G., Abuelo J.G. and Esparza A. Severe glomerulonephritis with late emergence of classic Wegener's granulomatosis. Report of 4 cases and review of the literature. *Medicine* 1987, 66: 181–191.

29. Guillevin L., Durand-Gasselin B., Cevallos R. *et al.* Microscopic polyangiitis: clinical and laboratory findings in eighty-five patients. *Arthritis Rheum* 1999, 42: 421–430.

30. Savage C.O., Winearls C.G., Evans D.J., Rees A.J. and Lockwood C.M. Microscopic polyarteritis: presentation, pathology and prognosis. *Q J Med* 1985, 56: 467–483.

31. Goldschmeding R., van der Schoot C.E., ten Bokkel Huinink D. *et al.* Wegener's granulomatosis autoantibodies identify a novel diisopropylfluorophosphate-binding protein in the lysosomes of normal human neutrophils. *J Clin Invest* 1989, 84: 1577–1587.

32. Jennette J.C., Hoidal J.R. and Falk R.J. Specificity of anti-neutrophil cytoplasmic autoantibodies for proteinase 3. *Blood* 1990, 75: 2263–2264.

33. Ludemann J., Utecht B. and Gross W.L. Anti-neutrophil cytoplasm antibodies in Wegener's granulomatosis recognize an elastinolytic enzyme. *J Exp Med* 1990, 171: 357–362.

34. Niles J.L., McCluskey R.T., Ahmad M.F. and Arnaout M.A. Wegener's granulomatosis autoantigen is a novel neutrophil serine proteinase. *Blood* 1989, 74: 1888–1893.

35. Jennette J.C., Wilkman A.S. and Falk R.J. Anti-neutrophil cytoplasmic autoantibody-associated glomerulonephritis and vasculitis. *Am J Pathol* 1989, 35: 921–930.

36. Bosch X., Mirapeix E., Font J., Borrellas X., Rodriguez R., Lopez-Soto A., Ingelmo M. and Revert L. Prognostic implication of anti-neutrophil cytoplasmic autoantibodies with myeloperoxidase specificity in anti- glomerular basement membrane disease. *Clin Nephrol* 1991, 36: 107–113.

37. Bosch X., Mirapeix E., Font J., Cervera R., Ingelmo M., Khamashta M.A., Revert L., Hughes G.R. and Urbano-Marquez A. Anti-myeloperoxidase autoantibodies in patients with necrotizing glomerular and alveolar capillaritis. *Am J Kidney Dis* 1992, 20: 231–239.

38. Jayne D.R., Marshall P.D., Jones S.J. and Lockwood C.M. Autoantibodies to GBM and neutrophil cytoplasm in rapidly progressive glomerulonephritis. *Kidney Int* 1990, 37: 965–970.

39. Short A.K., Esnault V.L. and Lockwood C.M. Anti-neutrophil cytoplasm antibodies and anti-glomerular basement membrane antibodies: two coexisting distinct autoreactivities detectable in patients with rapidly progressive glomerulonephritis. *Am J Kidney Dis* 1995, 26: 439–445.

40. Hellmark T., Niles J.L., Collins A.B., McCluskey R.T. and Brunmark C. Comparison of anti-GBM antibodies in sera with or without ANCA. *J Am Soc Nephrol* 1997, 8: 376–385.

41. Savige J., Gillis D., Davies D. *et al.* International consensus statement on testing and reporting of antineutrophil cytoplasmic antibodies (ANCA). *Am J Clin Pathol* 1999, 111: 507–513.
42. D'Cruz D., Chesser A.M., Lightowler C. *et al.* Antineutrophil cytoplasmic antibody-positive crescentic glomerulonephritis associated with anti-thyroid drug treatment. *Br J Rheum* 1995, 34: 1090–1091.
43. Dolman K.M., Gans R.O., Vervaat T.J. *et al.* Vasculitis and antineutrophil cytoplasmic autoantibodies associated with propylthiouracil therapy. *Lancet* 1993, 342: 651–652.
44. Vogt B.A., Kim Y., Jennette J.C., Falk R.J., Burke B.A. and Sinaiko A. Antineutrophil cytoplasmic autoantibody-positive crescentic glomerulonephritis as a complication of treatment with propylthiouracil in children. *J Pediatr* 1994, 124: 986–988.
45. Mathieson P.W., Peat D.S., Short A. and Watts R.A. Coexistent membranous nephropathy and ANCA-positive crescentic glomerulonephritis in association with penicillamine. [Review]. *Nephrol Dial Transplant* 1996, 11: 863–866.
46. Devogelaer J.P., Pirson Y., Vandenbroucke J.M. *et al.* D-penicillamine induced crescentic glomerulonephritis: report and review of the literature. *J Rheum* 1987, 14: 1036–1041.
47. Ntoso K.A., Tomaszewski J.E., Jimenez S.A. and Neilson E.G. Penicillamine-induced rapidly progressive glomerulonephritis in patients with progressive systemic sclerosis: successful treatment of two patients and a review of the literature. *Am J Kidney Dis* 1986, 8: 159–163.
48. Nassberger L., Johansson A.C., Bjorck S. and Sjoholm A.G. Antibodies to neutrophil granulocyte myeloperoxidase and elastase: autoimmune responses in glomerulonephritis due to hydralazine treatment. *J Intern Med* 1991, 229: 261–265.
49. Balow J.E. Renal vasculitis. *Cur Opin Nephrol Hypertension* 1993, 2: 231–237.
50. Adu D., Pall A., Luqmani R.A., Richards N.T., Howie A.J., Emery P., Michael J., Savage C.O. and Bacon P.A. Controlled trial of pulse versus continuous prednisolone and cyclophosphamide in the treatment of systemic vasculitis. *Q J Med* 1997, 90: 401–419.
51. Hoffman G.S., Kerr G.S., Leavitt R.Y. *et al.* Wegener's granulomatosis: an analysis of 158 patients. *Ann Intern Med* 1992, 116: 488–498.
52. Bacon P.A. Therapy of vasculitis. *J Rheumatol* 1994, 21: 788–790.
53. Nachman P.H., Hogan S.L., Jennette J.C. and Falk R.J. Treatment response and relapse in ANCA-associated microscopic polyangiitis and glomerulonephritis. *J Am Soc Nephrol* 1996, 7: 33–39.
54. Jindal K.K. Management of idiopathic crescentic and diffuse proliferative glomerulonephritis: evidence-based recommendations. *Kidney Int Suppl* 1999, 70: S33–40.
55. Falk R.J., Hogan S., Carey T.S. and Jennette J.C. Clinical course of anti-neutrophil cytoplasmic autoantibody-associated glomerulonephritis and systemic vasculitis. The Glomerular Disease Collaborative Network. *Ann Intern Med* 1990, 113: 656–663.
56. Gaskin G., Savage C.O., Ryan J.J. *et al.* Anti-neutrophil cytoplasmic antibodies and disease activity during long-term follow-up of 70 patients with systemic vasculitis. *Nephrol Dial Transplant* 1991, 6: 689–694.
57. Pusey C.D., Gaskin G. and Rees A.J. Treatment of primary systemic vasculitis. *APMIS* Suppl. 1990, 19: 48–50.
58. Pusey C.D. Microscopic polyangiitis. *Clin Exp Immunol* 2000, 120, Suppl. 1 32.

59. Choy D.S., Gearhart R.P., Gould W.J., Sauer J., Jacobson L. and Rosenthal B. Development of multiple carcinomas in a long term survivor of Wegener's granulomatosus treated with immunosupressive drugs. *N Y State J Med* 1989, 89: 680–682.

60. Tarlar-Williams C., Hijazi Y., Walther M. *et al.* Cyclophosphamide-induced cystitis and bladder cancer in patients with Wegener granulomatosis. *Ann of Internal Med* 1996, 124: 477–484.

61. Cole E., Cattran D., Magil A. *et al.* A prospective randomized trial of plasma exchange as additive therapy in idiopathic crescentic glomerulonephritis. The Canadian Apheresis Study Group. *Am J Kidney Dis* 1992, 20: 261–269.

62. Glockner W.M., Sieberth H.G., Wichmann H.E. *et al.* Plasma exchange and immunosuppression in rapidly progressive glomerulonephritis: a controlled, multi-center study. *Clin Nephrol* 1988, 29: 1–8.

63. Rifle G. and Dechelette E. Treatment of rapidly progressive glomerulonephritis by plasma exchange and methylprednisolone pulses. A prospective randomized trial of cyclophosphamide. Interim analysis. The French Cooperative Group. *Prog Clin Biol Res* 1990, 337: 263–267.

64. Pusey C.D., Rees A.J., Evans D.J., Peters D.K. and Lockwood C.M. Plasma exchange in focal necrotizing glomerulonephritis without anti-GBM antibodies. *Kidney Int* 1991, 40: 757–763.

65. Gianviti A., Trompeter R.S., Barratt T.M., Lythgoe M.F. and Dillon M.J. Retrospective study of plasma exchange in patients with idiopathic rapidly progressive glomerulonephritis and vasculitis. *Arch Dis Childhood* 1996, 75: 186–190.

66. Jayne D.R., Davies M.J., Fox C.J., Black C.M. and Lockwood C.M. Treatment of systemic vasculitis with pooled intravenous immunoglobulin. *Lancet* 1991, 337: 1137–1139.

67. Tuso P., Moudgil A., Hay J. *et al.* Treatment of antineutrophil cytoplasmic autoantibody–positive systemic vasculitis and glomerulonephritis with pooled intravenous gammaglobulin. *Am J Kidney Dis* 1992, 20: 504–508.

68. Richter C., Schnabel A., Csernok E., Reinhold-Keller E. and Gross W.L. Treatment of Wegener's granulomatosis with intravenous immunoglobulin. *Adv Exp Med Biol* 1993, 336: 487–489.

69. Hogan S.L., Nachman P.H., Wilkman A.S., Jennette J.C. and Falk R.J. Glomerular disease collaborative network: Prognostic markers in patients with ANCA-associated microscopic polyangiitis and glomerulonephritis. *J Am Soc Nephrol* 1996, 7: 23–32.

70. Luqmani R.A., Bacon P.A., Moots R.J. *et al.* Birmingham Vasculitis Activity Score (BVAS) in systemic necrotizing vasculitis. *Q J Med* 1994, 87: 671–678.

71. Exley A.R., Bacon P.A., Luqmani R.A., Kitas G.D., Gordon C., Savage C.O. and Adu D. Development and initial validation of the Vasculitis Damage Index for the standardized clinical assessment of damage in the systemic vasculitides. *Arthritis Rheum* 1997, 40(2): 371–380.

72. Bajema I.M., Hagen E.C., Hermans J., Noel L.H., Waldherr R., Ferrario F., Van Der Woude F.J. and Bruijn J.A. Kidney biopsy as a predictor for renal outcome in ANCA-associated necrotizing glomerulonephritis. *Kidney Int* 1999, 56: 1751–1758.

73. Franssen C.F., Gans R.O., Arends B. *et al.* Differences between anti-myeloperoxidase- and anti-proteinase 3-associated renal disease. *Kidney Int* 1995, 47: 193–199.

74. Cohen Tervaert J.W., Huitema M.G., Hene R.J. *et al.* Prevention of relapses in Wegener's granulomatosis by treatment based on antineutrophil cytoplasmic antibody titre. *Lancet* 1990, 336: 709–711.

75. Kerr G.S. and Hallahan T.S. Limited prognostic value of changes in antineutrophil cytoplasmic antibody titers in patients with Wegener's granulomatosis. *Adv Exp Med Biol* 1993, 336: 389–392.

76. Pettersson E.E., Sundelin B. and Heigl Z. Incidence and outcome of pauci-immune necrotizing and crescentic glomerulonephritis in adults. *Clin Nephrol* 1995, 43: 141–149.

77. Allen A., Pusey C. and Gaskin G. Outcome of renal replacement therapy in antineutrophil cytoplasmic antibody-associated systemic vasculitis. *J Am Soc Nephrol* 1998, 9: 1258–1263.

78. Steinman T.I., Jaffe B.F., Monaco A.P., Wolff S.M. and Fauci A.S. Recurrence of Wegener's granulomatosis after kidney transplantation Successful re-induction of remission with cyclophosphamide. *Am J Surg Pathol* 1980, 4: 191–196.

79. Grotz W., Wanner C., Rother E. and Schollmeyer P. Clinical course of patients with antineutrophil cytoplasm antibody positive vasculitis after kidney transplantation. *Nephron* 1995, 69: 234–236.

80. Yang C.W., Kim Y.S., Kim S.Y. and Bang B.K. Renal transplantation of ANCA-positive idiopathic crescentic glomerulonephritis: two-year follow-up [letter]. *Clin Nephrol* 1994, 42: 209.

81. Rosenstein E.D., Ribot S., Ventresca E. and Kramer N. Recurrence of Wegener's granulomatosis following renal transplantation. [Review]. *Br J Rheumatol* 1994, 33: 869–871.

82. Morin M.P., Thervet E., Legendre C., Page B., Kreis H. and Noel L.H. Successful kidney transplantation in a patient with microscopic polyarteritis and positive ANCA. *Nephrol Dial Transplant* 1993, 8: 287–288.

83. Boubenider S.A., Akhtar M., Alfurayh O., Algazlan S., Taibah K. and Qunibi W. Late recurrence of Wegener's granulomatosis presenting as tracheal stenosis in a renal transplant patient. *Clin Transplant* 1994, 8: 5–9.

84. Nachman P.H., Segelmark M., Westman K. *et al.* Recurrent ANCA-small vessel vasculitis after transplantation: a pooled analysis. *Kidney Int* 1999, 56: 1544–1550.

14

Polyarteritis nodosa: Clinical characteristics, outcome and treatment

Loïc Guillevin

Introduction

Polyarteritis nodosa (PAN) was the first vasculitis to be described by Küssmaul and Maier.[1] For decades, the term PAN served as an umbrella covering distinct vasculitides. The last to be separated from PAN were Churg-Strauss syndrome (CSS), a vasculitis occurring in asthmatic patients,[2] and microscopic polyangiitis (MPA), which were separated from PAN by Wohlwill,[3] and then redefined by Davson et al.[4] PAN is now a well-defined vasculitis that predominantly affects medium-sized vessels. Considering the etiologies of PAN, primary and secondary vasculitides can also be distinguished, since PAN can be the consequence of hepatitis B virus (HBV) infection[5-7] and sometimes of other etiological agents.[8-10] In this chapter, we review the main characteristics of PAN, its outcome and treatment. Histology and pathogenesis are addressed in detail in other chapters.

Classification

Classification criteria of PAN are reported in detail elsewhere, but we would like, nevertheless, to focus on some pertinent points. PAN and MPA were clearly distinguished in the Chapel Hill Nomenclature.[11] This distinction did not appear in the criteria for classification[12] developed in 1990 by the American College of Rheumatology (ACR) (Table 14.1) because some clinical manifestations are very similar. However, major differences exist between these two disorders. PAN primarily affects medium-sized vessels and MPA mainly small-sized vessels, especially arterioles, capillaries and venules. MPA is responsible for glomerulonephritis and lung capillaritis; PAN is characterized by vascular nephropathy and never affects the lung parenchyma.

Characteristics of PAN

Epidemiology

PAN is a rare disease. In a study[13] which considered only biopsy-proven forms, the annual incidence and prevalence of the disease were, respectively, 0.7 per

Table 14.1 1990 ACR criteria for the classification of polyarteritis nodosa [12]

Criterion	Definition
1. Weight loss > 4 kg	Loss of 4 kg or more of body weight since illness began, not due to dieting or other factors
2. Livedo reticularis	Mottled reticular pattern over the skin of portions of the extremities or torso
3. Testicular pain or tenderness	Pain or tenderness of the testicles, not due to infection, trauma, or other causes
4. Myalgias, weakness or polyneuropathy	Diffuse myalgias (excluding shoulder and hip girdle) or weakness of muscles or tenderness of leg muscles
5. Mononeuropathy or polyneuropathy	Development of mononeuropathy, multiple mononeuropathies, or polyneuropathy
6. Diastolic BP > 90 mm Hg	Development of hypertension with the diastolic BP higher than 90 mm Hg
7. Elevated BUN or creatinine	Elevation of BUN > 40 mg/dL (14.3 μmol/L) or creatinine > 1.5 mg/dL (132 μmol/L), not due to dehydration or obstruction
8. Hepatitis B virus	Presence of hepatitis B surface antigen or antibody in serum
9. Arteriographic abnormality	Arteriogram showing aneurysms or occlusions of the visceral arteries, not due to arteriosclerosis, fibromuscular dysplasia, or noninflammatory causes
10. Biopsy of small- or medium-sized artery	Histologic changes showing the presence of granulocytes or granulocytes and mononuclear leukocytes in the artery wall

For classification purposes, a patient with vasculitis shall be said to have PAN if at least 3 of these 10 criteria are present. The presence of any 3 or more criteria yields a sensitivity of 82.2% and a specificity of 86.6%. BP: blood pressure; BUN: blood urea nitrogen.

100,000 and 6.3 per 100,000 inhabitants. Estimates of the annual incidence rate for PAN-type systemic vasculitis in a general population range from 4.6 per 1,000,000 in England,[13] 9.0 per 1,000,000 in Olmsted County, Minnesota, to 77 per 1,000,000 in a hepatitis B-hyperendemic Alaskan Eskimo population.[14]

Etiology can be identified in only a minority of patients. In some cases, infections, mainly viral, have been recognized as being responsible for PAN. Indeed, a close relationship has been demonstrated between PAN and HBV infection.[5] In France, we have observed that HBV infection due to a contaminated blood transfusion has now disappeared, but that intravenous drug use is becoming an important cause of HBV-related PAN.[7] The development of vaccines against HBV and their administration to people at risk also explain the dramatic decrease of the number of new cases observed since 1989. Over the past few years, the frequency of PAN related to HBV has declined to 7.3%.[7] For the last 2 years, fewer than 10 patients a year have been identified throughout the country.

Some other viruses have been associated with the occurrence of PAN but could explain only a few cases of the disease. The prevalence of hepatitis C virus (HCV) in our patients was low, less than 10% and confirms our previous results.[15] HCV does not seem to be an important etiological factor for PAN.[15,16] GB virus-C, an HCV variant when sought in patients with PAN, has not been considered to be an etiological agent of the disease.[17] A few cases of parvovirus B19 infections have been described[9,18] but a systematic survey of patients with PAN did not show a higher prevalence of parvovirus B19 in patients than in the control population.[19] Other viruses have been suspected as agents of PAN and anecdotal cases of human immunodeficiency virus (HIV) infections have been published.[20–22]

In addition to infectious causes, PAN has been described in association with malignancies, mainly hemopathies. The closest relationship has been established with hairy-cell leukemia.[23–25]

Clinical features

Age and sex

PAN can be observed in any individual independently of age, but predominates between 40 and 60 years, and the sex ratio is around one. PAN can also occur in children and patients older than 65 (see Table 14.2).[23–32]

General symptoms

Early during the course of the disease, two-thirds of the patients are unwell. All types of fevers can be seen. Muscle biopsy performed at this time can provide the diagnosis.

An important clinical presentation is with pain from myalgia that can be intense, diffuse and spontaneous or induced by pressure. Arthralgias predominate in the major joints especially the knees, ankles, elbows and wrists. The shoulders and hips are not affected. Pain localized to nerve regions can be present. Amyotrophy reflects weight loss, sometimes greater than 20 kg, and palsy. Patients can be bedridden due to the intensity of pain and amyotrophy.

Neurological manifestations

Peripheral neurological symptoms are frequent and central nervous system (CNS) involvement is rare.

Peripheral neuropathy. Motor, sensory or sensory-motor peripheral neuropathies are the most frequent of the neurological manifestations of PAN. Mononeuritis multiplex is common and mainly distal and asymmetrical. The nerves involved include the superficial and deep peroneal nerves, sural nerves, radial, cubital and median nerves. Neuropathies occur early and abruptly during the course of the disease, usually during the first few months. Peripheral neuropathy is the first manifestation of PAN in 10% of the cases,[33] and is observed in 52 to 72% of the

Table 14.2 Clinical features of PAN, expressed as percentages of the studied population

	Frohnert and Sheps 1967 (26)	Leib* et al. 1979 (27)	Cohen* et al. 1980 (28)	Guillevin* et al. 1988 (30)	Guillevin** et al. 1992 (29)	Fortin* et al. 1995 (31)	Guillevin** et al. 1995 (32)
Patients (n)	130	64	53	165	182	45	62
Mean age (yr)		47	54	48		54	59
Range	6–75	17–80	17–78	11–65		22–86	
M/F	1.9	1.1	1.9	1.2	1	1.1	1
General symptoms	76						
Fever		36	31	69	65		56
Weight loss			16	66			76
Peripheral nerves	52	72	60	67	70	51	60
Muscles	30			53	54		45
Joints	58			44	46		27
Joints and muscles		73	55			51	
Cutaneous	58	28	58	46	49	44	40
Renal	8	63	66	29	36	44	42
Hypertension		25	14	31	33		32
Gastrointestinal tract	14	42	25	31	26	53	45
Respiratory	38	47	13	29	20	40	29
Central nervous system	3	25		17		24	2
Cardiac	10	30	4	23	9	18	8
Eyes		3	8				0
Ear, nose and throat		3	0	44			0

* Retrospective studies, ** prospective study.
N.B. All the series presented here comprised PAN, MPA and sometimes CSS patients (Guillevin et al.).

patients (see Table 14.2). Pain, paresthesias and, more rarely segmental oedema, may precede the occurrence of palsies.

Sensory symptoms can predominate, mostly hypoesthesia. Deep sensibility is never present. The electromyogram is characteristic of an axonal neuropathy. Usually, the electromyogram shows that the extent of neuropathy is greater than expected based on clinical manifestations. Symmetric neuropathy is observed less frequently.

Several flares of peripheral neuropathies may occur and they cannot be predicted. Neurological symptoms regress slowly under treatment. One year to 18 months are often necessary to obtain the optimal recovery and to evaluate the level of sequelae. Sensory symptoms persist longer, and sometimes indefinitively. Cranial nerve palsies are rare, and occurred in around 1% of our patients.[30] Cranial nerves III, VI, VII and VIII may be affected. Cerebrospinal fluid is usually normal but, in a few cases, the protein level can be elevated but no cells are present.[34]

Central nervous system involvement. CNS involvement is rare. Seizures, focal or generalized, hemiplegia and brain hemorrhage can be observed. CNS manifestations differ according to the location and mechanisms involved: brain arteritis, aneurysm rupture, hematoma. Cognitive dysfunction may also be present and improve with treatment. They can also be the first manifestation of angiitis. The computed tomography (CT) scan is usually normal but magnetic resonance imaging (MRI), indicates a T_2-weighted hypersignal localized to white matter. Although not specific, these hypersignals are highly indicative of the diagnosis. Brain angiography is performed less frequently but can show vessel-calibre irregularities that are suggestive of the diagnosis. Every brain region can be involved.

Ischemic or hemorrhagic seizures can also be the consequence of malignant hypertension. Distal obliteration of spinal vessels can be responsible for medullary symptoms.[35,36] Sphincter dysfunction may be observed and is probably underestimated.[37]

Renal manifestations

Ischaemic nephropathy can be responsible for renal insufficiency of variable intensity. Arterial hypertension may occur as a complication of ischaemic nephropathy and can be severe or malignant.[38]

Acute renal failure typically occurs during the early course of the disease or at the time of a flare. In some patients, renal dialysis can become necessary during the early phase or later, when renal failure occurs as a consequence of chronic renal ischemia. The outcome of renal insufficiency cannot be predicted and improvement may occur. Some patients may come off dialysis but end-stage renal failure may develop years after the early manifestations of the disease.

In patients with renal involvement, angiography, when performed, shows multiple stenoses and microaneurysms of branches of digestive and renal arteries. Renal infarcts are responsible for renal insufficiency. Microaneurysm rupture occurs rarely, either spontaneously or after renal biopsy.[39-44] Renal hematoma can be extensive and necessitates embolization[45] and, if this fails to control bleeding by a nephrectomy.[46]

Orchitis[7,47,48]

This manifestation is one of the most characteristic features of PAN and has been selected as one of the classification criteria established by the ACR.[12] Non-infectious orchitis is rarely the first manifestation of the disease. Involvement is usually unilateral and is the consequence of testicular artery ischemia. When treated immediately, orchitis may regress with steroids. Cases of isolated testicular involvement resemble a tumour or testicular torsion and histological examination provides the diagnosis.[47] We have observed orchitis in patients with PAN and, more specifically, HBV-related PAN,[7,49] but no close relationship could be demonstrated between the viral infection and testicular manifestations.

Skin manifestations

Vascular purpura is more common in PAN than MPA. Skin nodules can be present because the lesions contain medium-sized vessels.

Skin manifestations predominate on the lower limbs. Nodules are small, ranging in diameter from 0.5 to 2 cm. They occur and many disappear within a few days. They are dermal and hypodermal. Two types of livedo are observed: racemosa or reticularis. When such manifestations are observed in patients with atheroma, a differential diagnosis with cholesterol emboli should be considered. In the series reported in the literature,[26–28,30,50,51] half of the patients experienced at least one episode of skin involvement. However, in the majority of series, PAN and MPA were considered together and the majority of cutaneous manifestations should probably be attributed to MPA.

Peripheral vascular manifestations

Arterial obstruction is responsible for distal gangrene of toes or fingers. Angiography can demonstrate the presence of stenoses and/or microaneurysms. Raynaud's phenomenon, when present, can remain isolated or be complicated by necrosis. In some cases, type II or III cryoglobulinemia can be found. We do not know at present whether cryoglobulinemia is a biological symptom that rarely accompanies PAN or a symptom that orients the differential diagnosis towards PAN.

Lung manifestations

The lung parenchyma is not involved in PAN. Histological studies have shown that vasculitis of the bronchial arteries may be present but this is asymptomatic.[52] When pulmonary symptoms occur, infections should be looked for and are usually found.[53]

Gastrointestinal involvement

GI tract involvement is one of the most severe manifestations of PAN. Abdominal pain has been noted in one-quarter to one-third of the patients and can be the first symptom of vasculitis. In a majority of cases, ischemia is present in the small bowel, but rarely in the colon or stomach. Small intestine perforation and gastrointestinal bleeding[54,55] are the most severe manifestations of PAN. Gastric or esophageal perforations are rare.[56,57]

Relapses after surgery or medical treatment indicate a poor prognosis. Malabsorption and acute or chronic pancreatitis with pseudocysts have been described;[58] and the prognoses are extremely dismal. Vasculitis of the appendix or gallbladder[59-56] is sometimes the first manifestation of PAN. It is sometimes a pathological curiosity without any other clinical, histological and/or immunological involvement of vasculitis. Other cases develop cholecystitis[67] or appendicitis. The prognoses for these manifestations seem to differ depending upon whether the cholecystitis or appendicitis is the first manifestation of PAN or a complication of a previously diagnosed and treated PAN. In the former case, the prognosis remains good; however, when these symptoms occur during the course of PAN, they often precede other severe symptoms of GI involvement and the prognosis is poor. Liver involvement, such as infarction and hematomas[68,69] can exist even in the absence of HBV infection.

Cardiac manifestations

Cardiac manifestations are due to vasculitis of the coronary arteries or their branches, or to severe or malignant hypertension. In autopsy studies,[70,71] histological cardiac manifestations were found in 78% of the patients, and radiological and electrocardiographic abnormalities in 40% of cases. They affect mainly the myocardium. In our experience, despite coronary artery vasculitis, angina is rare and coronary angiography is usually normal.[72] Specific myocardial involvement is the consequence of coronary artery occlusions and stenoses of the main coronary arteries can be seen, as described by Küssmaul and Maïer[1] (nodular coronary arteritis). It was present in 25/66 patients autopsied by Holsinger *et al.*[70] Coronary aneurysms are sometimes present but ruptures are rare. Most cases have been described in infants[73,74] and, retrospectively, we can postulate that most cases could have been due to Kawasaki's disease. Arterioles can also be affected and foci of myocardial necrosis can be found.[70]

Left heart failure is the most frequent manifestation of cardiac involvement. When cardiac failure is present, it occurs early during the course of the disease.[72,75] Cardiac hypertrophy was observed in a quarter of the patients in one series.[72] Atria-ventricular block and severe ventricular rhythm disturbances are very rare. Supraventricular rhythm disturbances are more frequent than ventricular rhythm disturbances. The pericardium is less often affected by the vasculitic process and pericarditis is usually non-specific and secondary to myocardial involvement. Pericardial involvement is rare and asymptomatic. Pericarditis can be the first manifestation of PAN and the biopsy can provide the diagnosis.

Arterial hypertension

Hypertension is present in 40% of the patients and is usually mild; however, it should be kept in mind that it can be triggered or worsened by steroids.

Malignant hypertension was detected in 7/165 of our patients.[30,38] Hypertension is more frequent in HBV-related PAN. Treatment of hypertension with angiotensin-converting enzyme inhibitors improves the overall prognosis of PAN.

Miscellaneous

Periosteal modifications of leg bones can be seen rarely.[76,77] Ophthalmological signs have been described in PAN. Some of them are severe, like uni-or bilateral retinal detachment[78] and retinal vasculitis.[79–82] Splenic infarction[83] and splenic rupture[31] have also been described. Rare anecdotal descriptions of specific gingivitis, [84,85] breast[86,87] or uterine artery involvement[88] have been published.

HBV-related PAN

The immunological process responsible for PAN usually occurs less than 6 months after infection. Hepatitis is rarely diagnosed and remains silent before the development of PAN. Clinical manifestations are roughly the same as those commonly observed in PAN[7] but we found some differences: malignant hypertension (29.6%), renal infarction and orchiepididymitis (26%) were more often associated with HBV infection than with idiopathic PAN. These manifestations occur typically in patients under 40 years of age. The disease is acute. Seroconversion usually leads to recovery. Sequelae are the consequence of ischaemic nephropathy but, even in patients with renal insufficiency, it is possible to obtain recovery with little residual impairment of renal function. Regarding other symptoms, we frequently observed abdominal manifestations (46.3%) and especially surgical emergencies (17%). In contrast to our previous results obtained in patients treated with steroids and cyclophosphamide,[89] we did not observe in our recent studies[7,90,91] an increased mortality due to surgical emergencies. In the study by Sergent *et al.*,[92] 2 of the 3 deaths (among 9 patients), were related to colon vasculitis. Among the Eskimo patients described by McMahon *et al.*,[14] 31% of them died and 1 of the 4 early deaths was the consequence of bowel perforation. Hepatic manifestations of PAN during disease are clinically moderate. Hepatic necrosis is moderate in most cases and cholestasis is minor or absent. When liver biopsies were performed, they frequently showed signs of chronic hepatitis even in PAN which occurred only a few months after HBV infection.

Laboratory tests and angiographic investigations

Biological analyses

Inflammatory signs are found in more than 80% of the cases. Hypereosinophilia > 1500/mm^3, is observed in a few patients. Presence of HBs antigen should be systematically sought, although it is found in only 7 to 36% of the patients.[7,89]

Antineutrophil cytoplasm antibodies (ANCA) are found in less than 5% of the sera of patients with PAN (personal data) and we propose that, in the context of systemic vasculitides, the presence of a perinuclear ANCA pattern and antimyeloperoxidase detection by ELISA, should exclude 'classic-PAN', and be in favour of a diagnosis of MPA.[93] Others[93,95] have also found perinuclear ANCA labelling with myeloperoxidase reactivity in a small number of patients.

Angiography

Angiography shows the presence of microaneurysms and stenoses (narrowing or tapering) in medium-sized vessels. They are not pathognomonic but are commonly present in PAN. Arterial sacular or fusiform aneurysms range in size from 1 to 5 mm and are predominantly seen in the kidneys, mesentery and/or liver. The lesions may disappear with resolution of the arteritis.[96] Angiography is a useful diagnostic tool when other diagnostic examinations are negative, especially when abdominal pain and nephropathy are present. In our opinion, the presence of microaneurysms detected angiographically should be considered a criterion of PAN, and for MPA.

Outcome and prognosis

Relapses

PAN may be considered a self-limiting disease which tends not to recur once remission has been induced. In our series, 6% of the patients with HBV-related PAN relapsed,[7] and we can hypothesize a similar relapse rate for PAN without HBV markers. At present, it is not possible to predict the subgroup of patients who will relapse or to predict the severity of the relapses. The clinical pattern of relapse does not necessarily mimic the original presentation, in that previously unaffected organs can be involved at relapse.

Deaths

The causes of death can be divided into two categories: deaths related to vasculitis manifestations and deaths related to treatment side effects.

Deaths related to the vasculitis

In all vasculitides, when major organs are involved, lethal complications may occur. A few patients die early from multiple organ involvement and treatment is unable to control the disease. Death occurs during the course of a disease characterized by fever, rapid weight loss, diffuse pains and one or several major organ involvement. It often occurs in the first months of the disease and is frequently the consequence of GI involvement.[97]

Deaths related to treatment side effects

These causes of death are not rare and, although the deaths occurring during the first months of the disease are often due to uncontrolled vasculitis, those occurring in during the following years may be the consequence of treatment side effects. Infections are the primary cause of death and they are related to treatment with steroids and/or cytotoxic agents. Lowering doses and shortening treatment duration will probably lead to fewer such complications, but treatment intensity and duration should be calculated from prospective studies. Septicaemia occurs during the first months of treatment and is the consequence of the intensive initial therapy. Viral infections usually occur later. We would like to emphasize the occurrence of rare cases of *Pneumocystis carinii* pneumonia that have been described mainly in Wegener's granulomatosis[98,99] but which can also occur in MPA and PAN.

Treatment

At the beginning of this chapter, the reader was made aware that the reported results of nearly all series concerning the treatment and outcome of PAN considered in fact two separate diseases, PAN and MPA,[26-28] and sometimes CSS as well.[7,29,32,100]

To help the clinician choose the most effective therapy and avoid overtreatment, we devised a five-factors score (FFS)[51] which had significant prognostic value and whose parameters, defined as follows, were responsible for higher mortality: proteinuria > 1 g/day, renal insufficiency (creatininemia > 140 μmol/l), cardiomyopathy, GI manifestations and CNS involvement. When FFS = 0, mortality at 5 years was 12%; when FFS = 1, mortality was 26%; when FFS = 2, mortality was 46%. Although it has not been demonstrated that treatment should be chosen as a function of such criteria, it seems probable that the FFS should be considered in the therapeutic strategy.

Steroids were the first successful treatment of PAN, and they increased the 5-year survival rate from 10% for untreated patients to about 55% in the mid-to late-70s.[26-28] Survival was further prolonged by adding immunosuppressants, either azathioprine or cyclophosphamide,[27,101] to the treatment regimen, attaining a 5-year survival rate of 82% for patients given steroids and cyclophosphamide.[27] However, the benefit accorded by retrospective studies has not always been confirmed.[28] In the study by Fauci *et al.*,[102] who advocated the use of cyclophosphamide, the mean duration of corticosteroid treatment at the time of entry into the study was 22 months (range: 2–48 months).

Steroids

They are given to all patients with PAN. In the case of PAN related to HBV, steroids are prescribed for only few days. In the other cases, the treatment is prolonged to 12 months. High doses of corticosteroids may be useful at the time of diagnosis. The administration of methylprednisolone pulses (usually 10–15 mg/kg intravenously (IV) over 60 min repeated at 24-h intervals for 1 to 3 days) has become widely used at the initiation of therapy for severe systemic vasculitis because of its rapid action and relative safety,[103,104] especially in the presence of life-threatening organ involvement or the extension phase of mononeuritis multiplex. Oral corticosteroids are given at the dose of

1 mg/kg/day of prednisone or its equivalent of methyl-prednisolone. Therapy can be administered in a single morning dose or divided into 2 daily doses. As the patient's clinical status improves, the steroids dose should be tapered progressively in order to reach 5 to 10 mg at 1 year post onset.[29,105] This treatment is effective and can control the minor forms of the disease without the addition of cytotoxic agents. When prednisone is combined with cyclophosphamide, the prednisone dose should be tapered more rapidly to avoid infectious complications.

Cyclophosphamide

A low oral dose has conventionally been defined as 2 mg/kg/day or less for 1 year and, in combination with corticosteroids, represented the traditional treatment of PAN. Although this regimen is effective for the treatment of vasculitic disease, it has a low therapeutic/toxic index. Major side effects associated with daily cyclophosphamide administration include hemorrhagic cystitis,[106,107], bladder fibrosis, bone-marrow suppression, ovarian failure[100] and neoplasm (bladder cancer and haematological malignancies).[107] Severe infections represent a major cause of mortality in patients with systemic vasculitis, especially whilst receiving high doses of corticosteroids with adjunctive immunosuppressive drugs.[58,97] In an attempt to decrease the morbidity associated with daily cyclophosphamide administration, protocols utilizing intermittent treatment have been developed.[100,105,108] Pulse cyclophosphamide therapy is now being used increasingly in PAN and should be preferred to oral cyclophosphamide.[100,105] The cyclophosphamide content of each pulse, as well as both the total number and the frequency of the pulses, may be adjusted according to the patient's condition, renal function, haematological data and the disease's response to previous therapies, including previous cyclophosphamide pulses. Initial doses used vary from 0.5 to 2.5 g at intervals of 1 week to 1 month, and up to 3 months for maintenance therapy. In the protocols of the French Co-operative Study Group for PAN, the cyclophosphamide-pulse dose was 0.6 g/m^2 delivered monthly for 1 year.[109] High-dose IV cyclophosphamide may be particularly dangerous in patients with renal failure, suggesting that dose reduction according to renal function would be prudent. Intense hydration and the use of sodium 2-mercaptoethanesulfonate (mesna) should be recommended during pulse therapy. Pulse cyclophosphamide therapy allows a lower cumulative dose to be given and exposes the patient to potential toxicity for shorter periods.

In our opinion, cyclophosphamide should not be systematically prescribed as the first-line treatment in all cases of PAN, and the management decision must consider the anatomical localization of the involvement, its severity and the intensity of disease activity. When patients fail to respond to pulse cyclophosphamide, or in the case of relapse within the first 6 months of treatment[110] oral cyclophosphamide has been successfully introduced to control disease activity. Treatment duration with corticosteroids and cyclophosphamide should not exceed 1 year.

Other cytotoxic agents

Azathioprine, methotrexate and several other cytotoxic agents have been used. They are only indicated in patients in whom cyclophosphamide is contraindicated.

Plasma exchange

There is presently no argument to support the systematic prescription of plasma exchanges at the time of diagnosis of PAN without HBV infection,[105] even for patients thought to have poor prognosis.[32,111] However, plasma exchange may be a useful tool, as second-line treatment, for PAN refractory to conventional therapy.

Treatment of HBV-related PAN

In HBV-related PAN, conventional treatment with corticosteroids and cyclophosphamide jeopardize the patient's outcome by allowing the virus to persist, thereby favouring its replication and facilitating progression towards chronic hepatitis and liver cirrhosis. Thus, cyclophosphamide, like prolonged steroid treatment, are contraindicated. The rationale of combining plasma exchanges and antiviral treatment was as follows: initial corticosteroids to rapidly control the most severe life-threatening manifestations of PAN which are common during the first weeks of the disease, abrupt stoppage of corticosteroids to enhance immunological clearance of HBV-infected hepatocytes and favour HBe antigen to anti-HBe antibody seroconversion. Plasma exchange can control the course of PAN without the addition of corticosteroids or cyclophosphamide. In HBV-related PAN, the combination of antiviral agents (vidarabine or interferon alpha-2b) gave excellent overall therapeutic results[90,91] and should be preferred to conventional regimens that jeopardize the outcome. The efficacy of this strategy was confirmed in a series of 41 patients. Twenty-three (56.1%) no longer exhibit serological evidence of replication and 80.5% recovered.[7]

General considerations

Specific treatments for hypertension, pain, and motor rehabilitation are also important elements for optimal management of patients. Since maximal immunosuppression is given at the beginning of treatment, prevention of opportunistic infections, like *Pneumocystis carinii* pneumonia, may be necessary and should be prescribed on an individual basis.[53] In the case of GI involvement with permanent abdominal pain despite medical treatment, an exploratory surgical procedure should be performed to identify and treat potential bowel perforation. For the same group of patients, it seems reasonable to administer drugs intravenously to circumvent possibly impaired drug absorption. Rapid and severe weight loss due to severe GI involvement must be countered with parental nutrition. Despite the fact that weight loss has not been demonstrated to be a factor of poor prognosis,[51]

15

Vasculitis (ANCA negative): Henoch-Schönlein purpura

Rosanna Coppo and Alessandro Amore

Definition

Henoch-Schönlein purpura (HSP) is a small vessel vasculitis which presents clinically with multiorgan involvement variably affecting the skin, gastro-intestinal tract, joints and kidneys (Meadow *et al.* 1972; Mills *et al.* 1990). First described by Heberden, the purpuric and articular manifestations were described by Schönlein, and the gastro-intestinal and renal features by Henoch. The combination of various systemic and renal symptoms leads to different clinical patterns of presentation that often overlaps with other autoimmune diseases. HSP needs to be differentiated from cutaneous allergic reactions to drugs, and infectious agents. In the past this led to designations such as hypersensitivity angiitis, anaphylactoid and rheumatoid purpura or streptococcal rheumatic peliosis.

Clinical and laboratory features

Diagnostic criteria

Following the 1990 American College of Rheumatology classification (Mills *et al.* 1990), the criteria for distinguishing HSP from other vasculitides are palpable purpura, acute abdominal pain or gastro-intestinal bleeding, young age (< 20 years) at disease onset and a biopsy showing granulocytes in the walls of small arterioles or venules (leukocytoclastic vasculitis). Subsequently the role of IgA vascular deposits was defined by the 1994 Consensus Conference (Jennette *et al.* 1994), which defined HSP as a small vessels vasculitis (involving capillaries, arterioles, venules) with immune deposits predominantly formed by IgA.

Epidemiology and enhancing factors

HSP is a relatively uncommon disease, particularly in adults, whereas in children its incidence is about 14/100,000 cases/year. It has a 2:1 male preponderance. In children, HSP is the most frequent vasculitis (Meadow *et al.* 1972). The median age at onset is about 4 years, although it can affect the elderly.

Renal involvement is most common in the first and second decade of life (Levy *et al.* 1976; Rieu and Noel 1999). In unselected cohorts of children, the prevalence of renal involvement during the course of HSP varies from 20% to 54% (mean 33%), whereas in adults this frequency is much higher (mean 63%) (Rieu and Noel 1999). Despite the possibility that the mildest cases of renal involvement among children could be under-diagnosed and that some adult patients could be misdiagnosed as primary vasculitis, the more frequent development of renal disease in older cases remains unquestionable and unexplained. From the Italian register of renal biopsies the frequency of glomerulonephritis (GN) secondary to HSP is higher in children (11.6% of children undergoing renal biopsy) than in the whole cohort (3.5% of biopsies) (Coppo *et al.* 1997a).

The geographical distribution is similar to primary IgA nephropathy, or Berger's disease (IgAN), and HSP is common in the Mediterranean and Japanese patients. Triggering factors are reported in about two-thirds of the cases (Levy *et al.* 1976), mostly infections and particularly in children. *Streptococcus* β, *Yersina*, *Mycoplasma* and *Toxoplasma* have been sporadically recorded among the precipitating factors. A coincident role of allergic reactions to drugs or other allergens has been strongly suspected in some cases. Some familial cases and restricted epidemic clusters of HSP have been observed.

Systemic extra-renal manifestations

The skin lesions are characteristic and consist in red-purple slightly raised 'palpable' purpuric macules that do not disappear on pressure and are not related to thrombocytopenia. Fever and general malaise may accompany the rash. At the beginning the picture is hardly distinguishable from infectious purpura or allergic reactions. HSP purpura mainly involves, initially, the lower extremities and buttocks but may become generalized in some cases. The lesions consist of a leukocytoclastic vasculitis of dermal vessels. Relapses of purpura are very frequent, in almost a third of patients, and may occur up to 10 times during follow-up (Coppo *et al.* 1997b).

Abdominal manifestations include diffuse abdominal pain, increasing after meals, referred to as 'bowel angina' and often accompanied by vomiting, hematemesis and rectal bleeding or melena (Mills *et al.* 1990). In some cases, the pain is so severe to mimic a surgical emergency, although intussusception, intestinal infarction, bowel perforation are very rare events. Gastro-intestinal symptoms are reported in 50–70% of all cases (Meadow *et al.* 1972). Transient arthralgia, due to oligo-articular synovitis, mostly involving lower limb joints, are reported in 50–70% of all cases (Meadow *et al.* 1972). These lesions do not evolve into joint erosions or deformities. Children, more frequently than adults, present with a systemic extra-renal clinical picture of particular severity (Levy *et al.* 1976). The severity of extra-renal signs, including the purpuric rash, is generally unrelated with the severity of renal lesions.

Table 15.1   Classification of Henoch-Schönlein nephritis lesions according to Emancipator 1992

Class I	Minimal glomerular lesions and absence of crescents
Class II	No crescents IIa Pure mesangial proliferation IIb Focal-segmental endo-capillary proliferation IIc Diffuse endo-capillary proliferation
Class III	Presence of extra-capillary cellular proliferation in less than 50% of glomeruli IIIa In association with focal and segmental endo-capillary proliferation IIIb With diffuse endo-capillary proliferation
Class IV	Florid extra-capillary proliferation in 50–75% of glomeruli IVa In association with focal and segmental endo-capillary proliferation IVb With diffuse endo-capillary proliferation
Class V	Extra-capillary proliferation in more than 75% of glomeruli Va In association with focal and segmental endo-capillary proliferation Vb With diffuse endo-capillary proliferation
Class VI	Pseudo-membranoproliferative glomerulonephritis

The cohort of patients gathered by the Italian collaborative study (Coppo *et al.* 1997b) showed a few cases with important extra-capillary proliferation (Classes IV and V in Table 15.1). More than 50% of the biopsies of both adults and children did not have proliferative extra-capillary lesions (Classes I and II). When present, these lesions involved less than 50% of glomeruli (Class III). In two-thirds of cases the crescent formation was associated with endo-capillary proliferation. Polymorphonuclear glomerular infiltration was generally associated with extracapillary lesions. Necrosis of the capillary tuft was seldom present (in 10% of adults and 8% of children), coincident with extra-capillary proliferation. In some biopsies (2% of adults and 15% of children) periglomerular inflammatory infiltrates, mostly associated with crescents, were observed. Focal interstitial infiltrates were present in 10% of the cases. Tubular necrotic lesions were found in 15% of adults and 6% of children, as well as blood casts (in 30%).

In a very few biopsies there was a lympho-monocytic infiltrate in the vascular wall in the periarteriolar and perivenular area. In 30% of the biopsies (both adult and paediatric cases) atherosclerotic lesions and arteriolar hyalinosis lesions were present, a figure higher than in other series.

Immunohistochemistry

The characteristic feature is granular mesangial IgA deposition which, in contrast with the frequent focal and segmental proliferative changes, is always diffuse as in primary IgAN. IgA1 is the dominant subclass with equal distribution of light chains. The J chain is generally present indicating dimeric IgA, whereas the secretory component is absent. Extensive sub-endothelial deposits are associated with the most severe histologic forms with endocapillary proliferation and/or crescent formation.

As in idiopathic IgAN, C3 is co-deposited with IgA in 75–85% of the cases. The alternative complement pathway components and the membrane attack complex C5-C9, are regularly detected. IgG and IgM co-deposits are present in 40% of the cases (Emancipator 1992). Fibrin/fibrinogen is frequent both in mesangial and in parietal areas, often associated with mesangial proliferation.

In cases with severe glomerular changes deposits of IgA and C3 can be found in arterioles and/or peritubular capillaries.

Electronic microscopy

Mesangial matrix expansion and variable degree of cellular hyperplasia are evident together with electron-dense deposits (Emancipator 1992). These deposits are initially paramesangial and small in size (100–120 nm) and subsequently become larger (up to 800 nm) and in the mesangial matrix. Sometimes, electron-dense deposits 'humps' with a 'garland' shape or fluffy aspect are detectable. When deposited in the external rara lamina they are delimited by a thin layer of new basement membrane.

Extra-renal lesions

The typical leukocytoclastic vasculitis — with fragmented nuclei of leukocytes in and around arterioles, capillaries and venules, surrounded by infiltrating neutrophils and monocytes is detectable in the kidneys and in other tissues, particularly in the skin and gut. Fibrinoid accumulation and arteriolar and venular necrosis are rarely found. Deposits of IgA and C3 are present in dermal capillaries walls in purpuric lesions and uninvolved skin. Co-deposits of IgG and IgM can be present, while C1q and C4 are absent. Similar deposits have been reported in superficial dermal capillaries of IgAN patients. In dermatitis herpetiformis IgA deposits are found as well, but they are located on the top of the dermal papilla. In SLE the dermal-epidermal junction is mostly positive for IgG, C1q and C4.

Clinico-pathological correlations at onset

In our series (Coppo *et al.* 1997b) patients with minimal proteinuria had a higher prevalence of Class I and II lesions, without crescents. In patients with significant proteinuria more severe renal lesions were frequently found, but with low predictive value for the single case. In children, particularly, cases with non-nephrotic proteinuria often had extra-capillary proliferation. Gross haematuria at presentation was associated with crescent formation in 22% of the cases, independently of the patient's age. Renal functional impairment at onset had a predictive value for severe histologic lesions.

Clinical course

The course of HSP nephritis is generally benign and the progression towards renal failure is estimated at around 2% in non-selected children admitted into General Paediatric Hospitals (Farine *et al.* 1986). In improving or recovered patients, sequential biopsies show regression of lesions, glomerular repair and disappearance of IgA deposits. Conversely, reference centres report remission rates below 50% and a poor outcome in 10–25% of children. HSP nephritis accounts for 2–3% of children on dialysis in Europe. In a long-term follow-up study of selected children, averaging 23 years, late progression was observed in 25% of children, even after initial clinical improvement (Goldstein *et al.* 1992). The disease is more severe in adults, where the progression to renal failure is reported in 8–68% of cases (Fogazzi *et al.* 1989, Rieu and Noel 1999). The outcome of patients selected on the need for renal biopsy is much more severe, and long-term analyses show that 15–30% of patients progress to renal failure with wide variability depending on the initial selection criteria and follow-up duration (Rieu and Noel 1999).

The cohort of patients enrolled in the Italian collaborative study provided information on the subgroup of patients with a renal disease severe enough to warrant renal biopsy. After 1–20 years (mean 5) one-third of the cases were in remission, often complete and without significant urinary abnormalities (Table 15.2). In another third of patients only minimal or moderate proteinuria was left. The outcome was substantially similar in the adults and in children. The time of progression to dialysis varied from a few days to 20 years, with an average of 3 years in the adults and 10 years in children. The long-term renal survival of HSP nephritis in adults and children with an indication for a renal biopsy showed loss of renal function in 25% of the cases after 10 years.

Risk factors for the progression

As discussed above, in non-selected series of HSP nephritis older age is associated with a higher risk of progression, but not in biopsied patients. A good cor-

Table 15.2   Clinical outcome after 1–20 years follow-up (mean 5 years) in patients with Henoch-Schönlein nephritis

	Adults (%)	Children (%)
Clinical remission	32.5	31.6
Minimal or moderate proteinuria, normal GFR	32.7	42.1
Nephrotic proteinuria, normal GFR	3.2	1.7
Moderate functional impairment	13.7	12.2
Severe functional impairment	2.1	5.3
Dialysis	15.8	7

(Italian Group of Renal Immunopathology, Coppo *et al.* 1997b).

relation between the clinical presentation and the long-term outcome is reported in paediatric series (Blanco *et al.* 1997). In some reports nephrotic syndrome and/or renal insufficiency at onset were risk factors (44%) for renal failure after more than 25 years of follow-up (Goldstein *et al.* 1992). In the cohorts of biopsied patients of the Italian study (Coppo *et al.* 1997b) the most unfavourable prognostic factor was renal impairment at presentation: 45% of adults with severe renal failure and 18% of those with moderate functional impairment eventually required chronic dialysis, versus only 2% of adults with normal renal function at onset. This association was not found in children, who experienced progression to renal failure even in cases with normal renal function at onset. Hypertension was a negative prognostic factor particularly in adults, in whom it was more constant and associated with renal function impairment. The predictive value of proteinuria showed different results in adults and children. In both cohorts absent or mild proteinuria or, at the opposite, a nephrotic-range levels, were respectively associated with high frequency of remission or deterioration of renal function. However, adult patients with moderate proteinuria seldomly showed extra-capillary proliferation, while children with mild proteinuria frequently displayed severe histologic lesions, with extra-capillary proliferation. Among adults, proteinuria > 1.5 g/day predicted an unfavourable outcome. On the contrary, it was impossible to define a level of proteinuria in children associated with increased risk, as nephrotic and non nephrotic children had a similar outcome.

The extent and activity of extra-capillary proliferation are recognized risk factors (Yoshikawa *et al.* 1981). In the Italian cohort almost all patients presented with crescents involving less than 50% of glomeruli. The predictive value of mild extra-capillary proliferation (renal failure in 39% of adults and in 18% of children with crescents) was not of statistical significance, since cases without crescents also experienced an unfavourable outcome (19% of adults and 23% of children).

HSP nephritis and renal transplantation

IgA mesangial deposits may recur in allografts, particularly in living-related transplants. The risk for recurrence is 35% at 5 years, with a loss of grafts in 11% (Kessler *et al.* 1996).

Therapy

It is generally thought that corticosteroids are effective in controlling the extra-renal signs, particularly abdominal pain and arthritis, although they have been thought to be ineffective for HSP nephritis. A protective effect of prednisone on the development of nephritis is still discussed (Mollica *et al.* 1992). The most significant results have been obtained in paediatric patients with epithelial crescents involving more than 50% of glomeruli or with a nephrotic syndrome. In these cases pulses of methylprednisone, followed by several months of oral prednisone induced favourable results in 70% of patients versus 40% in untreated children (Niaudet and Habib 1998). It is of interest to notice that in the same cohort, no effect of treatment was found when crescents involved less than 50% of glomeruli. Positive results have been obtained in crescentic forms with a combination of prednisone, azathioprine or cyclophosphamide (Bergstein *et al.* 1998). Our group (Coppo *et al.* 1985) and more recently others (Hattori *et al.* 1999) successfully treated with plasma exchange, steroids and cytotoxic drugs patients with rapidly progressive HSP nephritis. Favourable results have been reported in potentially progressive patients with heavy proteinuria, by treatment with intravenous immunoglobulin infusions (Kasuda *et al.* 1999).

Pathogenesis

Since HSP nephritis is similar to idiopathic IgAN, a common pathogenesis has been envisaged for a long time and most nephrologists consider the two diseases as systemic or renal-limited forms of a single pathogenetic entity. Several reports support a common origin for the two diseases. These include the recurrence of IgAN in the transplanted kidneys of patients with HSP nephritis, the development of HSP in a twin of a primary IgAN patient, the finding of high levels of circulating IgAIC and IgA-fibronectin aggregates in both conditions, even though at higher levels in HSP nephritis (Coppo *et al.* 1982; Coppo *et al.* 1984; Jennette *et al.* 1991). Besides the mild and reversible form of HSP nephritis affecting children, when the disease become chronic and severe enough to warrant renal biopsy as in the Italian study, the histologic lesions and the clinical outcome are similar to primary IgAN.

HSP nephritis was ascribed to the accumulation of IgAIC within glomeruli, as idiopathic IgAN. Indeed the above mentioned studies revealed high levels of IgAIC during clinically active phases of HSP nephritis. Over the last years attention has been focused on the carbohydrate moieties of IgA, and several data support the hypothesis of defective immunoregulation leading to aberrant IgA glycosylation in patients with primary IgAN and, of interest, some of these defect have been reported also in HSP patients (Allen *et al.* 1998). Human IgA1, the predominant subclass deposited in both primary IgAN and HSP nephritis, is highly glycosylated and contains five short O-linked oligosaccharide chains composed of N-acetylgalactosamine, galactose and sialic acid. Serum IgA in patients with primary IgAN and HSP nephritis exhibit a reduced content of galactose, and a defective activity of $\beta 1$–3 galactosyltransferase in their B-cells has been detected. Although an imbalance in lymphocyte function, with a prevalence of Th2 over Th1 T cell subsets, can lead to altered IgA glycosylation, similar abnormalities could derive from a congenital defect, or from *de novo* somatic mutations.

The reason why some patients with IgAN develop a systemic vasculitis and present with the full expression of HSP, is the clue of the problem of the different pathogenesis of these two entities. Antineutrophil cytoplasm antibodies of the IgA isotype (IgA-ANCA) have been reported in adults with active HSP, but other reports were negative. Our group found that patients with HSP nephropathy had various abnormal reactivities of serum IgA due to its abnormal glycosyl-ation supporting an increased reactivity with the ANCA antigens, either crude neutrophil extract or purified myeloperoxidase (Coppo *et al.* 1997c). Since IgA-ANCA are likely to be due to lectin interactions, they may only be detected by some assays, and this may account for the different results. Of interest, this reactivity has not been observed in sera of patients with primary IgAN, even though they have aberrantly glycosylated IgA.

The pathogenetic meaning of aberrant IgA glycosylation or of reactivity towards lysosomal antigens of leucocytes is a matter of recent investigations. Such aberrantly glycosylated IgA molecules show a high tendency to self-aggregation, leading to macromolecules with a molecular weight similar to IgAIC and escape the hepatic asialoglycoprotein receptor clearance. In addition, by virtue of enhanced lectin reactivity with fibronectin, laminin, and collagen within the mesangial matrix (Coppo *et al.* 1993), abnormally glycosylated IgA might favour mesangial deposition. The interactions with mesangial cell Fcα receptors might enhance the synthesis of a variety of cytokines, vasoactive factors and chemokines in primary IgAN as well as in HSP nephritis.

In the pathogenesis of HSP nephritis a peculiar role could be played by complement activation as previously described. It is of interest that aberrantly glycosylated IgA can activate complement more efficiently than normal IgA. Moreover, the experimental model that most closely reproduces HSP systemic vasculitis and nephritis was obtained by using a complement activating carbohydrate antigen (Montinaro *et al.* 1991). Differences in complement activation by aberrantly glycosylated IgA might represent the distinct pathogenetic mechanism inducing the vasculitic lesions that differentiate patients with HSP from those with primary IgAN.

References

Allen A.C. *et al.* (1998). Abnormal IgA glycosylation in Henoch-Schönlein purpura re-stricted to patients with clinical nephritis. *Nephrology Dialysis Transplantation*, 13, 930–3.

Amoroso A. *et al.* (1997). Immunogenetics of Henoch-Schönlein disease. *European Journal Immunogenetics*, 24, 323–35.

Bergstein J. *et al.* (1998). Response of crescentic Henoch-Schönlein purpura nephritis to corticosteroid and azathioprine theraphy. *Clinical Nephrology*, 49, 9–14.

Blanco R. *et al.* (1997). Henoch-Schönlein purpura in adulthood and childhood: two different expressions of the same syndrome. *Arthritis and Rheumatism*, 40, 859–64.

Coppo R. *et al.* (1982). Circulating immune complexes containing IgA, IgG and IgM in patients with primary IgA nephropathy and with Henoch-Schönlein nephritis. Correlation with clinical and histologic signs of activity. *Clinical Nephrology*, 18, 230–9.

Coppo R. *et al.* (1984) IgA1 and IgA2 immune complexes in primary IgA nephropathy and Henoch-Schönlein nephritis. *Clinical Experimental Immunology*, 57, 583–90.

Coppo R. *et al.* (1985). Plasma exchange in primary IgA nephropathy and Henoch-Schönlein syndrome nephritis. *Plasma Therapy Transfusional Technology*, 6, 705–23.

Coppo R. *et al.* (1993). Serum IgA and macromolecular IgA reacting with mesangial matrix components. *Contributions to Nephrology*, 104, 162–71.

Coppo R. *et al.* (1997a). Frequency of renal diseases and clinical indications for renal biopsy in children (report of the Italian National Registry of Renal Biopsies in Children). *Nephrology Dialysis Transplantation*, 13, 293–97

Coppo R. *et al.* for the Italian Group of Renal Immunopathology. (1997b). Long-term prognosis of Henoch-Schönlein nephritis in adults and in children. *Nephrology Dialysis Transplantation*, 12, 2277–83.

Coppo R. *et al.* (1997c). Properties of circulating IgA molecules in Henoch-Schönlein purpura nephritis with focus on neutrophil cytoplasmic antigen IgA binding (IgA-ANCA): new insight into a debated issue. *Nephrology Dialysis Transplantation*, 12, 2269–76.

Coppo R. *et al.* (1999). Clinical features of Henoch-Schönlein purpura. *Annales Medicine Interne*, 150, 143–50.

Emancipator S.N. (1992) Primary and secondary forms of IgA nephritis, Schönlein-Henoch Syndrome. In: R.H. Heptinstall (ed.) *Pathology of the Kidney* (4th edn), pp. 389–476. Boston, Toronto, London: Little, Brown and Company.

Farine M. *et al.* (1986). Prognostic significance of urinary findings and renal biopsies in children with Henoch-Schönlein nephritis. *Clinical Pediatrics*, 25, 257–9.

Fogazzi G.B. *et al.* (1989). Long-term outcome of Schönlein-Henoch nephritis in the adult. *Clinical Nephrology*, 83, 60–6.

Goldstein A.R. *et al.* (1992). Long-term follow-up of childhood Henoch-Schönlein nephritis. *Lancet*, 339, 280–2.

Hattori M. *et al.* (1999). Plasmapheresis as the sole theraphy for rapidly progressive Henoch-Schönlein purpura nephritis in children. *American Journal Kidney Diseases*, 33, 427–33.

Jennette J.C. *et al.* (1991). Serum IgA-fibronectin aggregates in patients with IgA nephropathy and Henoch-Schönlein purpura: diagnostic value and pathogenic implications. The Glomerular Disease Collaborative Network. *American Journal Kidney Diseases*, 18, 466–71.

Jennette J.C. *et al.* (1994) Nomenclature of systemic vasculitides. Proposal of an International Consensus Conference. *Arthritis and Rheumatism*, 2, 187–92.

Jin D.K. *et al.* (1996). Complement 4 locus II gene deletion and DQA1*0301 gene: genetic risk factors for IgA nephropathy and Henoch Schönlein nephritis. *Nephron*, 73, 390–95.

Kasuda A. *et al.* (1999). Successful treatment of adult-onset Henoch-Schönlein purpura nephritis with high-dose immunoglobulins. *Internal Medicine*, 38, 376–9.

Kessler M. *et al.* (1996). Recurrence of immunoglobulin A nephropathy after renal transplantation in the cyclosporine era. *American Journal Kidney Diseases*, 28, 99–104.

Levy M. *et al.* (1976). Anaphylactoid purpura nephritis in childhood natural history and immunopathology. In: J. Hamburger, J. Crosnier and M.H. Maxwell (eds) *Advances in Nephrology Necker Hospital*, pp. 183–228. Chicago, Year Book Medical.

Meadow S.R. *et al.* (1972) Schönlein-Henoch nephritis. *Quarterly Journal Medicine*, 163, 241–58.

Mills J.A. *et al.* (1990) The American College of Rheumatology 1990 criteria for the classification of Henoch-Schönlein purpura. *Arthritis and Rheumatism*, 33, 1114–21.

Mollica F. *et al.* (1992). Effectiveness of early prednisone treatment in preventing the development of nephropathy in anaphylactoid purpura. *European Journal Pediatrics*, 151, 140–4.

Montinaro V. *et al.* (1991). Antigen as mediator of glomerular injury in experimental IgA nephropathy. *Laboratory Investigation*, 64, 508–19.

Niaudet P. and Habib R. (1998). Methylprednisone pulse therapy in the treatment of severe forms of Schönlein-Henoch purpura nephritis. *Pediatric Nephrology*, 12, 238–43.

Rieu P. and Noel L.H. (1999). Henoch-Schönlein nephritis in children and adults. *Annales Medicine Interne*, 150, 151–8.

Yoshikawa N. *et al.* (1981). Prognostic significance of the glomerular changes in Henoch-Schönlein nephritis. *Clinical Nephrology*, 5, 223–9.

16

Takayasu's arteritis

Vivekanand Jha and Kirpal S. Chugh

Takayasu's arteritis (TA) is a chronic inflammatory arteriopathy of unknown etiology that involves large vessels like aorta, its main branches and pulmonary artery. The condition was first reported in 1908 by Mikito Takayasu, a Japanese ophthalmologist who described ocular lesions characterized by circular anastomosis of the retinal vessels, in a young female suffering from this disease (Chugh and Sakhuja 1992). Schimizo and Sano recognized the clinical triad of absent radial pulses, hypersensitive carotid sinus and ocular fundal changes in 1948. The term *Takayasu's disease* was introduced by Cacamise and Whitman in 1952. Other synonyms of TA are pulseless disease, aortic arch syndrome, occlusive thromboarteriopathy, middle-aortic syndrome, idiopathic medial aortopathy, aortitis syndrome, primary arteritis of the aorta, brachiocephalic arteritis, panaortitis, non-specific aortoarteritis and Onishi's disease.

Epidemiology

TA is now recognized to have a worldwide distribution, but the prevalence in Asian and Central and South American countries like Japan, India, China, Korea, Thailand, Singapore, Israel, Peru, Columbia, Mexico, and Brazil far exceeds that in the rest of the world (Chugh and Sakhuja 1992). About 150 new cases are reported annually in Japan. Studies from Sweden and USA revealed incidence rates of 1.2 and 2.6 cases per million population per year. Regardless of geographic location, ethnicity plays a significant role in the development of this disease. TA is rare amongst Caucasians and Asian women are over-represented in the TA population in USA than their registered racial distribution (Hoffman 1996). Most patients in France are from North Africa and Antilles islands. A predominance of 'mestizo' race (partly of American Indian ancestry) has been reported amongst Mexican and Colombian patients (Canas *et al.* 1998; Dabague and Reyes 1996).

A geographic variation has also been noted in the gender distribution of TA. A marked female preponderance is encountered in Japan (8–24: 1), Mexico (7: 1), Korea (6: 1), Brazil (5: 1), Turkey (4: 1), and China and Colombia (3: 1), but the gender disparity is not so marked in India (1.5: 1), Israel (1.8: 1) and Thailand (2.2: 1). Differences are also noted in the pattern of arterial involvement in different geographic regions. Aortic arch and its branches are predominantly involved in Japanese patients whereas abdominal aortic disease including involvement of renal arteries is seen in a majority of Indian and Korean cases. The inflammation culminates in vascular stenosis in Japanese, American and European populations whereas aneurysm formation is more common in India, Thailand and Mexico.

Etiology and pathogenesis

The precise etiology of TA still remains unknown. Hereditary factors, infectious agents and hormonal and immunological perturbations have been implicated in the causation of this disease.

The geographic variation in the incidence and pattern of TA has led to evaluation of the role of hereditary factors in the genesis of this disease. Familial occurrence of TA including that in monozygotic twins has been reported from Japan, Brazil and India and has focused attention on the association of TA with a number of human lymphocyte antigen (HLA) alleles (Table 16.1). Linkage studies suggest the association to be stronger with B than D locus. One recent study has revealed sequence similarity between the Japanese and Mexican TA patients even when they did not share HLA alleles (Rodriguez-Reyna *et al.* 1998), suggesting that these sequences may be more important than the alleles *per se*. Recent studies of MHC class I chain related (MIC) gene, located on chromosome 6 near the B locus, revealed a close relationship with MICA type 1.2 (Kimura *et al.* 1998). MICA 1.2 has shown a significantly higher odds ratio of risk to TA in the absence of HLA B52. In addition to genetic factors, socioeconomic factors are also reported to influence the polymorphic symptoms, sign and arterial localization of this disease.

Infections like tuberculosis and syphilis were considered to play a pathogenic role in TA in earlier studies because of the histological similarity of this disease with granulomatous pathology of tuberculosis and syphilitic aortitis. Moreover, TA is frequently encountered in populations where *M. tuberculosis* infection is highly endemic. Tuberculin positivity was noted in 81% of TA patients compared to 66% of general population, and the aortic lesions were noted in close proximity to involved lymph nodes. In some studies, mycobacterial injection in

Table 16.1 HLA associations of Takayasu's arteritis in different countries

Japan	Bw52, Dw12, DQw1, DR2, C4A2, C4BQO
Korea	Bw52, DR7, DQw52
North America	DR4, Dw3
Canada	absent DR1
India	B5, B51, B52
Mexico	B21, DR6, DRB1*1301
Thailand	A31, B52

Data from Castro *et al.* 1982; Charoenwongse *et al.* 1998; Girona *et al.* 1996; Khraishi *et al.* 1992; Mehra *et al.* 1998; Park and Park 1992; Volkman *et al.* 1982; Yajima *et al.* 1994.

TA and pregnancy

TA has no effect on fertility. A worsening of hypertension with risk of superimposed pre-eclampsia is noted in a majority with pre-existing hypertension. In one study, however, 50% patients showed improvement in inflammatory indices (Matsumura *et al.* 1992). Low birth weight is common and may be related to poor placental circulation due to maternal aortic disease. Poor prognostic indicators include worsening of hypertension, aneurysmal disease, extensive disease of abdominal aorta and renal vessels and cardiac failure. Therapeutic abortion may be necessary during first trimester in high-risk patients. During labour, uterine contractions are associated with a surge in blood pressure, and shortening of second stage with a low forceps delivery may be required. Caesarian section is needed only for obstetric indications (Chugh and Sakhuja 1992).

Pathology

The arterial involvement is patchy, with areas of thickening alternating with skip areas giving rise to focal stenoses or aneurysms. Complete occlusion is rarely seen in abdominal aorta. Histology shows a panarteritis (Sharma *et al.* 1998). The thickening is produced by mucopolysaccharide accumulation in the intima. The adventitia and media show a mixed cellular infiltrate with giant cells and granuloma formation. This is prominent around the vasa vasora that also show endothelial proliferation and obliteration of their lumina. There is degeneration of internal elastic lamina, smooth muscle proliferation, adventitial fibrosis and neovascularization in later stages. Involved vessels may manifest secondary atherosclerosis or luminal thrombi. The changes are similar to those seen in giant cell arteritis or aortitis associated with seronegative arthropathies. The skip lesions help in differentiation from syphilitic aortitis which is diffuse and does not extend below the diaphragm.

Imaging studies

Conventional angiography remains the gold standard for imaging of involved arteries in TA and is the only method that allows evaluation of the full extent of the disease and determination of arterial pressure across the stenotic lesions. Abnormalities include irregularities in the wall and segmental stenosis/occlusion of aorta and its branches at their origin (Figs. 16.1, 16.2. 16.3). Aneurysms involve only the aorta and can be saccular or fusiform. The 1994 International Takayasu Conference classified TA into five types (Moriwaki *et al.* 1997) based on angiographic appearance of the arterial tree. Over 50% of both Indian and Japanese patients exhibit type V disease. Type IV disease is the next commonest amongst Indians (28%) whereas types I and IIa predominate amongst the re-

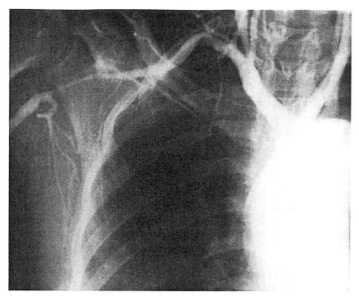

Fig. 16.1 Arch aortogram showing a long segment of stenosis involving the midportion of the right subclavian artery.

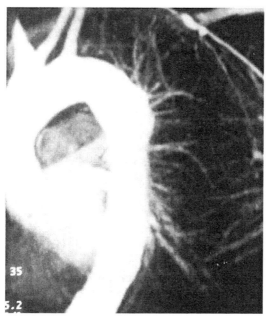

Fig. 16.2 Arch aortogram showing extensive involvement of the descending aorta.

promote endothelial cell activation, migration and proliferation have been characterized. These include vascular endothelial growth factor (VEGF), acidic and basic fibroblastic growth factors (FGF), hepatocyte growth factor (HGF), insulin–like growth factor, platelet–derived growth factor, placental growth factor and transforming growth factor-β. An increase in circulating VEGF and HGF levels has been demonstrated at sites of tissue ischaemia including in one case of TA (Harada *et al.* 1998). Recombinant VEGF, FGF and HGF have shown angiographically and histologically demonstrable increase in the number of collateral vessels in ischaemic limbs of experimental animals. Case reports have documented subjective and objective improvement in limb ischaemia in some patients. These proteins, however, have very short half-lives (3–5 minutes) and require repeated parenteral administration. Initial studies of arterial and intramuscular gene transfer in experimental animals and humans with atherosclerotic peripheral vascular disease and Buerger's disease have shown promising results in terms of protein expression and clinical improvement. Although the possibility of providing a 'biological bypass' seems exciting, a number of issues remain to be resolved before this approach can enter full-fledged clinical trials. These include choice of appropriate formulation of growth factor(s), selection of suitable vector, route of administration and long-term risk of increase in incidence of cancers.

References

Arend, W.P., Michel, B.A., Bloch, D.A., Hunder, G.G., Calabrese, L.H., Edworthy, S.M., Fauci, A.S., Leavitt, R.Y., Lie, J.T. and Lightfoot, R.W. Jr (1990). The American College of Rheumatology 1990 criteria for the classification of Takayasu arteritis. *Arthritis Rheum*, 33: 1129–34.

Bali, H.K., Jain, S., Jain, A. and Sharma, B.K. (1998). Stent supported angioplasty in Takayasu arteritis. *Int J Cardiol*, 66, Suppl. 1: S213–7.

Canas, C.A., Jimenez, C.A., Ramirez, L.A., Uribe, O., Tobon, I., Torrenegra, A., Cortina, A., Munoz, M., Gutierrez, O., Restrepo, J.F., Pena, M. and Iglesias, A. (1998). Takayasu arteritis in Colombia. *Int J Cardiol*, 66, Suppl. 1: S73–9.

Castro, G., Chavez-Peon, C., Sanchez-Torres, G. and Reyes, P.A. (1982). HLA A and B antigens in Takayasu's arteritis. *Rev Invest Clin*, 34: 15–17.

Charoenwongse, P., Kangwanshiratada, O., Boonnam, R. and Hoomsindhu, U. (1998). The association between the HLA antigens and Takayasu's arteritis in Thai patients. *Int J Cardiol*, 66, Suppl. 1: S117–20.

Chugh, K.S., Jain, S., Sakhuja, V., Malik, N., Gupta, A., Sehgal, S., Jha, V. and Gupta, K.L. (1992). Renovascular hypertension due to Takayasu's arteritis among Indian patients. *Q J Med*, 85: 833–43.

Chugh, K.S. and Sakhuja, V. (1992). Takayasu's arteritis as a cause of renovascular hypertension in Asian countries [editorial]. *Am J Nephrol*, 12: 1–8.

Dabague, J. and Reyes, P.A. (1996). Takayasu arteritis in Mexico: a 38-year clinical perspective through literature review. *Int J Cardiol*, 54, Suppl.: S103–9.

Desiron, Q. and Zeaiter, R. (2000). Takayasu's arteritis. *Acta Chir Belg*, 100: 1–6.

Deyu, Z., Lisheng, L., Ruping, D., Haiying, W. and Guozhang, L. (1998). Percutaneous transluminal renal angioplasty in aortoarteritis. *Int J Cardiol*, 66, Suppl. 1: S205–11.

Egido, J.A., Castrillo, C., Sanchez, M. and Rabano, J. (1996). Takayasu's arteritis: transcranial Doppler findings and follow-up. *J Neurosurg Sci*, 40: 121–4.

Flamm, S.D., White, R.D. and Hoffman, G.S. (1998). The clinical application of 'edema-weighted' magnetic resonance imaging in the assessment of Takayasu's arteritis. *Int J Cardiol*, 66, Suppl. 1: S151–9.

Fraga, A., Mintz, G., Valle, L. and Flores-Izquierdo, G. (1972). Takayasu's arteritis: frequency of systemic manifestations (study of 22 patients) and favorable response to maintenance steroid therapy with adrenocorticosteroids (12 patients). *Arthritis Rheum*, 15: 617–24.

Girona, E., Yamamoto-Furusho, J.K., Cutino, T., Reyes, P., Vargas-Alarcon, G., Granados, J. and Alarcon-Segovia, D. (1996). HLA-DR6 (possibly DRB1*1301) is associated with susceptibility to Takayasu arteritis in Mexicans. *Heart Vessels*, 11: 277–80.

Harada, M., Yoshida, H., Mitsuyama, K., Sakamoto, M., Koga, H., Matsuo, K., Teshima, Y., Ikeda, E., Sakisaka, S., Sata, M. and Tanikawa, K. (1998). Aortitis syndrome (Takayasu's arteritis) with cataract and elevated serum level of vascular endothelial growth factor. *Scand J Rheumatol*, 27: 78–9.

Hoffman, G.S. (1995). Treatment of resistant Takayasu's arteritis. *Rheum Dis Clin North Am*, 21: 73–80.

Hoffman, G.S. (1996). Takayasu arteritis: lessons from the American National Institutes of Health experience. *Int J Cardiol*, 54, Suppl.: S99–102.

Hoffman, G.S. and Ahmed, A.E. (1998). Surrogate markers of disease activity in patients with Takayasu arteritis. A preliminary report from The International Network for the Study of the Systemic Vasculitides (INSSYS). *Int J Cardiol*, 66, Suppl. 1: S191–4.

Hoffman, G.S., Leavitt, R.Y., Kerr, G.S., Rottem, M., Sneller, M.C. and Fauci, A.S. (1994). Treatment of glucocorticoid-resistant or relapsing Takayasu arteritis with methotrexate. *Arthritis Rheum*, 37: 578–82.

Ishikawa, K. (1988). Diagnostic approach and proposed criteria for the clinical diagnosis of Takayasu's arteriopathy. *J Am Coll Cardiol*, 12: 964–72.

Isner, J.M. (1999). Manipulating angiogenesis against vascular disease. *Hosp Pract (Off Ed)*, 34: 69–74, 76, 79–80 *passim*.

Ito, I., Saito, Y. and Nonaka, Y. (1975). Immunological aspects of aortitis syndrome. *Jpn Circ J*, 39: 459–62.

Kerr, G. (1994). Takayasu's arteritis. *Curr Opin Rheumatol*, 6: 32–8.

Kerr, G.S., Hallahan, C.W., Giordano, J., Leavitt, R.Y., Fauci, A.S., Rottem, M. and Hoffman, G.S. (1994). Takayasu arteritis. *Ann Intern Med*, 120: 919–29.

Khraishi, M.M., Gladman, D.D., Dagenais, P., Fam, A.G. and Keystone, E.C. (1992). HLA antigens in North American patients with Takayasu arteritis. *Arthritis Rheum*, 35: 573–5.

Kimura, A., Kobayashi, Y., Takahashi, M., Ohbuchi, N., Kitamura, H., Nakamura, T., Satoh, M., Sasaoka, T., Hiroi, S., Arimura, T., Akai, J., Aerbajinai, W., Yasukochi, Y. and Numano, F. (1998). MICA gene polymorphism in Takayasu's arteritis and Buerger's disease. *Int J Cardiol*, 66 Suppl. 1: S107–13.

Kiyosawa, M. and Baba, T. (1998). Ophthalmological findings in patients with Takayasu disease. *Int J Cardiol*, 66, Suppl. 1: S141–7.

Lagneau, P., Michel, J.B. and Vuong, P.N. (1987). Surgical treatment of Takayasu's disease. *Ann Surg*, 205: 157–66.

Lupi-Herrera, E., Sanchez-Torres, G., Marcushamer, J., Mispireta, J., Horwitz, S. and Vela, J.E. (1977). Takayasu's arteritis. Clinical study of 107 cases. *Am Heart J*, 93: 94–103.

Matsumura, A., Moriwaki, R. and Numano, F. (1992). Pregnancy in Takayasu arteritis from the view of internal medicine. *Heart Vessels Suppl*, 7: 120–4.

Matsunaga, N., Hayashi, K., Sakamoto, I., Matsuoka, Y., Ogawa, Y., Honjo, K. and Takano, K. (1998). Takayasu arteritis: MR manifestations and diagnosis of acute and chronic phase. *J Magn Reson Imaging*, 8: 406–14.

Mehra, N.K., Jaini, R., Balamurugan, A., Kanga, U., Prabhakaran, D., Jain, S., Talwar, K.K. and Sharma, B.K. (1998). Immunogenetic analysis of Takayasu arteritis in Indian patients. *Int J Cardiol*, 66, Suppl. 1: S127–32.

Moriwaki, R., Noda, M., Yajima, M., Sharma, B.K. and Numano, F. (1997). Clinical manifestations of Takayasu arteritis in India and Japan – new classification of angiographic findings. *Angiology*, 48: 369–79.

Numano, F. and Shimamoto, T. (1971). Hypersecretion of estrogen in Takayasu's disease. *Am Heart J*, 81: 591–6.

Park, M.H. and Park, Y.B. (1992). HLA typing of Takayasu arteritis in Korea. *Heart Vessels Suppl*, 7: 81–4.

Rodriguez-Reyna, T.S., Zuniga-Ramos, J., Salgado, N., Hernandez-Martinez, B., Vargas-Alarcon, G., Reyes-Lopez, P.A. and Granados, J. (1998). Intron 2 and exon 3 sequences may be involved in the susceptibility to develop Takayasu arteritis. *Int J Cardiol*, 66, Suppl. 1: S135–8.

Seko, Y. (2000). Takayasu arteritis: insights into immunopathology. *Jpn Heart J*, 41: 15–26.

Seko, Y., Minota, S., Kawasaki, A., Shinkai, Y., Maeda, K., Yagita, H., Okumura, K., Sato, O., Takagi, A., Tada, Y. and *et al.* (1994). Perforin-secreting killer cell infiltration and expression of a 65-kD heat-shock protein in aortic tissue of patients with Takayasu's arteritis. *J Clin Invest*, 93: 750–8.

Sharma, B.K. and Jain, S. (1998). A possible role of sex in determining distribution of lesions in Takayasu Arteritis. *Int J Cardiol*, 66, Suppl. 1: S81–4.

Sharma, B.K., Jain, S. and Radotra, B.D. (1998). An autopsy study of Takayasu arteritis in India. *Int J Cardiol*, 66, Suppl. 1: S85–90.

Sharma, B.K., Jain, S., Suri, S. and Numano, F. (1996). Diagnostic criteria for Takayasu arteritis. *Int J Cardiol*, 54, Suppl.: S141–7.

Sima, D., Thiele, B., Turowski, A., Wilke, K., Hiepe, F., Volk, D. and Sonnichsen, N. (1994). Anti-endothelial antibodies in Takayasu arteritis. *Arthritis Rheum*, 37: 441–3.

Sparks, S.R., Chock, A., Seslar, S., Bergan, J.J. and Owens, E.L. (2000). Surgical treatment of Takayasu's arteritis: case report and literature review. *Ann Vasc Surg*, 14: 125–9.

Subramanyan, R., Joy, J. and Balakrishnan, K.G. (1989). Natural history of aortoarteritis (Takayasu's disease). *Circulation*, 80: 429–37.

Ueda, H. (1971). Takayasu's disease – pulseless disease – aortitis syndrome. *Naika*, 27: 428–9.

Volkman, D.J., Mann, D.L. and Fauci, A.S. (1982). Association between Takayasu's arteritis and a B-cell alloantigen in North Americans. *N Engl J Med*, 306: 464–5.

Yajima, M., Numano, F., Park, Y.B. and Sagar, S. (1994). Comparative studies of patients with Takayasu arteritis in Japan, Korea and India – comparison of clinical manifestations, angiography and HLA-B antigen. *Jpn Circ J*, 58: 9–14.

Yamada, I., Nakagawa, T., Himeno, Y., Kobayashi, Y., Numano, F. and Shibuya, H. (2000). Takayasu arteritis: diagnosis with breath-hold contrast-enhanced three-dimensional MR angiography. *J Magn Reson Imaging*, 11: 481–7.

PART III

Systemic sclerosis: The spectrum, immunopathogenesis, clinical features, and treatment

Robert W. Simms and Joseph H. Korn

Introduction

Systemic sclerosis is a multisystem disease whose clinical manifestations result from vascular injury and obliteration, cutaneous and visceral fibrosis, and inflammation (Postlethwaite and Seyer 1990; Strehlow and Korn 1998). In some organs, such as the skin, fibrotic and inflammatory features predominate, whereas in others, particularly the kidney, vascular disease is preeminent. Raynaud's phenomenon, a triphasic vasospastic response to cold or other stimuli, is usually the first disease feature. Episodic vasoconstriction usually involves the hands and may progress to involve other acral areas including the face. While initially a functional disorder, structural occlusion of digital and other vessels is often seen in later disease.

Scleroderma, thickening and induration of the skin, is the hallmark feature of the disease. Skin changes begin distally, usually on the fingers, and progress proximally. Other common clinical features include intestinal hypomotility, particularly of the esophagus, pulmonary fibrosis, pulmonary hypertension, myocardial fibrosis and dysfunction, and renovascular ischemia with hypertension. Broadly, there are two forms of the disease: diffuse and limited. The former is characterized by diffuse skin disease involving the trunk and proximal extremities as well as more distal areas. The latter has involvement limited to the hands and occasionally forearms. Patients with limited disease, formerly called CREST (calcinosis, Raynaud's, esophageal hypomotility, sclerodactyly and telangiectasia) are at risk for intestinal involvement, a primary type of pulmonary hypertension and, to a lesser extent, pulmonary interstitial disease. Patients with diffuse systemic sclerosis are also at risk for renal disease, inflammatory interstitial lung disease progressing to fibrosis and myocardial small vessel disease with ischemia and fibrosis.

Pathogenesis of systemic sclerosis

Systemic sclerosis is characterized by evidence of T lymphocyte activation, autoimmunity and autoantibody formation, altered fibroblast metabolism, and as yet

PART IV

36. Targoff I.N. Humoral immunity in polymyositis/dermatomyositis. *J Investigative Dermatology* 1993, 100(1): 116S–123S.
37. Sloan M.F., Franks A.J., Exley K.A., and Davison A.M. Acute renal failure due to polymyositis. *Br Med J* 1978, 1(6125): 1457.
38. Dyck R.F., Katz A., Gordon D.A. *et al.* Glomerulonephritis associated with polymyositis. *J Rheumatology* 1979, 6(3): 336–344.

PART V

19

Amyloidosis: pathogenesis and diagnosis

H.J. Lachmann and P.N. Hawkins

Introduction

Amyloidosis is a disorder of protein folding in which normally soluble plasma proteins are deposited in the extracellular space in an abnormal insoluble fibrillar form (Pepys 1994; Pepys 1995). Accumulation of these fibrils causes progressive disruption of the structure and function of organs and tissues which, in systemic amyloidosis, can occur in virtually any site except the brain parenchyma. Without treatment systemic disease is usually fatal but measures that reduce the supply of amyloid fibril precursor proteins frequently lead to regression of amyloid deposits, prevention of organ failure and improved survival. However, since the regression of amyloid is relatively slow, early diagnosis can greatly improve the prognosis. Amyloid is remarkably diverse and can be hereditary or acquired, localized or systemic, and lethal or merely an incidental finding. It is certainly not rare, localized forms of the disease being associated with several extremely common disorders including type II diabetes mellitus and Alzheimer's disease.

Amyloid structure

Amyloid deposits consist mainly of protein fibrils, the different peptide sub-units of which constitute the basis for its classification (Table 19.1) (Husby 1992). In addition, all deposits contain some minor non-fibrillar common elements, most notably including restricted subsets of glycosaminoglycans and the normal plasma glycoprotein, serum amyloid P component (SAP). SAP has a highly characteristic pentameric structure and binds in a calcium dependent manner to a ligand that is evidently common to all types of amyloid fibril. The specific binding of SAP to amyloid fibrils is responsible for the universal presence of SAP in all amyloid deposits, and underlies the use of radiolabelled SAP as a diagnostic nuclear medicine tracer. This and the role of SAP in the pathogenesis of amyloidosis are discussed below.

The pathogenesis of amyloid centres around 'off-pathway' folding of the various fibril precursor proteins. About 20 different extremely heterogeneous proteins are known to form amyloid fibrils *in vivo* and other related and even completely unrelated proteins have lately been manipulated *in vitro* to undergo a similar transformation (Jiménez *et al.* 1999). Amyloid fibril proteins can evidently

Table 19.1 Classification of amyloidosis

Type	Fibril protein precursor	Clinical syndrome
AA	Serum amyloid A protein	Reactive systemic amyloidosis associated with acquired or hereditary chronic inflammatory diseases. Formerly known as secondary amyloidosis
AL	Monoclonal immunoglobulin light chains	Systemic amyloidosis associated with myeloma, monoclonal gammopathy, occult B cell dyscrasia. Formerly known as primary amyloidosis
ATTR	Normal plasma transthyretin	Senile systemic amyloidosis with prominent cardiac involvement
ATTR	Genetically variant transthyretin	Familial amyloid polyneuropathy, usually with systemic amyloidosis. Sometimes prominent amyloid cardiomyopathy or nephropathy
$A\beta_2M$	β_2-microglobulin	Periarticular and, occasionally, systemic amyloidosis associated with renal failure and long-term dialysis
$A\beta$	β-protein precursor (and rare genetic variants)	Cerebrovascular and intracerebral plaque amyloid in Alzheimer's disease. Occasional familial cases
AApoAI	Apolipoprotein AI	Autosomal dominant systemic amyloidosis. Predominantly non-neuropathic with prominent visceral involvement
AFib	Fibrinogen A α chain	Autosomal dominant systemic amyloidosis. Non-neuropathic with prominent visceral involvement
ALys	Lysozyme	Autosomal dominant systemic amyloidosis. Non-neuropathic with prominent visceral involvement
ACys	Cystatin C	Hereditary cerebral hemorrhage with cerebral and systemic amyloidosis
AGel	Gelsolin	Autosomal dominant systemic amyloidosis. Predominant cranial nerve involvement with lattice corneal dystrophy
AIAPP	Islet amyloid polypeptide	Amyloid in islets of Langerhans in type II diabetes mellitus and insulinoma

Amyloid composed of peptide hormones, prion protein, and unknown proteins, not included here.

exist as two radically different yet stable structures, i.e. the normal soluble form and a highly abnormal fibrillar conformation, and characterization of this has refuted the traditional dogma that amino acid sequence is the sole determinant of a protein's tertiary form. Amyloidogenic proteins are thought to transiently populate partly unfolded intermediate molecular states that expose β-sheet structure of the requisite type, which can interact with and bind to like molecules in a highly ordered fashion (Glenner 1980a; Glenner 1980b). Although amino acid sequence ultimately underlies the propensity for a protein to form amyloid, the propagation from low molecular weight protofilament cores into mature amyloid fibrils and their subsequent progressive accumulation is probably a self-perpetuating process that depends only on a sustained supply of the respective fibril precursor protein.

It has long been known that the ultrastructural morphology and histochemical properties of all amyloid fibrils, regardless of the precursor protein type, are remarkably similar, and their major component of cross-β secondary structure was identified some 25 years ago. Recent diffraction studies of a number of different *ex vivo* and synthetic amyloid fibrils confirmed that they all share a common core structure consisting of anti-parallel β-strands forming sheets lying with their long axes perpendicular to the long axis of the fibril (Sunde *et al.* 1997). This extremely abnormal but highly ordered conformation underlies the distinctive physicochemical properties of amyloid fibrils including their ability to bind molecules of the dye Congo red in a spatially organized manner, their relative resistance to proteolysis, and their capacity to bind SAP (Pepys 1995). In some instances the fibrils *in vivo* are composed of intact whole precursor molecules, for example in lysozyme, β$_2$-microglobulin and some forms of transthyretin amyloidosis (Pepys *et al.* 1993), (Saraiva *et al.* 1984; Gorevic *et al.* 1985), but more often, amyloid precursor proteins undergo partial cleavage, although it is not known whether this occurs before, during, or even after fibril formation (Husebekk *et al.* 1985; Mori *et al.* 1992).

In clinical practice amyloid deposition occurs in three different circumstances. Firstly when there is abnormal abundance of a structurally normal precursor protein, which is the case in both dialysis related amyloid in which the precursor is β$_2$-microglobulin, and in AA type in which the precursor is the acute phase reactant, serum amyloid A protein (SAA). The second situation arises when a normal but intrinsically amyloidogenic protein has been present in normal quantities for a very prolonged period of time. An example of this is senile cardiac amyloidosis in which wild type transthyretin is accumulated as amyloid in the myocardium of elderly individuals. The third and commonest situation with respect to systemic amyloidosis, is amyloid deposition involving a protein with an abnormal structure. Examples of this include acquired monoclonal immunoglobulin light chain (AL) amyloidosis in patients with clonal plasma cell dyscrasias, and the autosomal dominant hereditary amyloidosis syndromes associated with genetically variant forms of transthyretin, fibrinogen A α-chain, lysozyme, apolipoprotein A1, cystatin C and gelsolin.

Systemic amyloidosis associated with monoclonal immunocyte dyscrasias, AL amyloidosis (Chapter 21)

AL amyloidosis may potentially occur in association with any form of mono-clonal B cell dyscrasia. AL proteins are derived from the N-terminal region of monoclonal immunoglobulin light chains and consist of the whole or part of the variable (V_L) domain. Intact light chains may rarely be found, and the molecular weight therefore varies between about 8000 and 30,000 Da. The light chain of the monoclonal paraprotein is either identical to, or clearly the precursor of, AL isolated from the amyloid deposits. AL is more commonly derived from λ chains than from κ chains, despite the fact that κ chains predominate among both normal immunoglobulins and the paraprotein products of immunocyte dyscrasias. A new λ chain subgroup, λ_{VI}, was identified first as an AL protein in two cases of immunocyte dyscrasia-associated amyloidosis before it had been recognized in any other form, and it has subsequently been observed in many more cases of AL amyloidosis. Furthermore, there is increasing evidence from sequence analy-ses of Bence Jones proteins of both κ and λ type from patients with AL amyloi-dosis, and of AL proteins themselves, that these polypeptides contain unique amino acid replacements or insertions compared to non-amyloid monoclonal light chains. The inherent 'amyloidogenicity' of particular monoclonal light chains has been elegantly confirmed in an *in vivo* model in which isolated Bence Jones pro-teins are injected into mice. Animals receiving light chains from AL amyloid pa-tients developed typical amyloid deposits composed of the human protein whereas animals receiving light chains from myeloma patients without amyloid did not (Solomon 1991).

Dialysis related amyloidosis (DRA) (Chapter 31)

This is a potential complication of long-term renal replacement by either haemodialysis or, less often, chronic peritoneal dialysis. The amyloid fibrils are composed of β_2-microglobulin ($\beta_2 M$). This is the invariant light chain of Class I MHC antigens and is expressed by all nucleated cells. In health it is catabolized by the proximal renal tubules and it is not adequately cleared by dialysis. Persistently elevated levels of $\beta_2 M$ are universal in dialysed patients and the ma-jority of those receiving renal replacement for more than 10 years will develop symptomatic DRA (Bardin T 1986).

Senile systemic amyloidosis

This syndrome is not uncommon in the very elderly, and seemingly never occurs before the age of 60 years. The amyloid fibrils are composed of normal wild-type TTR (Westermark *et al.* 1990). The deposits are usually sparse and asympto-matic but occasionally, extensive infiltration of the myocardium causes congestive cardiac failure and may be fatal.

Hereditary systemic amyloidosis

Hereditary systemic amyloidosis caused by deposition of variant proteins as amyloid fibrils has been reported with the following proteins: transthyretin, cystatin C, gelsolin, apolipoprotein AI, lysozyme and fibrinogen A α-chain. These diseases are all inherited in an autosomal dominant pattern with variable penetrance, and may present clinically at any time from the teens to old age, though usually in adult life. By far the commonest hereditary amyloidosis is caused by transthyretin variants and usually presents as familial amyloid polyneuropathy with peripheral and autonomic neuropathy (Costa *et al.* 1978). Thus far more than 70 amyloidogenic TTR mutations have been described and there are almost certainly many more (Benson and Uemichi 1996). Cystatin C amyloidosis presents as cerebral amyloid angiopathy with recurrent cerebral haemorrhage and clinically silent systemic deposits, and has been reported only in Icelandic families. Gelsolin amyloidosis presents with cranial neuropathy but there are also systemic deposits; it is also extremely rare (Maury 1991). Hereditary non-neuropathic systemic amyloidosis was first described by Ostertag in 1932 (Ostertag 1932). It is now recognized to be caused by mutations in the apolipoprotein AI (Nichols *et al.* 1988; Soutar *et al.* 1992), lysozyme (Pepys *et al.* 1993) or α-fibrinogen (Benson *et al.* 1993) genes. The amyloid deposits in these syndromes can affect any or all the major viscera, with renal involvement usually being prominent, although apolipoprotein AI amyloid occasionally also manifests with neuropathy. Increasing numbers of kindreds of mutations affecting these three proteins have lately been reported, and we continue to discover more, indicating that these conditions are much less rare than previously thought.

Localized amyloidosis

Localized amyloid deposition occurs quite commonly and presumably results either from local production of fibril precursors, or from properties inherent to the particular microenvironment, which favour localization and fibril formation of a more widely distributed precursor protein. Most symptomatic deposits occur in the skin, respiratory or urogenital tracts and are of AL type. They are associated with extremely subtle focal monoclonal B cell proliferation and surgical resection of these localized 'amyloidoma's can be curative.

Cerebral amyloidosis

The brain and intracerebral blood vessels are usually spared in systemic amyloidosis but are important sites for local deposition of amyloid (Duchen 1992). The best characterized form of cerebral amyloid is that related to Alzheimer's disease, the commonest form of dementia world-wide. The fibril protein in the intracerebral and cerebrovascular amyloid of Alzheimer's disease, Down's syndrome and hereditary amyloid angiopathy of Dutch type is known as β-protein. This 39–43 residue sequence is cleaved from β-amyloid precursor protein (APP). There is now mounting evidence that cerebral amyloid deposition is directly neurotoxic but the exact mechanisms leading to neuronal degeneration have yet to be elucidated. There is mounting evidence that relatively low molecular amyloid aggregates, as opposed to mature fibrils, may have a major part in the pathogenesis of this disorder.

Diagnosis

Diagnosis of amyloid relies on a high index of clinical suspicion. Unfortunately amyloid is frequently asymptomatic until a relatively late stage and can then present with highly variable or non-specific symptoms. The protean manifesta-

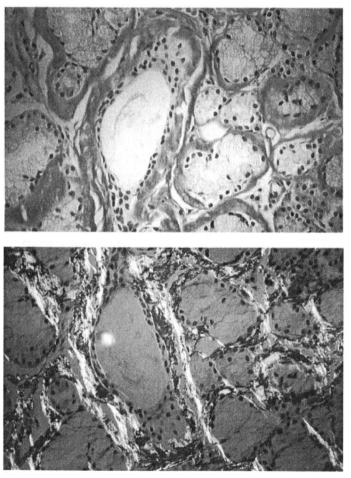

Fig. 19.1 Typical Congo red histology. The same tissue section viewed under conventional microscopy demonstrating Congophilic amyloid deposits and under cross light demonstrating the pathognomonic apple-green birefringence.

tions of systemic amyloid depend on the predominant organs affected and can include symptoms and signs referable to any system except the CNS.

Histology

The diagnosis of amyloid generally requires histological confirmation. Biopsy of a clinically affected visceral organ, e.g. the kidney, liver or heart, is usually diagnostic but gives no information about the total body amyloid load or the distribution of deposits in other organs. Biopsy can be hazardous as there is an increased risk of haemorrhage and significant bleeds have been reported in 5% of liver biopsies. This is attributable to the increased fragility of affected blood vessels, reduced elasticity of severely amyloidotic organs, and, very occasionally in AL type to an acquired deficiency of clotting factors IX and X. A less invasive alternative in suspected systemic disease is fine needle aspiration of subcutaneous fat, or rectal or labial salivary gland biopsy (Westermark and Stenkvist 1973; Delgado and Mosqueda 1989). In skilled hands these 'screening' biopsies can produce positive results in up to 80% of cases, but in routine practice sensitivity is only about 50%.

Amyloid fibrils stained with Congo red give pathognomonic red-green birefringence when viewed under crossed polarized light, and this tinctorial property remains the diagnostic gold standard (Puchtler *et al.* 1962). Congo red staining was first used to identify amyloid deposits in tissue sections in 1922 and the characteristic apple-green birefringence seen under crossed polarized filters was described in 1927. The alkaline-alcoholic Congo red method described by Puchtler *et al.* (1962) gives the most specific and consistent results as it reduces any non-specific background staining. The stain is unstable and must be prepared at least every 8 weeks. Congo red also stains collagen, elastic fibres and hyaline material quite strongly, although in these cases polarization studies give white birefringence and this can be a source of diagnostic confusion. The pathognomonic birefringence is dependent on a sufficient density of amyloid and reliable results are only obtained with tissue sections cut at 6–8 μm rather than the usual 2–3 μm.

There are a number of problems inherent in histological based diagnoses; tissue samples must be adequate and there is unavoidable element of sampling error. This means that biopsies cannot satisfactorily reveal the extent or distribution of amyloid, and failure to demonstrate amyloid cannot exclude the diagnosis. Many of these problems can be overcome by combining histological examination of biopsy material with whole body SAP scintigraphy.

Immunohistochemistry

Congo red histology should always be followed by immunohistochemical staining to further characterize the amyloid type. Antibodies against most known amyloid fibril proteins are commercially available but are more useful in some amyloid types than others. Immunohistochemistry gives reliable and specific results in AA and β_2M but should be interpreted with caution in AL type. In AL the fibrils are comprised of light chain fragments and these frequently contain unique epitopes from the N-terminal variable domain. These tend not to be recognized by commercial polyclonal antibodies which are largely directed against determinants in the constant domains of κ or λ chains, and consequently diagnostic results are obtained in only about half the cases of AL type. A few cases of immunoglobulin heavy chain amyloid deposition have been reported (Eulitz *et al.* 1990).

It is important to appreciate that amyloid fibrils are derived from circulating plasma proteins and that many potential amyloid precursor proteins are detectable as background staining in entirely normal tissue. The demonstration of amyloidogenic proteins in tissues does not, on its own, establish the presence of amyloid and the diagnosis must always be confirmed by concomitant Congo red staining.

Electron microscopy

The appearance of amyloid fibrils in tissues under the electron microscope is not always completely specific, and sometimes they cannot be convincingly identified. Although electron microscopy has been claimed to be more sensitive than light microscopy, it is not sufficient by itself to confirm the diagnosis of amyloidosis.

SAP scintigraphy

In 1988 SAP scintigraphy was introduced as a sensitive, specific and non-invasive means of quantitatively imaging amyloid deposits *in vivo* (Hawkins *et al.* 1988). Highly purified SAP is labelled with the medium-energy, short half-life, pure gamma emitter ^{123}I and injected intravenously. No localization or retention of labelled SAP occurs in individuals without amyloidosis, in whom the tracer is rapidly catabolized and excreted. However, in patients with amyloidosis, labelled SAP localizes rapidly and specifically to the amyloid deposits. It does so in proportion to the amount of amyloid present, and will persist there without breakdown or modification. This 'localization' of labelled SAP to amyloid is in fact a specific dilution phenomenon since circulating SAP is at all times in a dynamic equilibrium with the far greater quantity of SAP concentrated within amyloid deposits. The technique has 100% diagnostic sensitivity in patients with systemic AA amyloidosis, and approximately 90% in AL type and is the only method available for serial monitoring the progression or regression of amyloid throughout the body.

The doses of radioactivity are well within acceptable limits (effective dose equivalent ~3.5 mSv), and more than 2000 patient studies have now been performed without adverse effects at the National Amyloidosis Centre (Hawkins 1994). The technique has provided substantial new information, including the varied patterns of distribution in the different forms of the disease, the demonstration of amyloid in sites not normally available for biopsy, and evidence of frequent poor correlation between quantity of amyloid and degree of organ dysfunction. In addition, scintigraphy has permitted study of the natural history

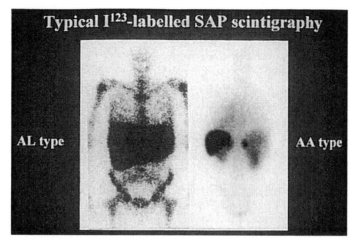

Fig. 19.2 Posterior whole body scintigraphic images following the intravenous injection of I^{123}-labelled human SAP showing the typical appearances of AL amyloidosis with abnormal tracer uptake into amyloid deposits in the liver, spleen and bone marrow and AA amyloid with deposits in the spleen, kidneys and adrenal glands.

of the various types of the disease, and turnover of amyloid deposits following treatment (Hawkins *et al.* 1993a; Hawkins *et al.* 1993b; Holmgren *et al.* 1993; Tan *et al.* 1994). SAP scintigraphy is eminently suitable as a screening test in patients thought to be at risk of systemic amyloid deposition, including those with chronic inflammatory conditions, monoclonal gammopathies or known amyloidogenic mutations, but unfortunately is not widely available.

Echocardiography

Significant cardiac amyloid deposition confers a poor prognosis. Unfortunately the heart is poorly visualized by SAP scintigraphy, probably reflecting cardiac motility, blood pool signal from the cardiac chambers, and relatively slow localization of labelled SAP across the non-fenestrated myocardial endothelium. Cardiac amyloidosis is best evaluated by a combination of echocardiography and ECG. Two-dimensional Doppler echocardiography classically reveals concentric biventricular wall thickening, 'sparkling' myocardial echodensity and thickened but pliable valves, and restrictive filling pattern. Amyloid causes diastolic dysfunction with well-preserved contractility until a very late stage. Other frequent findings are biatrial dilatation, pericardial effusions and, in end-stage disease right ventricular dilatation with evidence of pulmonary hypertension (Dubrey *et al.* 1998). The ECG may be normal in patients with substantial cardiac amyloidosis, but in advanced disease commonly shows small voltages, pathological 'Q' waves (pseudo-infarct pattern) in the anterior chest leads and conduction abnormalities.

DNA analysis

Hereditary amyloidoses are rare, and the diagnosis can all too easily be over-looked. Although all types are dominantly inherited, penetrance is highly variable, and successful immunohistochemical typing depends heavily on tissue fixation, antibody preparations, inclusion of comprehensive absorption and tissue controls and technical experience. In practice, definitive immunohistochemical typing of hereditary amyloidosis quite frequently cannot be obtained. Patient prognosis and treatment are entirely dependent on the nature of the precursor protein, and DNA analysis is now mandatory in all patients with non-AA systemic amyloidosis that cannot be confirmed absolutely to be AL type. Several, or indeed many, amyloidogenic mutations have been identified in most of the genes associated with hereditary amyloidosis and new variants are regularly identified. It is therefore best to carry gene sequencing rather than to use methods such as RFLP analysis which are directed at individual known mutations.

Protein sequencing

In cases in which it is not possible to identify the amyloid type by the various techniques described above, isolation of amyloid fibrils from fresh biopsy material enables amino acid sequencing of the fibril subunit peptide to be performed. This requires technical expertise and is time consuming but can be achieved using very small tissue samples. It is the method by which all amyloid proteins have been discovered.

Investigation of the underlying disease

The process underlying amyloid deposition needs to be sought and characterized in each case. AL amyloidosis is a complication of clonal B cell dyscrasias, but the spectrum of these is very wide: 15% of patients with AL amyloidosis have multiple myeloma and, at the other end of the spectrum in another 15% of cases conventional bone marrow examination and protein electrophoresis and immunofixation will fail to identify any evidence of clonal disease. In some such cases, immunoglobulin gene rearrangement analysis using Southern blotting or polymerase chain reaction (PCR) techniques may be informative (Vigushin *et al.* 1994).

The chronic inflammatory disorders that underlie AA amyloidosis are usually quite straightforward to classify clinically, but up to 5% of cases present without overt prior disease. More than half of such patients in our own series have had Castleman's disease tumours of the solitary plasma cell type, which are typically sited in the gut mesentery or mediastinum and are amenable to surgical excision.

References

Axelrad, M.A., Kisilevsky, R., Willmer, J., Chen, S.J. and Skinner, M. (1982). Further characterization of amyloid-enhancing factor. *Laboratory Investigation*, 47, 139–46.
Baba, S., Masago, S.A., Takahashi, T., Kasama, T., Sugimura, H., Tsugane, S., Tsutsui, Y. and Shirasawa, H. (1995). A novel allelic variant of serum amyloid A, SAA1g:

genomic evidence, evolution, frequency, and implication as a risk factor for reactive systemic AA-amyloidosis. *Human Molecular Genetics*, 4, 1083–7.

Bardin, T., Zingraff, J., Kuntz, D. and Drüeke, T. (1986). Dialysis related amyloidosis. *Nephrology, Dialysis, Transplantation*, 1, 151–4.

Benson, M.D. and Uemichi, T. (1996). Transthyretin amyloidosis. *Amyloid: The International Journal of Experimental and Clinical Investigation*, 3, 44–56.

Benson, M.D., Liepnieks, J., Uemichi, T., Wheeler, G. and Correa, R. (1993). Hereditary renal amyloidosis associated with a mutant fibrinogen a-chain. *Nature Genetics*, 3, 252–5.

Booth, D.R., Bellotti, V., Sunde, M., Robinson, C.V., Fraser, P.E., Radford, S.E., Blake, C.C.F., Hawkins, P.N. and Pepys, M.B. (1996). Molecular mechanisms of amyloid fibril formation: the lysozyme model. *Clinical Science*, 90 (Suppl. 34), 1P.

Booth, D.R., Sunde, M., Bellotti, V., Robinson, C.V., Hutchinson, W.L., Fraser, P.E., Hawkins, P.N., Dobson, C.M., Radford, S.E., Blake, C.C.F. and Pepys, M.B. (1997). Instability, unfolding and aggregation of human lysozyme variants underlying amyloid fibrillogenesis. *Nature*, 385, 787–93.

Booth, D.R., Booth, S.E., Gillmore, J.D., Hawkins, P.N. and Pepys, M.B. (1999). SAA$_1$ alleles as risk factors in AA amyloidosis. In: R.A. Kyle and M.A. Gertz (eds) *Amyloid and Amyloidosis 1998*, pp. 369–71. Parthenon Publishing, New York.

Botto, M., Hawkins, P.N., Bickerstaff, M.C.M., Herbert, J., Bygrave, A.E., McBride, A., Hutchinson, W.L., Tennent, G.A., Walport, M.J. and Pepys, M.B. (1997). Amyloid deposition is delayed in mice with targeted deletion of the serum amyloid P component gene. *Nature Medicine*, 3, 855–9.

The French FMF Consortium (1997). A candidate gene for familial Mediterranean fever. *Nature Genetics*, 17, 25–31.

The International FMF Consortium. (1997). Ancient missense mutations in a new member of the *RoRet* gene family are likely to cause familial Mediterranean fever. *Cell*, 90, 797–807.

Costa, P.P., Figueira, A.S. and Bravo, F.R. (1978). Amyloid fibril protein related to pre-albumin in familial amyloidotic polyneuropathy. *Proceedings of The National Academy of Sciences of the United States of America*, 75, 4499–503.

Delgado, A.W. and Mosqueda, A. (1989). A highly sensitive method for diagnosis of secondary amyloidosis by labial salivary gland biopsy. *Journal of Oral Pathology and Medicine*, 18, 310–14.

Dubrey, S.W., Cha, K., Anderson, J., Chamarthi, B., Skinner, M. and Falk, R.H. (1998). The clinical features of immunoglobulin light-chain (AL) amyloidosis with heart involvement. *Quarterly Journal of Medicine*, 91, 141–57.

Duchen, L.W. (1992). Current status review: cerebral amyloid. *International Journal of Experimental Pathology*, 73, 535–50.

Eulitz, M., Weiss, D.T. and Solomon, A. (1990). Immunoglobulin heavy-chain-associated amyloidosis. *Proceedings of The National Academy of Sciences of the United States of America*, 87, 6542–6.

Glenner, G.G. (1980a). Amyloid deposits and amyloidosis – the b-fibrilloses. I. *New England Journal of Medicine*, 302, 1283–92.

Glenner, G.G. (1980b). Amyloid deposits and amyloidosis – the b-fibrilloses. II. *New England Journal of Medicine*, 302, 1333–43.

Gorevic, P.D., Casey, T.T., Stone, W.J., DiRaimondo, C.R., Prelli, F.L. and Frangione, B. (1985). Beta-2 microglobulin is an amyloidogenic protein in man. *Journal of Clinical Investigation*, 76, 2425–9.

Hawkins, P.N. (1994). Studies with radiolabelled serum amyloid P component provide evidence for turnover and regression of amyloid deposits *in vivo*. *Clinical Science*, 87, 289–95.

Hawkins, P.N. (1995). Amyloidosis. *Blood Reviews*, 9, 135–42.

Hawkins, P.N., Myers, M.J., Epenetos, A.A., Caspi, D. and Pepys, M.B. (1988). Specific localization and imaging of amyloid deposits *in vivo* using 123I-labeled serum amyloid P component. *Journal of Experimental Medicine*, 167, 903–13.

Hawkins, P.N., Peters, A.M., Vigushin, D.M., Richardson, S., Seymour, A., Holmgren, G., Steen, L., Woo, P., Hall, A. and Pepys, M.B. (1993a). SAP scintigraphy and turnover studies demonstrate regression of amyloidosis. *Nuclear Medicine Communications*, 14, 259–60.

Hawkins, P.N., Richardson, S., Vigushin, D.M., David, J., Kelsey, C.R., Gray, R.E.S., Hall, M.A., Woo, P., Lavender, J.P. and Pepys, M.B. (1993b). Serum amyloid P component scintigraphy and turnover studies for diagnosis and quantitative monitoring of AA amyloidosis in juvenile rheumatoid arthritis. *Arthritis and Rheumatism*, 36, 842–51.

Holmgren, G., Ericzon, B.G., Groth, C.G., Steen, L., Suhr, O., Andersen, O., Wallin, B.G., Seymour, A., Richardson, S., Hawkins, P.N. and Pepys, M.B. (1993). Clinical improvement and amyloid regression after liver transplantation in hereditary transthyretin amyloidosis. *Lancet*, 341, 1113–16.

Husby, G. (1992). Nomenclature and classification of amyloid and amyloidoses. *Journal of Internal Medicine*, 232, 511–12.

Husebekk, A., Skogen, B., Husby, G. and Marhaug, G. (1985). Transformation of amyloid precursor SAA to protein AA and incorporation in amyloid fibrils *in vivo*. *Scandinavian Journal of Immunology*, 21, 283–7.

Jiménez, J.L., Guijarro, J.I., Orlova, E., Zurdo, J., Dobson, C.M., Sunde, M. and Saibil, H.R. (1999). Cryo-electron microscopy structure of an SH3 amyloid fibril and model of the molecular packing. *EMBO Journal*, 18, 815–21.

Lorenzo, A., Razzaboni, B., Weir, G.C. and Yankner, B.A. (1994). Pancreatic islet cell toxicity of amylin associated with type-2 diabetes mellitus. *Nature*, 368, 756–60.

Maury, C.P.J. (1991). Gelsolin-related amyloidosis. Identification of the amyloid protein in Finnish hereditary amyloidosis as a fragment of variant gelsolin. *Journal of Clinical Investigation*, 87, 1195–9.

Mori, H., Takio, K., Ogawara, M. and Selkoe, D.J. (1992). Mass spectrometry of purified amyloid b protein in Alzheimer's disease. *Journal of Biological Chemistry*, 267, 17082–6.

Nelson, S.R., Lyon, M., Gallagher, J.T., Johnson, E.A. and Pepys, M.B. (1991). Isolation and characterization of the integral glycosaminoglycan constituents of human amyloid A and monoclonal light-chain amyloid fibrils. *Biochemical Journal*, 275, 67–73.

Nichols, W.C., Dwulet, F.E., Liepnieks, J. and Benson, M.D. (1988). Variant apolipoprotein AI as a major constituent of a human hereditary amyloid. *Biochemical and Biophysical Research Communications*, 156, 762–8.

Ostertag, B. (1932). Demonstration einer eigenartigen familiaren paraamyloidose. *Zentralblatt Aug Pathologie*, 56, 253–4.

Pepys, M.B. (1994). Amyloidosis. In: M.M. Frank, K.F. Austen, H.N. Claman and E.R. Unanue (eds) *Samter's Immunologic Diseases*, pp. 637–55. Little, Brown and Company, Boston.

Pepys, M.B. (1995). Amyloidosis. In: D.J. Weatherall, J.G.G. Ledingham and D.A. Warrell (eds) *Oxford Textbook of Medicine*,pp. 1512–24. Oxford University Press, Oxford.

Pepys, M.B., Hawkins, P.N., Booth, D.R., Vigushin, D.M., Tennent, G.A., Soutar, A.K., Totty, N., Nguyen, O., Blake, C.C.F., Terry, C.J., Feest, T.G., Zalin, A.M. and

Hsuan, J.J. (1993). Human lysozyme gene mutations cause hereditary systemic amyloidosis. *Nature*, 362, 553–7.

Puchtler, H., Sweat, F. and Levine, M. (1962). On the binding of Congo red by amyloid. *Journal of Histochemistry and Cytochemistry*, 10, 355–64.

Saraiva, M.J.M., Birken, S., Costa, P.P. and Goodman, D.S. (1984). Amyloid fibril protein in familial amyloid polyneuropathy, Portuguese type. Definition of molecular abnormality in transthyretin (prealbumin). *Journal of Clinical Investigation*, 74, 104–19.

Schnitzer, T.J. and Ansell B.M. (1977). Amyloidosis in juvenile chronic polyarthritis. *Arthritis and Rheumatism*, 20, 245–52.

Simmons, L.K., May, P.C., Tomaselli, K.J., Rydel, R.E., Fuson, K.S., Brigham, E.F., Wright, S., Lieberburg, I., Becker, G.W., Brems, D.N. and Li, W.Y. (1994). Secondary structure of amyloid beta peptide correlates with neurotoxic activity *in vivo*. *Molecular Pharmacology*, 45, 373–9.

Solomon, A., Weiss, D.T. and Kattine, A.A. (1991). Nephrotoxic potential of Bence Jones proteins. *New England Journal of Medicine*, 324, 1845–51.

Soutar, A.K., Hawkins, P.N., Vigushin, D.M., Tennent, G.A., Booth, S.E., Hutton, T., Nguyen, O., Totty, N.F., Feest, T.G., Hsuan, J.J. and Pepys, M.B. (1992). Apolipoprotein AI mutation Arg-60 causes autosomal dominant amyloidosis. *Proceedings of The National Academy of Sciences of the United States of America*, 89, 7389–93.

Sunde, M., Serpell, L.C., Bartlam, M., Fraser, P.E., Pepys, M.B. and Blake, C. C.F. (1997). Common core structure of amyloid fibrils by synchrotron X-ray diffraction. *Journal of Molecular Biology*, 273, 729–39.

Tan, S.Y., Madhoo, S., Brown, E., Gower, P., Irish, A., Winearls, C., Clutterbuck, E.J., Pepys, M.B. and Hawkins, P.N. (1994). Effect of renal transplantation on dialysis-related amyloid deposits: Prospective evaluation by ^{123}I-SAP scintigraphy. *Nephrology Dialysis, Transplantation*, 9, 1017.

Tennent, G.A., Lovat, L.B. and Pepys, M.B. (1995). Serum amyloid P component prevents proteolysis of the amyloid fibrils of Alzheimer's disease and systemic amyloidosis. *Proceedings of The National Academy of Sciences of the United States of America*, 92, 4299–303.

Vigushin, D.M., Vulliamy, T., Kaeba, J.S., Hawkins, P.N., Luzzatto, L. and Pepys, M.B. (1994). Immunoglobulin gene rearrangement analysis in AL amyloidosis. In: R. Kisilevsky, M.D. Benson, B. Frangione, J. Gauldie, T.J. Muckle and I.D. Young (eds) *Amyloid and Amyloidosis* 1993, pp. 287–9. Parthenon Publishing, New York,

Westermark, P. and Stenkvist, B. (1973). A new method for the diagnosis of systemic amyloidosis. *Archives of Internal Medicine*, 132, 522–3.

Westermark, P., Sletten, K., Johansson, B. and Cornwell, G.G. (1990). Fibril in senile cardiac amyloidosis is derived from normal transthyretin. *Proceedings of the National Academy of Sciences of the United States of America*, 87, 2843–5.

20

Amyloidosis: Rheumatic disease and amyloid; clinical features and treatment

H.J. Lachmann and P.N. Hawkins

Introduction

Most of the clinical features of amyloid are non-specific; indeed malaise and weight loss are frequent early symptoms and, although a high index of suspicion may improve the diagnostic yield, the diagnosis of systemic amyloidosis, especially AL type, very often remains an unexpected finding at biopsy. Even after amyloidosis has been confirmed, subsequent identification of amyloid type is not always straightforward. Definitive diagnosis relies on a combination of clinical features, predisposing conditions, histology, immunohistochemistry and, where available, more specialized but highly informative investigations such as SAP scintigraphy and DNA analysis. It is unwise to rely on any of these particular findings in isolation given the limitations in their sensitivity and specificity, and the possibility that a condition which may be associated with amyloidosis, such as a monoclonal gammopathy or an amyloidogenic mutation, might just be an incidental finding. Clinical evaluation of a patient with amyloidosis must always extend to thorough characterization of the underlying disorder since treatment of the latter remains the prime objective of clinical management.

General treatment principles

Although amyloid deposits are not irreversible, as was widely believed until recently, they do turn over relatively slowly and the natural history of amyloidosis is that the rate of fibril deposition usually exceeds that of mobilization. As a result, the amyloid diseases tend to be progressive. Amyloid would regress if *either* its rate of deposition is slowed or its clearance is enhanced. Although novel therapies with the latter aim are on the horizon, at present the treatment of all types of amyloid centres on reducing the supply of the respective amyloid precursor protein and supporting or replacing compromised organ function. Self-evidently, treatment depends completely on precise identification of the amyloid fibril type.

Preservation and replacement of organ function

Organs that are extensively infiltrated by amyloid may fail precipitously with little or no warning, and seemingly without provocation, even when organ function has previously been entirely normal. Scrupulous attention needs to be paid to salt and water balance, maintenance of the circulating volume and prompt treatment of sepsis to reduce the risk of acute organ failure at all times, and even more so during chemotherapy and other types of treatment. For these reasons elective surgery and general anaesthesia are best avoided in patients with systemic amyloidosis unless there are compelling indications. Therapy that retards or halts amyloid deposition is frequently followed by the gradual recovery of organ function, but inexorably progressive organ failure is inevitable, particularly in the case of amyloidotic kidneys, once a certain level of organ dysfunction has occurred.

In some cases organs are so severely compromised that, without support or replacement of their function, patients will not survive treatment, or live long enough to derive benefit from it. The most frequent such problem encountered in the management of patients with systemic amyloidosis is renal failure. It is usually feasible to manage this with renal replacement therapy in the form of haemodialysis or peritoneal dialysis until there is clear evidence of a response to treatment of the underlying amyloidogenic condition. Although nephrotic syndrome and, to a lesser extent, moderately impaired renal function frequently improve and can even normalise when amyloid deposits regress, dialysis or renal transplantation will need to be considered in patients with more advanced renal damage. However, the outcome of amyloidosis patients on long-term dialysis is relatively poor, their two year survival being in the order of 80% that of non-amyloidotic patients. By contrast, the outcome of renal transplantation in these patients is more favourable (Brunner *et al.*, 1976). Although their early post transplant mortality is increased, due to sepsis and cardiac failure, long-term graft survival and rejection rates compare very well with patients with other systemic diseases, and may even be better. Most amyloid patients have a functioning graft until death (Jacob, 1982; Jacob *et al.*, 1979), and although amyloid deposition in the transplanted organ has been reported in up to 20% of patients with AA amyloidosis, this rarely compromises graft function, and is rarely responsible for graft loss (Pasternack *et al.*, 1986). In all other types of the disease, clinically significant graft amyloid occurs far less frequently than is widely supposed, particularly the hereditary forms which may be very slow to progress generally.

A small proportion of patients with systemic amyloidosis present with severely compromised liver or cardiac function but with otherwise well preserved vital organ function. Most of these patients will have AL type and may be suitable for lifesaving liver or heart transplantation before proceeding to chemotherapy (Merlini, 1997). Selection of such cases remains very difficult, particularly with respect to liver replacement because all patients with end-stage hepatic amyloidosis have substantial amyloid deposits in other organ systems even when those organs appear to retain adequate function.

Reactive systemic, AA, amyloidosis

Associated conditions

AA amyloidosis may occur in any patient who has a sustained acute phase response. The list of chronic inflammatory, infective and neoplastic disorders that can lead to this type of amyloid is almost without limit (Table 20.1), but the predominant aetiology varies among different populations. In the Western world the commonest predisposing conditions are adult and juvenile rheumatoid arthritis (Gertz et al., 1991). For reasons that are not clear the incidence of AA amyloid is lower in the United States and much higher in parts of central Europe and Scandinavia (Filipowicz-Sosnowska et al., 1978; Svantesson et al., 1983). In the UK up to 5% of patients with rheumatoid arthritis, juvenile inflammatory arthritis (JIA) or ankylosing spondylitis are eventually affected (Schnitzer and Ansell, 1977; Gratacos et al., 1997). The incidence of AA amyloidosis increases with duration and severity of the underlying inflammatory disorder, and although the median latency between onset of inflammation and diagnosis of amyloid is usually 8 to 14 years, some individuals develop clinically significant amyloid in less than 12 months and others only after many decades. Amyloidosis occurs exceptionally rarely in systemic lupus erythematosis and ulcerative colitis, reflecting the unusually modest acute phase response evoked by these particular conditions. Familial Mediterranean fever is a significant cause of amyloid in some populations, and is discussed below.

Clinical features

AA amyloid deposition can be extensive without causing symptoms (Hawkins et al., 1993). It presents most commonly with non-selective proteinuria or nephrotic syndrome and may be accompanied by renal insufficiency (Schnitzer and Ansell, 1977). Approximately 5% of cases will not have proteinuria despite extensive renal amyloid deposition. Haematuria, tubular defects, and diffuse renal calcification occur rarely (Luke et al., 1969). Kidney size is usually normal, but may be enlarged, or, in advanced cases, reduced. End-stage renal failure is the cause of death in 40 to 60% of patients although the clinical course is unpredictable and may be characterized by step-wise deterioration. Acute renal failure is readily precipitated by transient reduction of kidney perfusion, even in cases without pre-existing clinically evident disease. A few patients present with organomegaly, e.g. hepato/splenomegaly, sometimes without any accompanying renal dysfunction although, invariably, amyloid deposits are widespread at diagnosis. The spleen is the first site of substantial parenchymal deposition and is infiltrated in almost every case at presentation (Hawkins et al., 1993). Palpable splenomegaly is unusual but there is often evidence of functional hyposplenism. The adrenal glands are infiltrated extensively in at least one-third of cases, and the liver in one-quarter, but function of both organs is typically well preserved

Table 20.1 Conditions associated with AA type amyloidosis

Idiopathic chronic inflammatory diseases
Rheumatoid arthritis
Juvenile inflammatory arthritis
Ankylosing spondilitis
Psoriatic arthropathy
Reiter's syndrome
Adult Still's disease
Polyarteritis nodosa
Behcet's disease
Systemic lupus erythematosis
Crohn's disease

Periodic fevers
Familial Mediterranean fever
Muckle-Well's syndrome
Tumour necrosis factor associated periodic syndrome (TRAPS)

Chronic microbial infections
Leprosy
Tuberculosis
Bronchiectasis
Chronic cutaneous ulcers
Chronic pyelonephritis
Osteomyelitis
Subacute bacterial endocarditis
Whipple's disease

Neoplasia
Hodgkin's disease
Renal cell carcinoma
Adenocarcinoma of the lung, gut, urogenital tract
Basal cell carcinoma
Hairy cell leukaemia
Castleman's disease
Hepatic adenoma

Other
Hypogammaglobulinaemia
Cyclic neutropaenia
Cystic fibrosis
Kartagener's syndrome
Epidermolysis Bullosa
IV drug abuse

even at a late stage. Microscopic histological involvement of the heart and gut is usual and although clinical sequelae are rare, these may now be encountered more often than previously because active supportive measures mean that patients with AA amyloidosis are surviving for longer.

Prognosis is related to the degree of renal involvement and without treatment the outlook is bleak. Almost three-quarters of patients reach end-stage renal failure within five years of diagnosis (Ahlmen *et al.*, 1987) and once the serum creatinine is elevated beyond the normal range half the patients are dead within 18 months (Lindqvist *et al.*, 1989). Although AA amyloid is a relatively unusual complication of juvenile inflammatory arthritis it is responsible for 40 to 50% of all deaths in these patients with a five-year survival of 50%, and by 15 years a further 25% have died (Schnitzer and Ansell, 1977; Smith *et al.*, 1968; Baum and Gutowska, 1977).

Treatment

Successful therapy in AA amyloidosis depends on as complete as possible suppression of the acute phase response, and will therefore vary according to the nature of the underlying inflammatory disease. Given that amyloid is potentially fatal, it may be justified to employ aggressive treatment strategies that would otherwise be considered too toxic. Hence, cytotoxic drugs, especially alkylating agents, have been used to treat patients with AA amyloidosis secondary to rheumatic diseases. Limb amputation may be required in cases of osteomyelitis that have not responded to antimicrobial drugs. There have been several case reports describing resolution of nephrotic syndrome following surgical resection of cytokine secreting lesions such as solitary Castleman's tumours of the plasma cell type (Vigushin *et al.*, 1994; Perfetti *et al.*, 1994; Ordi *et al.*, 1993). Patients with Crohn's disease have responded to medical therapy, elemental diet and occasionally in resistant disease to colectomy.

In the UK, chlorambucil has been used extensively in patients with AA amyloidosis due to rheumatoid arthritis and juvenile inflammatory arthritis. It was first used in children with JIA in the late 1960s and dramatically improved the prognosis both in terms of survival and renal function (Ansell *et al.*, 1971). Since then treatment has been extended to adults with a substantial benefit in about two-thirds of cases. Long-term survival is now frequent and reversal of nephrotic syndrome and stabilization or recovery of renal function are commonly recognized (Berglund *et al.*, 1987). Among a series of 80 patients with AA amyloidosis under long-term follow-up in our own unit, the 10-year survival of those in whom the plasma SAA had been suppressed to near normal levels was more than 95%, compared with 60% among those whose inflammatory disease did not remit. The majority of these 80 patients had RA or JIA, and most received chlorambucil following the diagnosis of amyloid. However, its use must be considered very carefully in each patient since it is not licensed for this indication, it is potentially carcinogenic, and it causes infertility.

AA amyloid deposits gradually regress in the majority of patients whose inflammatory disease remains in remission, but the rate varies substantially between different individuals. These differences suggest that the amyloid deposits are more stable in some patients than in others, or that individuals simply differ in their capacity to mobilize amyloid. Renal function however, especially proteinuria, often improves even when the amyloid deposits only remain stable, and vice versa. Residual amyloid deposits may be present to a substantial extent in some patients who appear to have been in complete clinical remission for decades. This should be borne in mind since these patients often have rather brittle organ function and are at increased risk of acute renal failure in association with intercurrent stresses including hypovolaemia, surgery and pregnancy. In addition, the presence of even a small amount of amyloid may serve as a template for further rapid amyloid accumulation should there be a recrudescence of inflammatory activity.

Familial Mediterranean fever

FMF is an autosomal recessively inherited disorder, characterized by recurrent self-limiting episodes of fever, peritonitic abdominal pain, pleurisy, pericarditis or arthritis in association with marked migration of neutrophils into serosal spaces and a very intense acute phase response (Livneh *et al.*, 1997) (Table 20.2). Most cases present in childhood, and the attacks rarely start after the age of 20 years. Physical or psychological stress, a high fat diet and menstruation or pregnancy have been reported to precipitate attacks, but the majority of attacks appear to be triggered by sub-clinical stimuli. The sterile peritonitis of FMF typically lasts 12–72 hours, and is often severe enough to suggest a surgical acute abdomen. In some series 30 to 40% of patients underwent laparotomy for presumed appendicitis or cholecystitis before the diagnosis of FMF was made (Ben-Chetrit and Levy, 1998b). Although the disorder may occur in all populations it predominantly affects non-Ashkenazi Jews, Armenians, Turks and Levantine Arabs, and without treatment is complicated by typical systemic AA amyloidosis in as many as 90% of cases (Sohar *et al.*, 1967). A very small proportion of patients with FMF develop AA amyloidosis before they have experienced clinical FMF symptoms, presumably as a result of mounting an acute phase response to sub-clinical inflammatory disease.

Table 20.2 Tel-Hashomer criteria for the diagnosis of familial Mediterranean fever

	Major criteria	Minor criteria
1.	Recurrent febrile episodes accompanied by serositis or synovitis	1. Recurrent febrile episodes
2.	AA amyloidosis without a predisposing cause	2. Erysipelas like erythema
3.	Response to continuous colchicine prophylaxis	3. FMF in a first degree relative

Definite diagnosis: 2 major or 1 major and 2 minor criteria
Probable diagnosis: 1 major and 1 minor criteria

The gene associated with FMF, named *MEFV*, is located on the short arm of chromosome 16 and was identified by linkage studies and positional cloning by two groups in 1997 (Consortium, 1997a, Consortium, 1997b). The 10 exon gene is expressed only in cells of myeloid lineage, predominantly neutrophils, and it encodes a hitherto uncharacterized protein called pyrin or marenostrin. Analysis of *MEFV* has already greatly enhanced the diagnosis of FMF. More than 25 mutations in *MEFV* have now been associated with FMF, and pairs of *MEFV* mutations, presumed to involve both alleles, can be found in most FMF patients consistent with autosomal recessive inheritance. Most pathogenic mutations are in exon 10 but a number have been described in exons 2, 3, 5 and 9 (Livneh *et al.*, 1999). A few kindreds with autosomal dominantly inherited FMF have been described. FMF in successive generations usually has a pseudo–dominant basis due to a high frequency of healthy carriers in some populations, but certain compound mutations on a single *MEFV* allele, or simple heterozygous deletion of pyrin residue M694, are associated with genuine dominant transmission with variable penetrance. Notably, the mutation encoding this latter deletion has only been identified in the British population (Booth *et al.*, 2000).

Pyrin is thought to have a role in preventing neutrophil activation, or downregulating established neutrophil activity as part of a negative feedback process involved in the resolution of inflammation. It is likely that the *MEFV* mutations which cause FMF disrupt the structure of pyrin sufficiently to reduce its function leading to neutrophil activation and migration in situations that would not normally produce these effects. The recurrent acute nature of the clinical attacks along with massive influx of neutrophils into serosal and synovial linings would be consistent with bursts of relatively uncontrolled neutrophil activity. Patients with FMF often have prolonged periods of apparently normal health between their attacks suggesting that reduced pyrin function has clinical consequences only in certain circumstances.

One pyrin variant merits particular attention. The allele encoding pyrin E148Q occurs in up to 20% of the Mediterranean populations in which FMF is frequent, but has lately been shown to occur with a similar frequency in Indian and Chinese populations in which FMF is not well recognized. Indeed, pyrin E148Q has been identified in almost every population in which it has been sought, including at low levels in the British population. Although pyrin E148Q homozygotes do not suffer from FMF, the variant can cause the disease when it is coupled with more disruptive exon 10 *MEFV* mutations on the opposing allele. In addition, individuals with pyrin E148Q who have rheumatoid arthritis appear to be at substantially greater risk of developing AA amyloidosis, suggesting that it may augment the inflammatory response non-specifically. Recognition that pyrin E148Q occurs in hundreds of millions of individuals in different ethnic groups world–wide, coupled with the suggestion of an enhanced inflammatory response, suggests that the FMF trait may have conferred survival benefit during evolution.

Colchicine was serendipitously found to be a very effective treatment for FMF in 1972 (Goldfinger, 1972). Prophylactic use of the drug substantially inhibits the disease process in most cases, and prevents the risk of developing amyloidosis. Colchicine is concentrated in neutrophils and presumably inhibits the neutrophil migration which occurs during attacks (Bar-Eli *et al.*, 1981). A dose of 1 to 2 mg per day is sufficient in most patients, and the commonest cause of a poor response is non–compliance. It is remarkably safe in the long term at these doses, although can occasionally cause troublesome diarrhoea (Ben-Chetrit and Levy, 1998a). Colchicine therapy can lead to regression of amyloid in FMF, and improvement in renal function so long as renal failure is not too advanced (Livneh *et al.*, 1994). The dose of colchicine in FMF patients with amyloidosis should be titrated against frequent measurements of the plasma SAA concentration to ensure as complete suppression of inflammation as possible.

Systemic amyloidosis associated with plasma cell dyscrasia, AL amyloidosis

Associated conditions

AL amyloid fibrils are derived from monoclonal immunoglobulin light chains and AL amyloidosis can complicate most clonal B cell dyscrasias, including myeloma, lymphomas, macroglobulinaemia. AL amyloidosis develops in up to 15% of patients with myeloma, and although it occurs at a very much lower frequency among individuals with low grade and otherwise 'benign' monoclonal gammopathies, the latter are much more prevalent and underlie the majority (~80%) of cases. Indeed, the plasma cell dyscrasias in most cases of AL amyloidosis are much more subtle than those in the typical patient with so-called monoclonal gammopathy of undetermined significance. A monoclonal component can be identified in the serum or urine of 65% and 86% of AL patients respectively provided that very sensitive techniques such as immunofixation of concentrated urine are utilized. Sub-normal levels of some or all serum immunoglobulins ('immune paresis'), or increased numbers of marrow plasma cells may provide less direct clues to the underlying aetiology. However, in 14% of patients with confirmed AL amyloid no other evidence of the monoclonal gammopathy can be detected and this can lead to diagnostic confusion. On the other hand, low grade

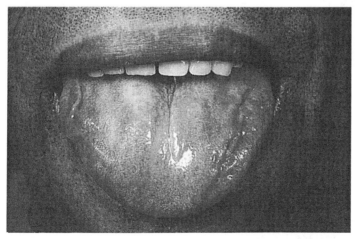

Fig. 20.1 Infiltration of soft tissues by AL amyloid producing macroglossia.

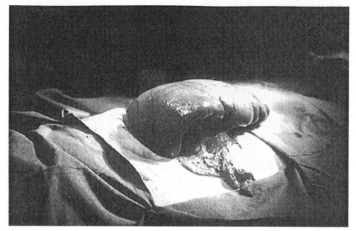

Fig. 20.2   A massively enlarged amyloidotic spleen.

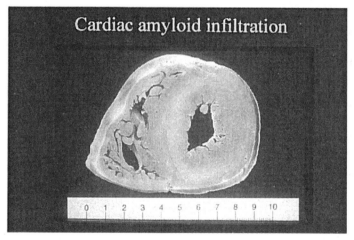

Fig. 20.3   AL amyloid infiltration of the heart with a thickened, pseudohypertrophied myocardium.

monoclonal gammopathies occur in up to 10% of the older population, and their presence in a patient with amyloidosis may be completely incidental.

Clinical features

AL amyloid usually occurs over age 50 years, although it can present in very young adults. Clinical manifestations are extremely variable since almost any organ other than the brain can be directly involved. Although certain clinical features are very strongly suggestive of AL amyloidosis, and multiple vital organ dysfunction is common, many patients present with non-specific symptoms such as malaise and weight loss. The outlook of untreated AL amyloid is far worse than AA type, with a 5-year survival of approximately 10% and a 10-year survival of less than 5%. Most affected individuals die of heart failure, uraemia, or some other effect of amyloid within 2 years of diagnosis. In most cases there is substantial histological cardiac involvement. Restrictive cardiomyopathy is the presenting feature in up to one-third of patients and causes death in one-half. Such patients may deteriorate dramatically if given venodilators and are best managed with diuretic based therapy. Although increased sensitivity to digoxin has been reported, possibly through the drug binding to amyloid fibrils, this is rarely a cause of clinical problems. Conduction defects may require cardiac pacing, and although arrhythmias are presumed to account for many cases of sudden death, rhythm disturbances beforehand are rarely documented, and evidence supporting the use of prophylactic anti-arrhythmic drugs is lacking. Renal involvement is frequent in AL amyloidosis and presents in the same manner as renal AA amyloid. Gut involvement can cause motility disturbances (often secondary to autonomic neuropathy), malabsorption, perforation, haemorrhage, or obstruction. Hyposplenism, usually in association with splenomegaly, is an occasional feature. Peripheral neuropathy occurs in one-fifth of cases and typically presents with a painful sensory polyneuropathy followed later by motor deficits. Carpal tunnel syndrome is present in 40%. Autonomic neuropathy causing orthostatic hypotension, impotence, and gastrointestinal disturbances may occur in isolation or with a peripheral neuropathy. Cutaneous involvement takes the form of papules, nodules, and plaques usually on the face and upper trunk, and involvement of dermal blood vessels results in purpura characteristically around the eyes. Macroglossia is infrequent, but is almost pathognomonic of AL type. Articular amyloid usually occurs in association with myeloma and may mimic rheumatoid or an asymmetric seronegative synovitis. Infiltration of peri-articular structures can cause large painful soft tissue masses, and glenohumeral joint involvement occasionally produces the distinctive 'shoulder pad' sign. A rare but potentially serious manifestation of AL amyloid is an acquired bleeding diathesis that may be associated with deficiency of factor X and sometimes also factor IX, or with increased fibrinolysis. SAP scan appearances are much more heterogeneous than those seen in AA type and any pattern of organ distribution may be seen. The only distinctive feature is bone marrow involvement which occurs in approximately 30% of cases and is pathognomonic of AL type. In contrast, the pattern of radiolabelled SAP uptake into the spleen, kidneys and adrenal glands, which occurs frequently in AA amyloidosis, occurs in less than 5% of patients with AL type.

Although AL amyloid is a progressive systemic disease, its clinical course is often punctuated by step-wise deteriorations, often terminating in multi-system failure. The lack of obvious disease progression from one clinic visit to the next may be falsely reassuring. In the very extensive Mayo Clinic experience (Kyle and Bayrd, 1975; Kyle and Greipp, 1983), comprising over 400 cases of AL amyloidosis, median survival was only 12–15 months and was even less when associated with multiple myeloma. Median survival is only about 6 months in cases where heart failure is evident at presentation (Kyle and Greipp, 1978). Other very poor prognostic factors include hyperbilirubinaemia, autonomic neuropathy, and a large whole body amyloid load on SAP scintigraphy.

Treatment

The aim of treatment in AL amyloidosis is to suppress proliferation of the underlying B-cell clone and, therefore, production of the amyloid fibril precursor protein. There are, however, many difficulties. Chemotherapy regimes are based on those used in multiple myeloma, but the plasma cell dyscrasias in most AL patients are relatively low grade and may be less chemosensitive. Diagnosis is difficult and can be delayed, and many patients have advanced multi-system disease which limits their options for chemotherapy. Regression of amyloid is a gradual process which may not lead to measurable clinical improvement or re-

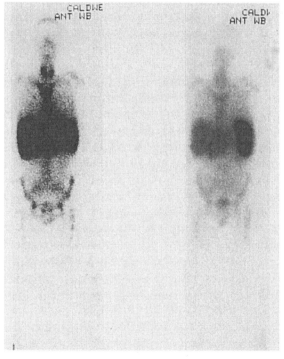

Fig. 20.4 Serial anterior whole body scintigraphic images following the injection of I[123]-labelled human SAP showing regression of AL amyloid following 4 cycles of intravenous chemotherapy. The initial scan shows extensive uptake in the bone marrow, liver and spleen (obscuring the renal deposits). Six months later following successful treatment with 'VAD' the liver deposits have dramatically decreased with less regression from the spleen and bone marrow.

covery of organ function for many months, or even years, after successful suppression of the causative plasma cell dyscrasia. Mobilization of amyloid from the heart is much slower than from the liver or kidneys, and many patients with cardiac or multi-system dysfunction do not live long enough to benefit from chemotherapy, even when it has suppressed their clonal disease. Moreover, it can be impossible to determine at an early stage whether the underlying plasma cell dyscrasia has been suppressed by treatment because of its subtle nature. However, despite these problems, many patients with AL amyloidosis do benefit substantially from chemotherapy. Prolonged low intensity cytotoxic regimes such as oral melphalan and prednisolone are beneficial in about 20% of patients (Kyle *et al.*, 1997), and dose intensive infusional chemotherapy regimes such as vincristine, doxorubicin (adriamycin) and dexamethasone ('VAD') (Wardley *et al.*, 1998; Persey *et al.*, 1996), and autologous peripheral blood stem-cell transplantation show far more promising early results (Gillmore *et al.*, 1998; Gertz *et al.*, 2000). However, very rigorous patient selection for high dose chemotherapy is essential because the procedure mortality is high in individuals with multiple organ involvement, especially patients with autonomic neuropathy, severe cardiac amyloidosis, or a history of gastrointestinal bleeding, and in those aged over 55 years.

Dialysis related amyloidosis (DRA), β₂-microglobulin amyloidosis

Associated conditions

The amyloid fibril precursor protein is β₂-microglobulin which is the invariant chain of the MHC class 1 molecule, and is expressed by all nucleated cells. It is synthesized at an average rate of 150 to 200 mg per day and in normal circumstances is freely filtered at the glomerulus and then reabsorbed and catabolized by the proximal tubular cells (Karlsson *et al.*, 1980). Decreasing renal function causes a proportionate rise in levels. β₂-microglobulin amyloidosis was first described in 1980 (Assenat *et al.*, 1980) and occurs only in patients who have been on dialysis for several years, or very occasionally in individuals with long-standing severe chronic renal impairment. DRA is better recognized in the haemodialysis population but also occurs in patients on CAPD. Relatively few patients have yet been maintained on peritoneal dialysis for the 5 to 10 years required to develop symptomatic β₂-microglobulin amyloid, but histological studies of early sub-clinical deposits suggest that the incidence of DRA is similar among patients receiving the two modalities of dialysis. Indeed, β₂-microglobulin amyloid deposits are present in 20 to 30% of patients within three years of commencing dialysis for end-stage renal failure (Jadoul *et al.*, 1998).

Clinical features

β₂-microglobulin amyloidosis is preferentially deposited in articular and peri-articular structures, and its manifestations are largely confined to the locomotor system (Drüeke, 2000). Carpal tunnel syndrome is usually the first clinical manifestation of β_2-microglobulin amyloidosis. Some individuals develop symptoms within 3 to 5 years and by 20 years the prevalence is almost 100% (Bardin *et al.*, 1986). Older patients appear to be more susceptible to the disease, and tend to exhibit symptoms more rapidly (Jadoul, 1998). Amyloid arthropathy tends to occur a little later but eventually affects most patients on dialysis (Drüeke, 1998). The arthalgia of β_2-microglobulin amyloidosis affects the shoulders, knees, wrists, and small joints of the hand and is associated with joint swelling, chronic tenosynovitis and, occasionally, haemarthroses. Spondylarthropathies are also well recognized, as is cervical cord compression. β_2-microglobulin amyloid deposition within the periarticular bone produces typical appearances of sub-chondral erosions and cysts, which can contribute to pathological fractures particularly of the femoral neck, cervical vertebrae and scaphoid. Although β_2-microglobulin amyloidosis is a systemic form of amyloid, manifestation outside the musculoskeletal system is rare, but there have been reports of β_2-microglobulin amyloidosis causing congestive cardiac failure, gastrointestinal bleeding, perforation or pseudo-obstruction and macroglossia (Maher *et al.*, 1988; Zhou *et al.*, 1991; Sethi *et al.*, 1989).

Treatment

The only really effective treatment for DRA is successful renal transplantation. Serum levels of β_2-microglobulin fall rapidly following transplantation and this is usually accompanied by a very rapid and substantial improvement in symptoms. Although prospective SAP scintigraphy has shown that β_2-microglobulin amyloid deposits can gradually regress, the resolution of DRA symptoms within days or weeks of renal transplantation implicates other factors. This probably includes the anti-inflammatory properties of immunosuppression after transplantation, and some effect of discontinuation of the dialysis procedure itself. In contrast to the symptoms, radiological bone cysts heal very slowly indeed (Tan *et al.*, 1996), and unsurprisingly amyloid can be demonstrated histologically many years after renal transplantation. Symptoms of DRA may reappear very rapidly if the graft is lost, providing further evidence that dialysis is required for the clinical expression of disease associated with β_2-microglobulin amyloid deposits. Possible explanations of this phenomenon are that newly deposited β_2-microglobulin amyloid is more damaging than old, or that the cytokine modulating effects of dialysis are involved. Certainly, β_2-microglobulin amyloid deposits are unusual in that they are often associated with a degree of inflammation and macrophage infiltration.

Attempts have been made to reduce β_2-microglobulin levels and DRA by altering the dialysis prescription. There is some evidence that the risks of DRA are increased in patients dialysed using less 'biocompatible' cuprophane membranes, and that use of the more permeable membrane systems is relatively protective (Miyata *et al.*, 1998). Greater removal of β_2-microglobulin is attained in patients undergoing high flux haemodiafiltration, and in the long term these patients may be less prone to DRA.

Drug treatment of established DRA includes non-steroidal anti-inflammatory analgesics, systemic and intra-articular corticosteroid therapy; but none of these are especially effective and long-term steroid therapy is particularly undesirable in this population of patients. Surgery may be required to relieve carpal tunnel compression, to stabilize the cervical spine or to treat bone fractures.

Hereditary amyloidosis

Familial amyloidotic polyneuropathy (FAP)

This is caused by point mutations in the gene encoding the plasma protein transthyretin (TTR) and is an autosomal dominant syndrome with peak onset between the third and sixth decades. The disease is characterized by progressive and disabling peripheral and autonomic neuropathy and varying degrees of visceral amyloid involvement. Severe cardiac amyloidosis is common. Deposits within the vitreous of the eye are recognized, but renal, thyroid, spleen, and adrenals deposits are usually asymptomatic. There are well-recognized foci in Portugal, Japan and Sweden and FAP has been reported in most ethnic groups throughout the world. There is considerable phenotypic variation in the age of onset, rate of progression, involvement of different systems and disease penetrance generally, although within families the pattern is often quite consistent. More than 70 variant forms of TTR are associated with FAP, the most frequent of which is the substitution of methionine for valine at residue 30.

Treatment

Until recently, the treatment of FAP was limited to supportive measures to help with malnutrition, bladder and bowel dysfunction, hypotension and renal and cardiac complications. Most patients died within 5–15 years of diagnosis. However, the situation has improved dramatically following the introduction of orthotopic liver transplantation in 1991 (Holmgren *et al.*, 1991). The procedure results in a rapid and near total replacement of the variant protein by donor wild type TTR, since almost all circulating TTR is produced by the liver. Most FAP patients who have liver transplants experience a symptomatic improvement within 6–12 months (Holmgren *et al.*, 1993), and successful liver transplantation has now been reported in hundreds of patients with this condition world-wide. Although the peripheral neuropathy usually only stabilizes, autonomic function can improves substantially and the associated visceral amyloid deposits have been shown by serial SAP scintigraphy to regress in most cases (Hawkins *et al.*, 1996; Rydh *et al.*, 1998). Important questions remain about the timing of the procedure but, so far, early intervention seems advisable.

Disappointingly in a few cases, there is evidence that wild-type TTR may continue to be deposited after liver transplantation, on the existing 'template' of

Generic therapies for amyloidosis

Inhibition of fibrillogenesis

Improved understanding of the protein folding mechanisms underlying amyloid fibrillogenesis, and the recognition that relative instability of the precursor molecules is a key factor in amyloidogenesis, strongly support therapeutic strategies based on inhibition of fibril formation. Many groups and companies are active in this area, exploring small molecules, peptides, and glycosaminoglycan analogues that bind to fibril precursors and stabilize their native fold, or interfere with refolding and/or aggregation into the cross-β core structure common to amyloid fibrils, or bind to mature amyloid fibrils and promote their refolding back towards the native conformation (Kisilevsky *et al.*, 1995; Merlini *et al.*, 1995; Peterson *et al.*, 1998; Soto, 1999). Some of these agents are reported to interfere with experimental murine AA amyloidosis and we look forward to evaluating them in patients with systemic amyloidosis.

Enhancement of amyloid regression: targeting SAP

Our own efforts to develop specific therapy for amyloidosis have focused on SAP, based on the long-standing observation that it is universally present in all types of amyloid deposit. SAP may provide a normal, autologous protein coat masking the abnormal amyloid fibrils from the scavenging processes that usually clear the tissues of abnormal material so efficiently, and the avid multivalent binding of SAP to amyloid fibrils must also stabilize the fibrils and assist their persistence. Furthermore, SAP itself is highly resistant to proteolysis (Kinoshita *et al.*, 1992), and we showed that binding of SAP to amyloid fibrils *in vitro* protects the fibrils from degradation by proteinases or phagocytic cells (Tennent, 1995). Finally, the role of SAP in amyloidogenesis was confirmed in SAP knockout mice, which failed to develop experimental AA amyloidosis normally (Botto *et al.*, 1997). These observations all support the idea that stripping SAP from amyloid deposits should facilitate their clearance, and we have been able to identify a drug compound that successfully achieves this objective *in vitro* and in animal models. The effect of this compound in patients with amyloidosis will be tested shortly and the results are eagerly awaited.

References

Ahlmen, M., Ahlmen, J., Svalander, C. and Bucht, H. (1987) *Clinical Rheumatology*, 6, 27–38.

Ansell, B.M., Eghtedari, A. and Bywaters, E.G. (1971) *Annals of the Rheumatic Diseases*, 30, 331.

Assenat, H., Calemard, E., Charra, B., Laurent, G., Terrat, J.C. and Vanel, T. (1980) *Nouvelle Presse Medicale*, 9, 1715.

Bardin, T., Zingraff, J., Kuntz, D. and Drüeke, T. (1986) *Nephrology, Dialysis, Transplantation*, 1, 151–4.

Bar-Eli, M., Ehrenfeld, M., Levy, M., Gallily, R. and Eliakim, M. (1981) *American Journal of the Medical Sciences*, 281, 15–18.

Baum, J. and Gutowska, G. (1977) *Arthritis and Rheumatism*, 20, 253–5.

Ben-Chetrit, E. and Levy, M. (1998a) *Seminars in Arthritis and Rheumatism*, 28, 48–59.

Ben-Chetrit, E. and Levy, M. (1998b) *Lancet*, 351, 659–64.

Benson, M.D., Liepnieks, J., Uemichi, T., Wheeler, G. and Correa, R. (1993) *Nature Genetics*, 3, 252–5.

Berglund, K., Keller, C. and Thysell, H. (1987) *Annals of the Rheumatic Diseases*, 46, 757–62.

Booth, D.R., Gillmore, J.D., Lachmann, H.J., Booth, S.E., Bybee, A., Soytürk, M., Akar, S., Pepys, M.B., Tunca, M. and Hawkins, P.N. (2000) *QJM*, 93, 217–21.

Booth, D.R., Tan, S.Y., Booth, S.E., Hsuan, J.J., Totty, N.F., Nguyen, O., Hutton, T., Vigushin, D.M., Tennent, G.A., Hutchinson, W.L., Thomson, N., Soutar, A.K., Hawkins, P.N. and Pepys, M.B. (1995) *QJM*, 88, 695–702.

Botto, M., Hawkins, P.N., Bickerstaff, M.C.M., Herbert, J., Bygrave, A.E., McBride, A., Hutchinson, W.L., Tennent, G.A., Walport, M.J. and Pepys, M.B. (1997) *Nature Medicine*, 3, 855–9.

Brunner, F.P., Giesecke, B., Gurland, H.J., Jacobs, C., Parsons, F.M., Scharer, K., Seyffart, G., Spies, G. and Wing, A.J. (1976) *Proceedings of the European Dialysis and Transplant Association*, 12, 2–64.

Consortium, T.F.F. (1997a) *Nature Genetics*, 17, 25–31.

Consortium, T.I.F. (1997b) *Cell*, 90, 797–807.

de la Chapelle, A., Tolvanen, R., Boysen, G., Santavy, J., Bleeker-Wagemakers, L., Maury, C.P.J. and Kere, J. (1992) *Nature Genetics*, 2, 157–60.

Drüeke, T. (2000) *Nephrology, Dialysis and Transplantation*, 15, 17–24.

Drüeke TB (1998) *Nephrology, Dialysis, Transplantation*, 13, 58–64.

Filipowicz-Sosnowska, A.M., Rostropowicz-Denisiewicz, K., Rosenthal, C.J. and Baum, J. (1978) *Arthritis and Rheumatism*, 21, 699–703.

Gertz, M.A., Kyle, R.A. and Greipp, P.R. (1991) *Blood*, 77, 257–62.

Gertz, M.A., Lacy, M.Q. and Dispenzieri, A. (2000) *Bone Marrow Transplantation*, 25, 465–70.

Gillmore, J.D., Booth, D.R., Rela, M., Heaton, N.D., Williams, R.S., Harrison, P. *et al.* (1999). In: R.A. Kyle and M.A Gertz (eds) *Amyloid and Amyloidosis 1998*, pp. 336–8, Parthenon Publishing, New York, Pearl River.

Gillmore, J.D., Davies, J., Iqbal, A., Madhoo, S., Russell, N.H. and Hawkins, P.N. (1998) *British Journal of Haematology*, 100, 226–8.

Goldfinger, W.E. (1972) *New England Journal of Medicine*, 287, 1302.

Gratacos, J., Orellana, C., Sanmarti, R., Sole, M., Collado, A., Gomez-Cassanovas, E., de Dios Canete, J. and Munoz-Gomez, J. (1997) *Journal of Rheumatology*, 24, 912–15.

Hamidi Asl, L., Fournier, V., Billerey, C., Justrabo, E., Chevet, D., Droz, D., Pecheux, C., Delpech, M. and Grateau, G. (1998) *Amyloid*, 5, 279–84.

Hamidi Asl, L., Liepnieks, J.J., Uemichi, T., Rebibou, J.M., Justrabo, E., Droz, D., Mousson, C., Chalopin, J.M., Benson, M.D., Delpech, M. and Grateau, G. (1997) *Blood*, 90, 4799–805.

Hawkins, P.N., Persey, M.R., Lovat, L.B., Madhoo, S., Stangou, A., McCarthy, M., Heaton, N., Williams, R. and Pepys, M.B. (1996) *Neuromuscular Disorders*, 6 (Suppl. 1), S77.

Hawkins, P.N., Richardson, S., Vigushin, D.M., David, J., Kelsey, C.R., Gray, R.E.S., Hall, M.A., Woo, P., Lavender, J.P. and Pepys, M.B. (1993) *Arthritis and Rheumatism*, 36, 842–51.

Holmgren, G., Ericzon, B.G., Groth, C.G., Steen, L., Suhr, O., Andersen, O., Wallin, B.G., Seymour, A., Richardson, S., Hawkins, P.N. and Pepys, M.B. (1993) *Lancet*, 341, 1113–16.

Holmgren, G., Steen, L., Ekstedt, J., Groth, C.G., Ericzon, B.G., Eriksson, S., Andersen, O., Karlberg, I., Norden, G., Nakazato, M., Hawkins, P., Richardson, S. and Pepys, M. (1991) *Clinical Genetics*, 40, 242–6.

Jacob, E.T. (1982) *Transplant Proceedings*, 14, 41.

Jacob, E.T., Bar-Nathan, N., Shapira, Z. and Gafni, J. (1979) *Archives of Internal Medicine*, 139, 1135–8.

Jadoul, M. (1998) *Nephrology, Dialysis, Transplantation*, 13, 61–4.

Jadoul, M., Garbar, C., Vanholder, R., Sennesael, J., Michel, C., Robert, A., Noel, H. and van Ypersele de Strihou, C. (1998) *Kidney International*, 54, 956–9.

Jones, L.A., Harding, J.A., Cohen, A.S. and Skinner, M. (1991). In: J.B. Natvig, Ø. Førre, G. Husby, A. Husebekk, B. Skogen, K. Sletten, and P.Westermark (eds) *Amyloid and Amyloidosis 1990*, pp. 385–8. Kluwer Academic Publishers, Dordrecht.

Karlsson, F.A., Groth, T., Sege, K., Wibell, L. and Peterson, P.A. (1980) *European Journal of Clinical Investigation*, 10, 293–300.

Kinoshita, C.M., Gewurz, A.T., Siegel, J.N., Ying, S.-C., Hugli, T.E., Coe, J.E., Gupta, R.K., Huckman, R. and Gewurz, H. (1992) *Protein Science*, 1, 700–9.

Kisilevsky, R., Lemieux, L.J., Fraser, P.E., Kong, X., Hultin, P.G. and Szarek, W.A. (1995) *Nature Medicine*, 1, 143–8.

Kyle, R.A. and Bayrd, E.D. (1975) *Medicine*, 54, 271–99.

Kyle, R.A., Gertz, M.A., Greipp, P.R., Witzig, T.E., Lust, J.A., Lacy, M.Q. and Therneau, T.M. (1997) *The New England Journal of Medicine*, 336, 1202–7.

Kyle, R.A. and Greipp, P.R. (1983) *Mayo Clinic Proceedings*, 58, 665–83.

Kyle, R.A. and Greipp, R.R. (1978) *Blood*, 52, 818–27.

Lindqvist, B., Andersen, S., Isacsson, B. and Lundberg, E. (1989) *International Urology and Nephrology*, 21, 555–9.

Livneh, A., Langevitz, P., Shinar, Y., Zaks, N., Kastner, D.L., Pras, M. and Pras, E. (1999) *Amyloid: International Journal of Experimental and Clinical Investigation.*, 6, 1–6.

Livneh, A., Langevitz, P., Zemer, D., Zaks, N., Kees, S., Lidar, T., Migdal, A., Padeh, S. and Pras, M. (1997) *Arthritis and Rheumatism*, 40, 1879–85.

Livneh, A., Zemer, D., Langevitz, P., Laor, A., Sohar, E. and Pras, M. (1994) *Arthritis and Rheumatism*, 37, 1804–11.

Luke, R.G., Allison, M.E., Davidson, J.F. and Duguid, W.P. (1969) *Annals of Internal Medicine*, 70, 1211–17.

Maher, E.R., Dutoit, S.H., Baillod, R.A., Sweny, P. and Moorhead, J.F. (1988) *BMJ*, 297, 265–6.

Merlini, G. (1997) *Amyloid: International Journal of Experimental and Clinical Investigation*, 4, 296–9.

Merlini, G., Ascari, E., Amboldi, N., Bellotti, V., Arbustini, E., Perfetti, V., Ferrari, M., Zorzoli, R., Marinone, M.G., Garini, P., Diegoli, M., Trizio, D. and Ballinari, D. (1995) *Proceedings of the National Academy of Sciences of the United States of America*, 92, 2959–63.

Miyata, T., Jadoul, M., Kurokawa, K. and van Ypersele de Strihou, C. (1998) *Journal of the American Society of Nephrology*, 9, 1723–35.

Ordi, J., Grau, J.M., Junque, A., Nomdedeu, B., Palacin, A. and Cardesa, A. (1993) *American Journal of Clinical Pathology*, 100, 394–7.

Ostertag, B. (1932) *Zentralblatt. Aug. Pathologie*, 56, 253–4.

Pasternack, A., Ahonen, J. and Kuhlback, B. (1986) *Transplantation*, 42, 598–601.

Pepys, M.B., Hawkins, P.N., Booth, D.R., Vigushin, D.M., Tennent, G.A., Soutar, A.K., Totty, N., Nguyen, O., Blake, C.C.F., Terry, C.J., Feest, T.G., Zalin, A.M. and Hsuan, J.J. (1993) *Nature*, 362, 553–7.

Perfetti, V., Bellotti, V., Maggi, A., Arbustini, E., De Benedetti, F., Paulli, M., Marinone, M.G. and Merlini, G. (1994) *American Journal of Hematology*, 46, 189–93.

Persey, M.R., Booth, D.R., Booth, S.E., van Zyl-Smit, R., Adams, B.K., Fattaar, A.B., Tennent, G.A., Hawkins, P.N. and Pepys, M.B. (1998) *Kidney International*, 53, 276–81.

Persey, M.R., Lovat, L.B., Apperley, J.F., Madhoo, S., Pepys, M.B. and Hawkins, P.N. (1996) *British Journal of Rheumatology*, 35 (Suppl. 1), 12.

Peterson, S.A., Klabunde, T., Lashuel, H.A., Purkey, H., Sacchettini, J.C. and Kelly, J.W. (1998) *Proceedings of the National Academy of Sciences of the United States of America*, 95, 12956–60.

Rydh, A., Suhr, O., Hietala, S.O., Åhlström, K.R., Pepys, M.B. and Hawkins, P.N. (1998) *European Journal of Nuclear Medicine*, 25, 709–13.

Schnitzer, T.J. and Ansell, B.M. (1977) *Arthritis and Rheumatism*, 20, 245–52.

Sethi, D., Cary, N.R., Brown, E.A., Woodrow, D.F. and Gower, P.E. (1989) *Nephrology, Dialysis, Transplantation*, 4, 1054–9.

Smith, M.E., Ansell, B.M. and Bywaters, E.G. (1968) *Annals of the Rheumatic Diseases*, 27, 137–45.

Sohar, E., Gafni, J., Pras, M. and Heller, H. (1967) *American Journal of Medicine*, 43, 227–53.

Soto, C. (1999) *Molecular Medicine Today*, 5, 343–50.

Soutar, A.K., Hawkins, P.N., Vigushin, D.M., Tennent, G.A., Booth, S.E., Hutton, T., Nguyen, O., Totty, N.F., Feest, T.G., Hsuan, J.J. and Pepys, M.B. (1992) *Proceedings of the National Academy of Sciences of the United States of America*, 89, 7389–93.

Svantesson, H., Akesson, A., Eberhardt, K. and Elborgh, R. (1983) *Scandinavian Journal of Rheumatology*, 12, 139–44.

Tan, S.Y., Irish, A., Winearls, C.G., Brown, E.A., Gower, P.E., Clutterbuck, E.J., Madhoo, S., Lavender, J.P., Pepys, M.B. and Hawkins, P.N. (1996) *Kidney International*, 50, 282–9.

Tennent, G.A. (1995). PhD Thesis, pp. 191. University of London, London, .

Uemichi, T., Liepnieks, J.J., Alexander, F. and Benson, M.D. (1996a) *QJM*, 89, 745–50.

Uemichi, T., Liepnieks, J.J., Yamada, T., Gertz, M.A., Bang, N. and Benson, M.D. (1996b) *Blood*, 87, 4197–203.

Uemichi, T., Liepnieks, J.J. and Benson, M.D. (1994) *Journal of Clinical Investigation*, 93, 731–6.

Uemichi, T., Liepnieks, J.J., Gertz, M.A. and Benson, M.D. (1998) *Amyloid*, 5, 188–92.

Vigushin, D.M., Pepys, M.B. and Hawkins, P.N. (1994) In: R. Kisilevsky, M.D. Benson, B. Frangione, J. Gauldie, T.J Muckle and I.D. Young (eds) *Amyloid and Amyloidosis 1993*, pp. 48–50. Parthenon Publishing, New York.

Wardley, A.M., Jayson, G.C., Goldsmith, D.J., Venning, M.C., Ackrill, P. and Scarffe, J.H. (1998) *British Journal of Cancer*, 78, 774–6.

Zhou, H., Pfeifer, U. and Linke, R. (1991) *Virchows Archiv – A, Pathology Anatomy and Histopathology*, 419, 349–53.

21

Primary amyloidosis

Robert A. Kyle

Although amyloid appears homogeneous and amorphous under the light microscope, it actually consists of rigid, linear, nonbranching, aggregated fibrils 7.5–10 mm wide and of indefinite length. The unique staining and optical features are due to arrangement of the fibrils in an anti-parallel or cross beta-pleated sheet configuration. Congo red is considered the most specific stain, which when viewed with a polarized light source, produces apple-green birefringence. Electron microscopy reveals a fibrillar pattern. The amyloid fibrils which are deposited extracellularly generally resist proteolytic digestion. This leads to loss of normal tissue elements and ultimately organ failure. Excellent reviews of amyloidosis have been published (1)(2).

All types of amyloidosis appear the same with Congo red staining and upon electron microscopy. However, the fibrils in primary amyloidosis (AL) consist of the variable portion of a monoclonal light chain (kappa or lambda); secondary amyloidosis (AA) fibrils consist of protein A, a nonimmunoglobulin; familial amyloidosis fibrils are usually composed of mutated transthyretin (prealbumin); senile systemic amyloid fibrils consist of normal transthyretin and amyloid associated with long-term dialysis consists of beta-2-microglobulin (β_2-M) (Table 21.1). The remainder of this chapter will be limited to primary amyloidosis.

Table 21.1 Systemic amyloidosis: immunohistochemical identification

	Congo red	Kappa/ Lambda	Protein A	β_2M	Transthyretin (Prealbumin)
AL	+	+	−	−	−
AA	+	−	+	−	−
FMF	+	−	+	−	−
AD	+	−	−	+	−
AF	+	−	−	−	+
SSA	+	−	−	−	+

Abbreviations: FMF, familial Mediterranean fever; AD, dialysis amyloidosis; AF, familial amyloidosis; SSA, senile systemic amyloidosis; AL, light chain amyloidosis; AA, secondary amyloidosis.

Clinical features

The incidence of AL is 0.9 per 100,000/year. AL accounts for 89% of our amyloid practice (Fig. 21.1). The median age is 65 years with only 1% younger than age 40 at diagnosis. Weakness, fatigue and loss of weight are the most common symptoms. The median weight loss is over 10 kg; some patients lose 20–25 kg without apparent cause. Purpura, particularly in the periorbital and facial areas, is present in one-sixth of patients. Occasionally amyloid involvement of the hands mimics seronegative rheumatoid arthritis. Deposits of amyloid in periarticular areas of the shoulders may produce pain, swelling and prominence (shoulder pad sign). Extensive deposits of amyloid may produce pseudohypertrophy of skeletal muscles. Dyspnoea, pedal edema, paresthesias, light-headedness and syncope may be troublesome. Impotence may occur. Hoarseness or weakness of the voice may be a prominent feature.

The liver is palpable at diagnosis in one-fourth of patients while splenomegaly is present initially in only 5%. Macroglossia occurs in about 10%. Generalized lymphadenopathy is infrequent. The skin is fragile and easily traumatized. Edema from nephrotic syndrome or congestive heart failure is common. Paresthesias and jaw or hip claudication may be distressing. Signs and symptoms of nephrotic syndrome, renal failure, congestive heart failure, peripheral neuropathy, carpal tunnel syndrome and orthostatic hypotension must be sought during the history and physical examination.

Nephrotic syndrome or renal insufficiency is the presenting symptom in more than one-fourth of patients while carpal tunnel syndrome occurs in one-fifth. Congestive heart failure is the major feature at diagnosis in one-sixth of patients while peripheral neuropathy is present as the major manifestation in about 15%.

Laboratory features

Anemia is not a prominent feature unless the patient has renal failure, multiple myeloma or gastrointestinal bleeding. Thrombocytosis occurs in 10% of patients. Renal insufficiency is found in almost one-half at diagnosis and the serum creatinine is > 2 mg/dL in 20% (3).

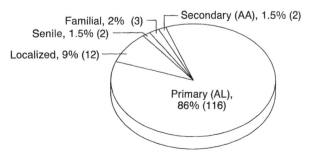

Fig. 21.1 Types of amyloidosis seen at the Mayo Clinic in 1999.

The serum protein electrophoretic pattern shows a localized band or spike in one-half but the size of the M-protein is modest (1.4 g/dL). Immunofixation of the serum shows a monoclonal protein in 70%. Approximately 25% have only free monoclonal light chains (Bence Jones proteinemia). Lambda light chains are twice as common as kappa. Immunofixation of the serum and urine reveals a monoclonal protein in almost 90% of patients.

About a fifth of patients have bone marrow plasmacytosis of 20% or more but the median value is only 7%. The electrocardiogram shows low voltage or loss of typical anterior septal forces mimicking the findings of myocardial infarction. The echocardiogram is abnormal in two-thirds of patients at diagnosis. The major features are increased thickness of the ventricular walls, abnormal myocardial texture, atrial enlargement, valvular thickening and regurgitation, pericardial effusion, and abnormal diastolic function. Ultimately reduced systolic ventricular function occurs.

Renal involvement

Nephrotic syndrome or renal failure was present in 30% of 474 patients at diagnosis (3). Many patients present with nephrotic-range proteinuria, hypercholesterolemia and edema but with a normal creatinine level. Hypoalbuminemia is common and results in low serum oncotic pressure with loss of fluid from the intravascular space into the extravascular space producing edema. The extent of amyloid deposits in the kidney biopsy specimen correlates poorly with the degree of proteinuria (4). Although the earlier literature suggests that the kidneys are enlarged in amyloid, most patients have normal-sized kidneys by ultrasonography. The adult Fanconi syndrome, renal vein thrombosis, retroperitoneal fibrosis and priapism have been reported.

Diagnosis

The possibility of AL must be considered in every patient who has an M-protein in the serum or urine and who also has an unexplained nephrotic syndrome, renal insufficiency, congestive heart failure, sensorimotor peripheral neuropathy, carpal tunnel syndrome, hepatomegaly or malabsorption. In fact the presence of a monoclonal light chain in the urine of a patient with nephrotic syndrome is almost always due to AL or light-chain deposition disease.

The diagnosis requires the demonstration of amyloid deposits. Congo red staining of tissue produces an apple-green birefringence under polarized light (5). The use of antisera to kappa, lambda, protein A, transthyretin and beta-2-microglobulin is the best approach for diagnosis and a proper classification.

An abdominal fat aspirate is positive in 70% of patients. The specimen must be stained properly with Congo red and interpreted by an experienced pathologist. Extraction of amyloid from the abdominal fat biopsy may be utilized for chemical characteristic of the amyloid type (6). A bone marrow aspirate and biopsy should be performed initially to determine the number of plasma cells and document whether they are monoclonal. The bone marrow biopsy is positive for amyloid in 55% of patients. Almost 90% of patients with AL will have a positive result with subcutaneous fat biopsy or bone marrow. If these tissues are negative, rectal biopsy including the submucosa may be done. If these sites are negative and the physician is still suspicious of amyloidosis, tissue should be obtained from a suspected organ. Biopsy of the kidney, liver, sural nerve, carpal ligament, endomyocardium or small intestine are all associated with a high percentage of positivity (3). I^{123}-labelled serum amyloid P component (I^{123}-SAP) scintigraphy can be used for identifying and monitoring the extent of systemic amyloidosis but it is not readily available (2).

Because minimal histologic evidence of amyloid can be associated with nephrotic syndrome, the biopsy specimens must be viewed carefully for the presence of Congo red deposits. The increased uptake of ^{99m}Tc-pyrophosphate is not a reliable diagnostic approach.

The differential diagnosis includes immunotactoid glomerulopathy (7). In this condition the width of the fibrils is twice that found in AL. Furthermore, extrarenal disease never develops and the deposits are not Congo red positive. Proteinuria is common but no M-protein is found. Light-chain deposition disease is characterized by the presence of non amyloid light chains which appear under electron microscopy as granules in the kidney. It can produce nephrotic syndrome and renal insufficiency. Occasionally the heart and liver may be involved from the light chain deposits.

Therapy

Because amyloid fibrils consist of monoclonal immunoglobulin light chains, treatment with alkylating agents which are effective against plasma cell neoplasms is warranted. Results of a randomized, placebo controlled, double blind study of 55 patients with primary systemic amyloidosis suggested treatment with melphalan and prednisone was of some benefit (8). In a prospective randomized study of 220 patients conducted at our institution, patients were randomized to receive: 1) colchicine, melphalan and prednisone; 2) melphalan and prednisone; or 3) colchicine alone. Patients were stratified according to their major clinical manifestation, age and sex. The median duration of survival was 8.5 months for the colchicine treated group, 18 months for the melphalan and prednisone group, and 17 months for the melphalan, prednisone, and colchicine group ($p < 0.001$). Among patients who had a reduction in serum or urine monoclonal protein at 12 months, the overall length of survival was 50 months, whereas among those without a reduction at 12 months, the overall length of survival was 36 months ($p = 0.03$). Thirty-four patients (15%) survived for five years or longer.

Measurement of response included improvement in renal function as demonstrated by a 50% decrease in the 24-hour urine protein excretion in the absence of progressive renal insufficiency when the patient presented with nephrotic syndrome; a reduction in the size of the liver by at least 2 cm and a 50% decrease in serum alkaline phosphatase; disappearance of serum monoclonal protein or a reduction of more than 50%; disappearance of urinary monoclonal protein or a decrease of more than 50%; an increase of at least 1 g/dL in serum albumin given an initial value of < 3 g/dL, and improvement in the echocardiogram with a 2 mm reduction in the thickness of the interventricular septum or an increase of 20 percentage points in the ejection fraction (9). In an effort to determine if more intensive therapy was beneficial, 101 patients were randomized to either melphalan and prednisone or a combination of drugs (vincristine, BCNU, melphalan, cyclophosphomide and prednisone) (VBMCP). Therapy with the multiple alkylating agents did not result in a higher response rate or longer survival time when compared with standard melphalan and prednisone (10). In addition, treatment with alkylating agents may be associated with myelodysplastic syndrome or acute leukemia. High-dose dexamethasone produces some benefit in 15–20% of patients. Vitamin E and alpha-2 interferon have not been beneficial. The use of 4′-iodo-4′-deoxydoxorubicin, which has an affinity for amyloid deposits, may aid in their dissolution (11).

The use of dose-intensive melphalan (200 mg/m^2) followed by peripheral blood stem cell transplant is a promising approach. At a median follow-up of 24 months, 68% of 25 patients were alive. Almost two-thirds evaluated at three months post-transplant had a response (12). The use of a smaller dose of melphalan (100 mg/m$_2$) for older patients or those with reduced renal function appears to be well tolerated and beneficial (13). The role of autologous stem cell transplantation for AL amyloidosis has recently been reviewed (14). Selection of patients for autologous stem cell transplant plays a significant role in survival. In a review of 1288 patients with AL, 234 met eligibility criteria (biopsy proof of AL, clinical absence of multiple myeloma, age < 70 years, cardiac interventricular septal thickness < 15 mm, cardiac ejection fraction > 55%, creatinine < 2 mg/dL, alkaline phosphatase < three times normal and direct bilirubin < 2 mg/dL. The 234 patients who fulfilled the criteria were treated with conventional alkylating agent therapy. The median survival was 45.6 months (15). Thus, selection of AL patients plays a major role in survival.

General treatment measures

The nephrotic syndrome should be treated with salt restriction and diuretics as needed. Furosemide is usually satisfactory but occasionally the addition of metolazone is helpful. Albumin infusions are not useful for long-term treatment of edema because they are of only transient benefit and are very expensive. Diuretic therapy can produce volume contraction and a decrease in cardiac output as well as orthostatic syncope.

Long-term dialysis is necessary when azotemia develops. Hypotension may be a problem with hemodialysis and the rapid fluid shifts can be intolerable for patients with associated congestive heart failure. Long-term ambulatory peritoneal dialysis may be useful in this setting. Neither type of dialysis is superior to the other. The median duration of survival for patients who begin dialysis is less than one year. The most common cause of death is cardiac rather than renal failure (16). Renal transplantation has been a benefit in a number of patients but there is a serious shortage of organ donors. Amyloid will often deposit in the transplanted kidney. Rarely, bilateral embolization of the renal artery has been performed for therapy-resistant nephrotic syndrome.

The management of cardiac amyloidosis is mainly with diuretics such as furosemide. Diuretic therapy is frequently limited by hypotension, low ejection fraction or autonomic insufficiency. Patients with cardiac amyloidosis may be very sensitive to calcium-channel blockers and consequently these agents should be avoided. Digoxin should be limited to the control of supraventricular tachycardias or arrhythmias but not for congestive heart failure. A pacemaker is required for symptomatic bradyarrhythmias.

Sensorimotor peripheral neuropathy is generally not benefited by alkylating agent therapy. The neurologic symptoms and findings usually continue to worsen in most patients. Dysthesias tend to disappear as the sensory involvement worsens. Analgesics and sedatives may be needed, depending on kind and severity of symptoms. Amitriptyline and fluphenazine have been helpful for some patients. The dysthesias may be sufficiently distressing to require narcotics for control. Codeine is useful and the long-term risks of habituation and tolerance are modest.

Treatment of orthostatic hypotension is challenging. Patients should rise slowly and sit on the edge of the bed for a few minutes before assuming an upright position. Elastic support extending to the waist (leotards) may be of some help. Fludrocortisone is often associated with increased fluid retention. Midodrine or L-THREO-3, 4-dihydroxyphenylserine (L-THREO-DOPS) may be of some benefit. Octreotide may be of help in the management of both autonomic induced diarrhoea and orthostatic hypotension. Decompression of the carpal ligament relieves the pain of carpal tunnel syndrome but residual sensory loss is frequent.

Patients with macroglossia frequently have obstructive sleep apnea and this may be treated with nasal continuous positive airway pressure. Airway obstruction can be managed by permanent tracheostomy. Resection of the tongue is not advised because of bleeding. Furthermore, the remaining tongue frequently enlarges following surgery. Gastrointestinal bleeding or perforation may occur. Patients with intestinal pseudo-obstruction must not be treated surgically because resection does not relieve the obstructive symptoms and complications are common.

References

1. Falk R.H., Comenzo R.L., Skinner M. The systemic amyloidosis. *N Eng J Med* 1997, 337: 898–909.
2. Gillmore J.D., Hawkins P.N., Pepys M.B. Amyloidosis: A review of recent diagnostic and therapeutic developments. *Br J Haem* 1997, 99: 245–56.
3. Kyle R.A. and Gertz M.A. Primary systemic amyloidosis: clinical and laboratory features in 474 cases. *Sem Hemat* 1995, 32: 45–59.

4. Watanabe T., Saniter T. Morphological and clinical features of renal amyloidosis. *Virchows Arch A Pathol Anat Histopathol* 1975, 366: 125.
5. Westermark G.T., Johnson K.H. and Westermark P. Staining methods for identification of amyloid in tissue. *Meth Enzymol* 1999, 309: 3–25.
6. Kaplan B., Hrncic R., Murphy C., Gallo G., Weiss D.T., Solomon A. Microextraction and purification techniques applicable to chemical characterization of amyloid proteins in minute amounts of tissue. *Meth Enzymol* 1999, 309: 67–81.
7. Korbert S.M., Schwartz M.M., Rosenberg B.E. *et al.* Immunotactoid glomerulopathy. *Medicine (Baltimore)* 1985, 64: 228.
8. Kyle R.A., Greipp P.R. Primary systemic amyloidosis: comparison of melphalan and prednisone versus placebo. *Blood* 1978, 52: 818–27.
9. Kyle R.A., Gertz M.A., Greipp P.R., Witzig T.E., Lust J.A., Lacy M.Q. *et al.* A trial of three regimens for primary amyloidosis: colchicine alone, melphalan and prednisone, and melphalan, prednisone, and colchicine. *N Engl J Med* 1997, 336: 1202–7.
10. Gertz M.A., Lacy M.Q., Lust J.A., Greipp P.R., Witzig T.E., Kyle R.A. Prospective randomized trial of melphalan and prednisone versus vincristine, carmustine, melphalan, cyclophosphamide and prednisone in the treatment of primary systemic amyloidosis. *J Clin Oncol* 1999, 17: 262–7.
11. Merlini G., Anesi E., Garini P., Perfetti V., Obici L., Ascari E. *et al.* Treatment of AL amyloidosis with 4′-iodo-4′-deoxydoxorubicin: An update. *Blood* 1999, 93: 1112–13.
12. Comenzo R.L., Vosburgh E., Falk R.H., Sanchorawala V., Reisinger J., Dubrey S. *et al.* Dose-intensive melphalan with blood stem-cell support for the treatment of A.L. (amyloid light-chain) amyloidosis: survival and responses in 25 patients. *Blood* 1998, 91: 3662–70.
13. Comenzo R.L., Sanchorawala V., Fisher C., Akpek G., Farhat M., Cerda S. *et al.* Intermediate-dose intravenous melphalan and blood stem cells mobilized with sequential GM+G-CSF or G-CSF alone to treat AL (amyloid light chain) amyloidosis. *Br J Haem* 1999, 104: 553–9.
14. Moreau P. Autologous stem cell transplantation for AL amyloidosis: a standard therapy? *Leukemia* 1999, 13: 1929–31.
15. Dispenzieri A., Lacy M.Q., Kyle R.A., Greipp P.R., Witzig T.E., Lust J.A. *et al.* Eligibility for PBSCT for AL amyloidosis is a favorable independent prognostic factor for survival: Survival of 234 patients with primary systemic amyloidosis (AL) functionally eligible for peripheral blood stem cell transplantation. *Proceed Am Soc Clin Oncol* 1999, 18: 20a.
16. Gertz M.A., Kyle R.A., O'Fallon W.M. Dialysis support of patients with primary systemic amyloidosis. A study of 211 patients. *Arch Intern Med* 1992, 152: 2245–50.

22

Light-chain and heavy-chain deposition diseases

Pierre Ronco

Definition

It was known from the late 1950s that nonamyloidotic forms of glomerular disease 'resembling the lesion of diabetic glomerulosclerosis', could occur in multiple myeloma. The presence of monoclonal light chains (LC) in these lesions was recognized in 1973 by Antonovych *et al.*, and confirmed in 1976 by Randall and associates (Randall *et al.* 1976) who published the first description of light-chain deposition disease (LCDD).

Monoclonal heavy chains were found together with light chains in the tissue deposits from some patients, thus defining light and heavy-chain deposition disease (LHCDD). More recently, deposits containing monoclonal heavy chains only were observed in patients affected with otherwise typical Randall's disease (Aucouturier *et al.* 1993); they define heavy-chain deposition disease (HCDD), which must be differentiated from heavy chain disease, a lymphoproliferative disorder in which renal involvement has infrequently been reported.

In clinical and pathological terms, LCDD, LHCDD, and HCDD are basically similar, and are therefore also referred to as monoclonal immunoglobulin deposition disease (MIDD). They differ from amyloidosis by the lack of affinity for Congo red and of fibrillar organization.

Epidemiology

MIDD occurs in a wide range of ages (26 to 79 years) with a slight male preponderance. It is found in 5% of myeloma patients at autopsy, while the prevalence of AL-amyloidosis is about 11% (Ivanyi *et al.* 1990). However, myeloma accounts for only 45% of LCDD, but as in amyloidosis, a monoclonal plasma cell proliferation can be demonstrated in virtually all patients by immunofluorescence examination of the bone marrow. We are aware of 20 patients with HCDD, so far, but it is likely that diagnosis of HCDD is markedly underestimated.

Pathogenesis

MIDD is characterized by kidney deposition of monoclonal immunoglobulin components, followed by a dramatic accumulation of extracellular matrix. That light-chain deposition involves unusual light-chain properties is supported by the absence of detectable monoclonal free light chain in the serum and the urine in 15% to 30% of LCDD patients, the recurrence of the disease in the transplanted kidney, the biosynthesis of abnormal (short or apparently large) light chains by bone marrow cells (Preud'homme *et al.* 1980), and the fact that discrete changes in the variable region (V_L) sequence are responsible for light-chain deposition in a mouse experimental model. However, light-chain deposition does not mean pathogenicity since after mouse injection, one-third (14/40) of light chains from patients with myeloma or AL-amyloidosis become deposited in basement membranes (Solomon *et al.* 1991). Thus, singular properties of light chain are most likely required for completion of the pathogenetic process leading to kidney fibrosis.

The following properties of monoclonal light chain may contribute to MIDD pathogenesis. The first is the restricted usage of three κ germline genes. Second, size abnormalities of light chains have been documented in 9 out of 22 patients by bone marrow biosynthesis experiments (Preud'homme *et al.* 1994). Third, there is a tight correlation between the absence of detectable circulating and urinary light chains, and their glycosylation that most likely increases their propensity to precipitate in tissues. Fourth, unusual amino-acid substitutions have been identified in primary structures of LCDD light chains, mostly in peptide loops corresponding to complementarity determining regions (CDRs), i.e. parts of the molecules normally implicated in antigen binding.

In the nine HCDD patients in whom a structural analysis of the heavy chain was performed, a deletion of the first constant domain $C_H 1$ was observed and associated in two cases with a larger deletion involving the hinge region and the $C_H 2$ (Moulin *et al.* 1999). In the blood, the deleted heavy chain was associated with light chains, mostly of the λ isotype, or circulated in small amounts as a free unassembled subunit. It is likely that the $C_H 1$ deletion facilitates the secretion of free unassembled or partially assembled heavy chains that are rapidly cleared from the circulation by organ deposition. In addition, sequence analysis of two HCDD proteins showed unusual residues in CDR and framework regions of the V_H (Khamlichi *et al.* 1995). Conformational singularities of the V_H probably contribute to heavy-chain deposition and are also most likely responsible for the granular aspect or fibrillar organization of the deposits found in HCDD and the rare patients with heavy-chain amyloidosis, respectively.

Another common feature shared by LCDD and HCDD is the dramatic accumulation of a qualitatively normal extracellular matrix. A role for TGF-β is supported by its strong expression in glomeruli of MIDD patients, and by *in vitro* experiments using cultured mesangial cells (Zhu *et al.* 1995). Because of the similarities between MIDD- and diabetes-induced nodular glomerulosclerosis, including the strong periodic acid-Schiff reagent (PAS) reactivity of the lesions, it has been suggested that immunoglobulin chains might stimulate mesangial cells in a similar manner to advanced glycosylation end-products.

Pathology

Light microscopy

In virtually all patients with MIDD, tubular lesions are characterized by the deposition of a refractile, eosinophilic, PAS-positive, ribbon-like material along the outer part of the tubular basement membrane. The deposits predominate around the distal tubules, loops of Henle, and, in some instances, around the collecting ducts. The epithelia of involved tubules are flattened and atrophied. In advanced stages, a marked interstitial fibrosis including refractile deposits is frequently associated with tubular lesions.

Glomerular lesions are more heterogeneous; nodular glomerulosclerosis resembling diabetic glomerulosclerosis the most characteristic (Fig. 22.1a), but it is found in only two-thirds of LCDD patients. Nodules are composed of membrane-like material with nuclei at the periphery. The capillary loops stretch at the periphery of florid nodules and may undergo aneurysmal dilatation. Milder glomerular forms simply show an increase in mesangial matrix and sometimes in mesangial cells, and a modest thickening of the basement membranes.

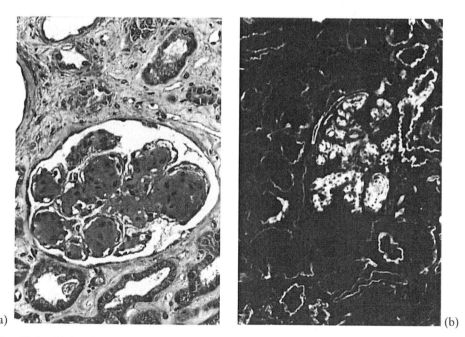

(a)　　　　　　　　　　　　　　　　　　　　(b)

Fig. 22.1 Light-chain deposition disease. (a) Nodular glomerulosclerosis with mesangial matrix accumulation ((Masson trichrome staining, ×312). (b) Bright staining of mesangial nodules and tubular basement membranes with anti-κ antibody (immunofluorescence, ×125), (Béatrice Mougenot's personal collection).

Glomerular lesions may also not be detected by light microscopy but require ultrastructural examination.

Arteries, arterioles and peritubular capillaries all may contain deposits in close contact with their basement membranes.

Immunofluorescence

A key step in the diagnosis of the various forms of MIDD is immunofluorescence examination of biopsy specimens which all show evidence of monotypic light (Fig. 22.1b) and/or heavy chain (Fig. 22.2) fixation along basement membranes. These criteria are mandatory for the diagnosis of MIDD. In contrast with AL-amyloidosis, the κ isotype is more frequent and detected in about 80% of patients with LCDD. In addition, examination with anti-heavy-chain antisera of biopsy specimens that did not stain for light chain has permitted both the identification of HCDD as a separate entity and heavy chain C-domain deletions (Fig. 22.2).

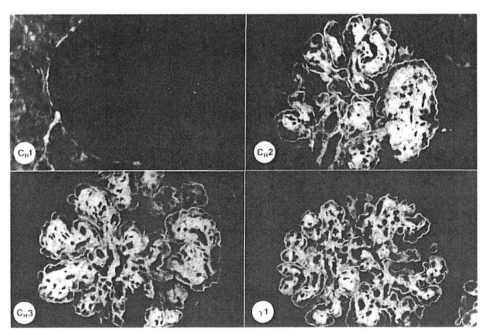

Fig. 22.2 Heavy-chain deposition disease. Nodular glomerulosclerosis. Mesangial and parietal deposits stain with a monoclonal antibody specific for the γ1 isotype in the absence of detectable light chain (bottom right). Immunofluorescence with a panel of monoclonal antibodies directed to the various constant domains of the γ heavy chain shows that glomerular deposits are stained with anti-C_H2 and anti-C_H3 but not with anti-C_H1 antibodies (×312), (Béatrice Mougenot's personal collection).

The tubular deposits stain strongly (Fig. 22.1b) and predominate along the loops of Henle and the distal tubules. In contrast, the pattern of glomerular immunofluorescence displays marked heterogeneity. In patients with nodular glomerulosclerosis, deposits of monotypic immunoglobulin chains are usually found along the peripheral glomerular basement membranes and to a lesser extent in the nodules themselves (Fig. 22.1b). In some cases, glomerular immunofluorescence is negative despite the presence of large amounts of granular glomerular deposits as seen by electron microscopy. Deposits of immunoglobulin chains are constantly found in vascular walls.

In the 20 patients with HCDD studied so far, immunofluorescence with anti-light-chain antibodies was negative despite typical nodular glomerulosclerosis. Kidney deposits were of the $\gamma 1$, $\gamma 4$, $\gamma 3$ and $\gamma 2$ subclasses, and the α class in seven, five, four, one, and three patients, respectively. In the eight biopsy specimens studied with monoclonal antibodies specific for γ-chain constant domains, the $C_H 1$ domain epitopes were undetectable (Fig. 22.2) in agreement with immunochemical analysis of the patients' serum and urine.

Electron microscopy

The most characteristic ultrastructural feature is the presence of finely or coarse granular electron-dense deposits that delineate the outer aspect of the tubular basement membranes. Glomerular lesions are characterized by the deposition of a nonfibrillar electron-dense material in the mesangial nodules and along the glomerular basement membrane.

Clinical manifestations

There are a number of clinical manifestations of MIDD (Ganeval *et al.* 1982; Confalonieri *et al.* 1988; Buxbaum *et al.* 1990; Heilman *et al.* 1992) because LCDD involves deposition of immunoglobulin light chains along basement membranes of a variety of organs. Light-chain deposition in these organs may be, however, totally asymptomatic. In HCDD, extrarenal deposits have only been described in two out of 20 patients, in the liver, the thyroid follicles, the skin, and the muscle (Aucouturier *et al.* 1993; Rott *et al.* 1988). A third patient presented with seronegative rheumatoid arthritis and $\gamma 3$-chain deposits in synovial tissue (Husby *et al.* 1998).

Renal manifestations

Renal involvement is a constant feature of MIDD, and renal symptoms, mostly proteinuria and renal failure, often dominate the clinical presentation. In 23% to 67% of LCDD patients, albuminuria is associated with the nephrotic syndrome. In 25%, the albumin loss is less than 1 g/day, and these patients exhibit mainly a tubulointerstitial syndrome. Haematuria is more frequent (44%) than one would expect for a nephropathy in which cell proliferation is usually modest.

Renal failure is remarkable for its high prevalence (89%), early appearance and severity, irrespective of urinary albumin output. It may present in the form of a subacute tubulointerstitial nephritis or a rapidly progressive glomerulonephritis, respectively. The prevalence of hypertension is variable, but it must be interpreted according to associated medical history.

Extrarenal manifestations

Liver and cardiac involvement are the most common extrarenal features of LCDD. Liver deposits are constant. They are either discrete and confined to sinusoids and basement membranes of biliary ductules without associated parenchymal lesions or they are massive with marked dilatation and multiple ruptures of sinusoids, resembling peliosis. Hepatomegaly and mild alterations of liver function are the most usual symptoms, but patients may also develop life-threatening hepatic insufficiency and portal hypertension.

Heart involvement also appears to be frequent, and may be responsible for cardiomegaly and severe heart failure. As in the kidney and liver, monotypic light-chain deposits in the vascular walls and perivascular areas of the heart were seen in all autopsy cases when examined with immunofluorescence.

Deposits may also occur along the nerve fibres and in the choroid plexus, as well as in the lymph nodes, bone marrow, spleen, pancreas, thyroid gland, submandibular glands, adrenal glands, gastrointestinal tract, abdominal vessels, lungs and skin.

Haematologic findings

The most common underlying disease in MIDD is myeloma. MIDD is often the presenting disease leading to the discovery of myeloma at an early stage. Some patients who presented with common myeloma and with normal-sized monoclonal immunoglobulin in the absence of kidney disease developed LCDD and immunoglobulin structural abnormalities when the myeloma relapsed after chemotherapy. MIDD can rarely complicate Waldenström's macroglobulinemia. It often occurs in the absence of a detectable malignant process, even after prolonged (more than 10 years) follow-up. In such 'primary' forms, a monoclonal bone marrow plasma cell population is easily detected by cytoplasmic immunofluorescence and bone marrow biosynthesis experiments. It is worth noting that in 15% to 30% of patients with LCDD, there is no detectable monoclonal immunoglobulin in the serum and urine, although an immunoglobulin light chain is deposited in those patients' tissues.

Among the 20 patients with HCDD (reviewed in Moulin *et al.* 1999, and Kambham *et al.* 1999), only four had a myeloma and at least two had no detectable monoclonal component in the serum and in the urine. The latter two patients did have renal monotypic γ3 and γ4 deposits, respectively, which suggests that these γ chains were rapidly cleared from the circulation.

Outcome and treatment

The natural history of MIDD remains uncertain, mainly because extrarenal deposits of light chains observed in various organs can be totally asymptomatic or can cause severe organ damage leading to death. This may explain why the survival time from the onset of symptoms varies from one month to 10 years; by comparison, the prognosis of a related disease, AL-amyloidosis, is much more homogeneous. The 5-year actuarial rates for patient survival and survival free of end-stage renal disease under chemotherapy are 70% and 37%, respectively (Heilman *et al.* 1992).

Two retrospective studies have shown the potential renal benefits of chemotherapy in MIDD (Ganeval 1988; Heilman *et al.* 1992). Prospective randomized controlled trials are obviously warranted but they are hampered by the relatively small number of MIDD patients. In the meantime, one could adopt the following pragmatic approach. MIDD patients over 60 years of age with myeloma should be treated with conventional chemotherapy, but intensive therapy with blood stem cell autografting should be considered in younger patients. As in AL-amyloidosis, deposited light chains have disappeared in isolated instances with the latter treatment. Treatment of non-myeloma patients should be discussed according to clinical presentation. Patients with rapidly progressive renal failure and life-threatening extrarenal complications should be treated.

Kidney transplantation has been performed in a few patients with MIDD. Recurrence of the disease is usually observed on the graft.

Renal diseases associated with MIDD

Amyloid deposits are found in one or more organs in about 7% of LCDD patients. Because amyloid deposits are focal, the true incidence of the association may be markedly underestimated.

It is generally considered that myeloma cast nephropathy and MIDD occur in mutually exclusive fashion. In fact, a few myeloma casts are identified in about 20% of patients with typical MIDD. Conversely, in typical cast nephropathy, light-chain deposits are not infrequent along glomerular and tubular basement membranes; however, these do not usually show the ribbon-like thickening characteristic of MIDD. Whether these light-chain deposits corespond to an early stage of MIDD cannot be established yet.

References

Aucouturier P., Khamlichi A.A., Touchard G., Justrabo E., Cogné M., Chauffert B., Martin F. and Preud'homme J.L. (1993). Brief report: heavy-chain deposition disease. *New England Journal of Medicine*, 329: 1389–93.

Buxbaum J.N., Chuba J.V., Hellman G.C., Solomon A. and Gallo G.R. (1990). Monoclonal immunoglobulin deposition disease: light chain and light and heavy chain deposition diseases and their relation to light chain amyloidosis. Clinical features, immunopathology, and molecular analysis. *Annals of Internal Medicine*, 112: 455–64.

Confalonieri R., Di Belgiojoso G.B., Banfi G., Ferrario F., Bertani T., Pozzi C., Casanova S., Lupo A., De Ferrari G. and Minetti L. (1988). Light chain nephropathy: histological and clinical aspects in 15 cases. *Nephrology, Dialysis and Transplantation*, 2: 150–6.

Ganeval D. (1988). Kidney involvement in light chain deposition disease. In *The kidney in plasma cell dyscrasia* (ed. L. Minetti, G. D'Amico and C. Ponticelli), pp. 221–8, Kluwer Academic Publishers, Dordrecht.

Ganeval D., Mignon F., Preud'homme J.L., Noël L.H., Morel-Maroger L., Droz D., Brouet J.C., Méry J.P. and Grünfeld J.P. (1982). Visceral deposition of monoclonal light chains and immunoglobulins: a study of renal and immunopathologic abnormalities. *Advances in Nephrology*, 11: 25–63.

Heilman R.L., Velosa J.A., Holley K.E., Offord K.P. and Kyle R.A. (1992). Long-term follow-up and response to chemotherapy in patients with light-chain deposition disease. *American Journal of Kidney Diseases*, 20: 34–41.

Husby G., Blichfeldt P., Brandtzaeg P., Mellbye O.J., Sletten K. and Stenstad T. (1998). Chronic arthritis and gamma heavy chain disease: coincidence or pathogenic link? *Scandinavian Journal of Rheumatology*, 27: 257–64.

Ivanyi B. (1990). Frequency of light chain deposition nephropathy relative to renal amyloidosis and Bence Jones cast nephropathy in a necropsy study of patients with myeloma. *Archives of Pathology and Laboratory Medicine*, 114: 986–7.

Kambham N., Markowitz G.S., Appel G.B., Kleiner M.J., Aucouturier P., and D'agati V.D. (1999). Heavy chain deposition disease: the disease spectrum. *American Journal of Kidney Diseases*, 33: 954–62.

Khamlichi A.A., Aucouturier P., Preud'homme J.L. and Cogné M. (1995). Structure of abnormal heavy chains in human heavy chain deposition disease. *European Journal of Biochemistry*, 229: 54–60.

Moulin B., Deret S., Mariette X., Kourilsky O., Imai H., Dupouët L., Marcellin L., Kolb I., Aucouturier P., Brouet J.C., Ronco P.M. and Mougenot B. (1999). Nodular glomerulosclerosis with deposition of monoclonal immunoglobulin heavy chains lacking C_H1. *Journal of the American Society of Nephrology*, 10: 519–28.

Preud'homme J.L., Aucouturier P., Touchard G., Striker L., Khamlichi A.A., Rocca A., Denoroy L. and Cogné M. (1994) Monoclonal immunoglobulin deposition disease (Randall type). Relationship with structural abnormalities of immunoglobulin chains. *Kidney International*, 46: 965–72.

Preud'homme J.L., Morel-Maroger L., Brouet J.C., Cerf M., Mignon F., Guglielmi P. and Seligmann M. (1980). Synthesis of abnormal immunoglobulins in lymphoplasmacytic disorders with visceral light chain deposition. *American Journal of Medicine*, 69: 703–10.

Randall R.E., Williamson W.C., Jr Mullinax F., Tung M.Y. and Still W.J. (1976). Manifestations of systemic light chain deposition. *American Journal of Medicine*, 60: 293–9.

Rott T., Vizjak A., Lindic J., Hvala A., Perkovic T. and Cernelc P. (1998). IgG heavy-chain deposition disease affecting kidney, skin, and skeletal muscle. *Nephrology, Dialysis Transplantation*, 13: 1825–8.

Solomon A., Weiss D.T., Kattine A.A. (1991). Nephrotoxic potential of Bence Jones proteins. *New England Journal of Medicine*, 324: 1845–51.

Zhu L., Herrera G.A., Murphy-Ullrich J.E., Huang Z.Q. and Sanders P.W. (1995). Pathogenesis of glomerulosclerosis in light chain deposition disease. *American Journal of Pathology*, 147: 375–85.

PART VI

23

Hepatitis C associated mixed cryoglobulinemia

Giuseppe D'Amico and Alessandro Fornasieri

Definition of cryoglobulinemia

Cryoglobulins are immunoglobulins which precipitate reversibly in the cold, usually at 4°C, but sometimes at an even higher temperature. According to the classification proposed by Brouet *et al.* (1) there are three types of cryoglobulinemia. In type I the cryoprecipitate is composed of a single monoclonal immunoglobulin without any antibody activity. This condition can be found in patients with mutiple myeloma, Waldenstrom macroglobulinemia or idiopathic monoclonal gammopathy. Both type II and III are mixed cryoglobulinemias, as they are composed by at least two immunoglobulins. In type II, the cryoglobulins are composed by a monoclonal immunoglobulin (usually an IgMk) with rheumatoid activity toward polyclonal IgG. In type III all the components are polyclonal (with one of them having a rheumatoid activity).

Mixed cryoglobulinemias constitute 60–75% of all mixed cryoglobulinemias, and type III is frequently found associated to connective tissue diseases, leukaemia, hepato-biliary diseases, infectious diseases and post-infectious glomerulonephritis. In these cases they are called secondary mixed cryoglobulinemias.

In the absence of such associated diseases and in the presence of the clinical syndrome originally described by Meltzer *et al.* in 1966 (2), the pathological condition was called 'essential mixed cryoglobulinemia'. The clinical syndrome is characterized by purpura, weakness and arthralgia and, in some patients, is associated with glomerulonephritis (3).

Now, the term 'essential' cannot be used for the majority of cases. In fact, over the past eight years anti-hepatitis C virus (HCV) antibodies and HCV RNA have been detected in a great number of patients with 'essential' mixed cryoglobulinemia of both type II and III (4–14). Polymerase chain reaction techniques (PCR) could demonstrate HCV in the sera of 63–86% of cases and within the cryoprecipitate of 75–93% of cases. Moreover several authors could demonstrate a hundredfold virus enrichment within cryoprecipitate compared to the corresponding serum (10, 13, 15, 16).

Cryoglobulinemia and hepatitis C Virus

The association between the cryoglobulinemic syndrome and HCV has been confirmed by several investigators. The relationship between hepatitis C and the presence of serum cryoglobulins has also been investigated in infected patients; it was 54 and 46% in two large series of patients with hepatitis C (17, 18), a prevalence much higher than that in control patients with HBV-associated chronic active hepatitis, in whom only 15% and 5% of patients had circulating cryoglobulins. Wong and co-workers found mixed cryoglobulins in 19% of 113 consecutive patients referred because of the presence of anti-HCV antibodies (not necessarily associated with liver involvement). In 91% of them cryoglobulins were of type III (19).

The prevalence of HCV genotypes in cryglobulinemic syndrome in Europe is commonly of type 1b, although genotype subgroup prevalences seems to be influenced by ethnic differences (20, 21). The genotype 1b is associated with higher levels of transaminases, higher viral load, worsened hepatic lesions, resistance to treatment, more frequent progression toward cirrhosis and relapse of the disease after liver transplantion.

The hepatitis C virus

The hepatitis C virus is part of the *Flaviridae* family. Its genome is composed of a single chain of RNA made of 10,000 nucleotides. Within the genome there is a single coding sequence which is translated into single polyprotein made up of 3010 aminoacids. This polyprotein is then cut into several functional proteins. Among these, there are structural proteins (one nucleocapside protein and two envelope proteins) and five non-structural proteins with enzymatic property (including RNA polymerase). The coding sequences of the pericapside glycoproteins are characterized by a certain variability. This has allowed the identification of at least six viral genotypes: type 1 and 2 are more frequent in USA and Europe, type 3 is prevalent in Asia, type 4 in North Africa, type 5 in South Africa and type 6 in Hong Kong.

HCV replication is exclusively cytoplasmic and its RNA has a messenger polarity, so after losing the capside, it can directly transfer upon ribosomes and subsequently begin the synthesis of the viral proteins. As a consequence, hepatitis C virus does not need preformed enzymes in order to enter the host cell and purified RNA is also infective (22).

Hepatitis C infection is usually silent in 70 to 80% of cases. About 80% of acute infections turn into chronic hepatitis, from mild hepatitis to overt cirrhosis, sometimes developing into liver cancer. About 50% of patients with chronic HCV infection have increasing levels of transaminasis, even though patients with normal levels of transaminases could also develop progressive liver damage (23).

Pathogenesis of cryoglobulinemia

Hepatitis C virus is not able to integrate its genome within the DNA of host cells. This is a condition that other viruses, such as HBV, use to defend themselves against the host immunologic repertoire, which develops a kind of immunotolerance. Hepatitis C virus has a great mutagenic capacity, as indicated by the frequency of mutations found in the hypervariable region in the NH2 extremity of the surface protein E2 (24). This condition is relevant for HCV persistence within the host. Moreover, E2 protein binds the CD81 receptor expressed on liver cells and B lymphocytes. The interaction between HCV and B lymphocytes modulates both lymphotropism and antibody synthesis (25). This is an important example of interaction between viral infection and immunological disorder that might induce a shift to the abnormal proliferation of a clone of B cells producing a monoclonal IgMk rheumatoid factor, thus inducing a type II mixed cryoglobulinemia. This hypothesis, which considers mixed cryoglobulinemia a benign lymphoproliferative disorder, might explain why overt B-cell malignancy occurs in some of these patients (26–30).

The intravenous injection of a 37°C solubilized type II cryoglobulins from patients with cryoglobulinemic glomerulonephritis into mice induces a pattern of mesangiocapillary lesions and immunodeposits very similar to those found in humans (31). In this model, the purified IgMk rheumatoid factor from mixed cryoglobulins (but not the IgMk from patients with Waldenstrom's disease, polyclonal IgM from patients with rheumatoid arthritis, or polyclonal IgM from normal subjects) binds to cellular fibronectin, a known constituent of mesangial matrix (32). These experiments suggest that monoclonal IgMk rheumatoid factor might deposit alone in the glomerular structures with subsequent *in situ* deposition of the polyclonal IgG, or else that the circulating mixed cryoglobulins could deposit as such or be already bound to viral antigens. Demonstration of HCV RNA or virus antigens in the glomeruli has remained elusive (9, 10, 13), and only recently have specific HCV-related proteins been detected in glomerular and tubulo-interstitial vascular structures by indirect immunohistochemistry, using electroelution of tissue sections to enhance the sensitivity of the method (33). However, the evidence that immune complexes containing intact virion are the main component of the glomerular deposits is inconclusive, while complexes containing HCV capsular antigens cannot be excluded.

Clinical manifestations of cryoglobulinemic disease

Symptoms

Mixed cryoglobulinemic patients present almost constantly with purpuric skin lesions, showing a leucocytoclastic vasculitis on biopsy. These lesions are usually found on the legs, but they can appear virtually anywhere. Sometimes they are confluent and can show necrotizing aspects with ulcers and even with mutilation of fingers or ears. Other frequent symptoms are asthenia, fever, arthralgias, and Raynaud's phenomenon. Peripheral neuropathy is also frequent and it presents usually with dysaesthesia and parasthesia but also with motor insufficency. Abdominal pain is also frequent during acute flare-up of the disease; it can simulate a surgical abdomen and is due to mesenteric vasculitic lesions. *Liver enlargement* and *splenomegaly* are also frequently found, and are a consequence of HCV infection. Increased levels of transaminases are frequently found (2). *Lung fibrosis* was recently reported to be associated with mixed cryoglobulinemia.

Examination of bone marrow biopsy often reveals a pattern of slight lymphoproliferative disorder with such frequency that several authors consider type II mixed cryoglobulinemia as a non-Hodgkin lymphoma with low grade malignancy (35). This assessement is consistent with the relatively frequent occurrence of a B-cell malignancy (in our experience 6% after an average observation of 10 years in 65 patients) and in a recent Italian multicentre study of 146 patients with cryoglobulinemic glomerulonephritis (unpublished data).

Renal disease usually occurs in the fifth to sixth decades of life and is slightly more frequent in women (60%). General symptoms of mixed cryoglobulinemia frequently manifest themselves an average of 2–3 years before the renal diagnosis is made, but sometimes renal and extrarenal signs appear at the same time. The most frequent syndrome in cryoglobulinemic glomerulonephritis is proteinuria with microscopic hematuria, often with evidence of moderate chronic renal failure (35–55% of cases). An acute nephritic syndrome is the first renal manifestation in 17–25% of cases; this acute syndrome is complicated by oliguria in approximately 5% of cases. Progression toward renal failure seems to be associated with gender (male) and age (old). Nephrotic syndrome affects another 20% of patients (36–38). Arterial hypertension is observed in more than 80% of patients at the time of the onset of renal disease. This is frequently severe and difficult to control, predisposes to cardiovascular and cerebrovascular accidents, and is often responsible for death (36, 37).

The clinical course can vary remarkably, with frequent fluctuation and exacerbation of extrarenal signs (purpura, other signs of systemic vasculitis, arthralgia, fever), usually associated with acute flare-ups of the renal disease (recurrent episodes of nephritic or nephrotic syndrome), although partial or total prolonged remission can occur spontaneously or after treatment in 10% to 15% of patients independently of the course of the systemic disease. On the contrary, the renal disease can flare in the absence of extrarenal exacerbation. In the majority of patients, the renal disease has an indolent course and does not progress to uremia despite the persistence of urinary abnormalities. End-stage renal failure requiring regular dialysis is relatively rare, involving 15% of patients studied by us after a mean follow-up of 11 years; but it is important to realize that during this time of follow-up, 40% of patients died because of extrarenal complications (37). In a study involving 105 consecutive patients, after 11 months of follow-up, 12 died because of cardiovascular complications, infections (9 patients), liver failure

(8 patients) and neoplasia mainly of hematologic origin (4 patients). The 10-year probability of surviving without dialysis was 49% (37).

It is important to search for cryoprecipitate very accurately, because they are sometimes present in small amounts in patient sera. It is crucial to keep the blood samples at 37° in each phase of the process, before obtaining sera. Sometimes it is useful to dilute the serum with distilled water in order to reveal cryoprecipitate. The amount of circulating cryoglobulins may vary between patients, and in the same patients with time. It tends to be higher in patients with type II cryoglobulinemia. Correlation of cryocrit with disease manifestations is scanty, but it has some utility in monitoring the disease of the same patients submitted to immunosuppressive therapy and plasma exchange.

The serum complement pattern is rather specific. Early complement components (C1q, C4) and CH50 are usually very low, usually lower than that seen in lupus nephritis. The high levels of complement breakdown products, including C3a and C5a, suggest that the presence of C4 binding protein in patients with cryoglobulinemic syndrome leads to continuous activation of the C3 convertase pathway (39). Frequently C3 is found to be slightly low. The behaviour of serum C3 is unpredictable. Often, flare-ups are characterized by a reduction of the level of C3, which heralds new disease activity despite the persistently depressed C4 level.

Rheumatoid factor titres are constantly high and, together with very low C4 levels, are the immunological hallmark of the disease. Monoclonal IgMk is frequently found at serum electrophoresis in type II mixed cryoglobulinemias: in such cases urinary k light chain is a common finding.

The HCV syndrome

The prevalence of antibodies against HCV in the USA population is about 1.5%. In an Italian blood donors population, the prevalence of HCV is lower than 1%, while in patients admitted to surgical departments it is about 4% (40). It is known that a minority of patients with hepatitis B infection develop chronic liver disease. On the contrary, the majority of patients with acute HCV infection will develop a chronic liver disease. Often this pathological condition is associated with several immunological abnormalities besides cryoglobulinemia (such as anti-tissue, anti-nuclear, anti-smooth muscle, anti-microsome, anti-thyroid and anti-thyroglobulin antibodies) which are independent of HCV genotype (41). Some patients develop extrahepatic clinical manifestations, sometimes variably associated together, such as *porphyria cutanea tarda*. This disease is characterized by a reduced decarboxylase activity of uroporphyirinogen and, in its sporadic form, is associated in 80% of cases with HCV infection (42) as are 57% of patients with *lymphocytic sialoadenitis* (equivalent to a *sicca syndrome* in Sjogren disease) (43). In addition, other still not well characterized pathological conditions that are associated frequently to HCV infection include: *autoimmune thyroiditis, lichen planus, Mooren's corneal ulcers* and *idiopathic lung fibrosis* (44).

Moreover, HCV infection is significantly higher in patients with non–Hodgkin lymphoma (45).

Histologic characteristics of cryoglobulinemic glomerulonephritis

Cryoglobulinemic glomerulonephritis is a peculiar type of membranoproliferative glomerulonephritis almost exclusively associated with type II mixed cryoglobulinemia, composed of monoclonal or oligoclonal IgMk with rheumatoid activity against polyclonal IgG. The pattern of glomerular involvement differs from that of idiopathic type I membranoproliferative glomerulonephritis and from that of the diffuse proliferative glomerulonephritis of systemic lupus erythematosus because of some characteristics:

(a) the particularly intense infiltration of leukocytes, prevalently monocytes/machrophages, which is the major constituent of endocapillary proliferation (36, 46–48) (Fig. 23.1).
(b) the frequent presence, especially during episodes of acute nephritic syndrome of the so-called '*intraluminal thrombi*', which are amorphous, eosinophilic, PAS positive deposits of variable size and diffusion, lying against the inner side of the glomerular capillary wall and often filling completely the capillary lumen. Sometimes these huge intraluminal deposits and the subendothelial deposits are revealed by electron microscopy as having a specific microtubular structure that is identical to that of the *in-vitro* cryoprecipitate of the same patients. This structure consists of cylinders that are 100 to 1000 μm long

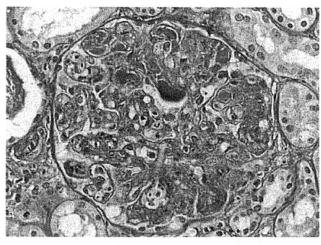

Fig. 23.1 The glomerulus shows a marked endocapillary hypercellularity, mainly an infiltration of inflammatory mononuclear leukocytes. The majority of loops show a thickened glomerular capillary wall. Several amorphous, huge deposits ('intraluminal thrombi') fill the capillary lumina (Masson trichrome ×190).

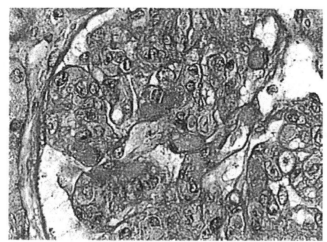

Fig. 23.2 Portion of a glomerulus showing a double contoured appearance of the glomerular basement membrane (Silver staining ×304).

and have an allow axis, appearing in cross-section like anular bodies (49–51). The identity of the deposits with the circulating IgG-IgMk cryoglobulins has been confirmed by demonstration in renal biopsy specimens of the same idiotype of the circulating monoclonal rheumatoid factor (52).

(c) the double contoured appearance of the glomerular basement membrane (Fig. 23.2) which, at electron microscopy examination, appears to be due to the interposition of monocyte/macrophages between the basement membrane and the endothelial cells or the newly formed basement membrane-like material. Double contours are more diffuse and evident than in idiopathic membranoproliferative glomerulonephritis in which they are due to the prevalent interposition of mesangial cells. This difference in the composition of double contour might explain why it can disappear in cryoglobulinemic glomerulonephritis in a later stage of less clinical activity. Moreover, this milder mesangial involvement might explain why glomerular segmental and global sclerosis is less severe than in other types of idiopathic or secondary membranoproliferative glomerulonephritis (36). Electron microscopy also shows that monocyte/macrophages in close contact with the subendothelial and intraluminal deposits are involved in their degradation.

Mesangial sclerosis is found in late stages in the central area of the glomerular lobules (lobular glomerulonephritis) in a minority of patients. In other cases mesangial sclerosis is a late and usually mild feature. In some cases, the typical pattern of cryoglobulinemic glomerulonephritis is lacking, the monocyte infiltration is less consistent, intraluminal thrombi are absent, and a picture of mild segmental mesangial proliferation is found in 20% of patients. This pattern can be found at presentation of renal disease or later when a re-biopsy is performed after intensive immunosuppressive therapy.

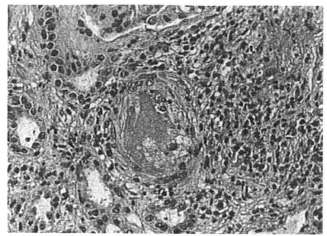

Fig. 23.3 The medium-sized renal artery presents diffuse fibrinoid necrosis of the vessel wall and intraparietal and perivascular leukocyte infiltration (Masson trichrome ×190).

Finally, about 30% of patients with cryoglobulinemic glomerulonephritis have acute vasculitis of small- and medium-size arteries, characterized by fibrinoid nerosis of the arteriolar wall and infiltration of monocytes in and around the wall (37) (Fig. 23.3). This renal vasculitis is often associated with other signs of systemic vasculitis, such as purpura or mesenteric vasculitis and can appear in the absence of clear glomerular involvement. Even when the fibrinoid necrosis of renal arterial walls is severe, focal necrosis of the capillary loops is never present and crescentic extracapillary proliferation is a rare observation (37).

When subendothelial deposits prevail, the immunofluorescence pattern is similar to that found in idiopathic membranoproliferative glomerulonephritis: intense granular, diffuse subendothelial staining of IgM, IgG and C3 (Fig. 23.4).

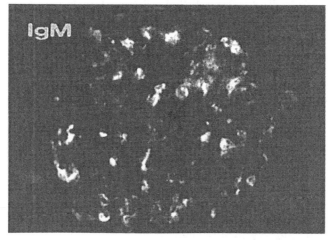

Fig. 23.4 Intense massive staining of some of the deposits filling the capillary lumina. Faint and irregular parietal deposits (IgM, ×190).

The pattern at immunofluorescence microscopy, when massive intraluminal deposits can be seen by light microscopy, is characterized by intense staining of such deposits prevalently by IgM and IgG, commonly associated with faint irregular segmental subendothelial staining of some peripheral loops. In mild segmental mesangial proliferation, only faint, irregular, segmental, parietal staining of some peripheral loops is found by immunofluorescence.

Therapy

In the past, before the close relationship between cryoglobulinemic syndrome and HCV infection became evident, steroids (with or without cyclophosphamide) were used by the majority of investigators to treat severe vasculitic complications of the cryoglobulinemic syndrome and acute exacerbations of cryoglobulinemic glomerulonephritis and renal vasculitis. High dose steroids, usually starting with intravenous pulses of methylprednisolone (1 g/day for three days), were usually found to be effective, especially when given in association with cyclophosphamide. Plasmapheresis or cryoapheresis was used with this therapy in more acute phases. Plasmapheresis removes circulating cryoglobulins, thus preventing deposition in vessel walls and in glomeruli, but should be administered only in association with steroids and possibly cyclophosphamide, to avoid rebound effects, with increase of cryocrit and severe vasculitis after discontinuation. Low doses of oral steroids are used to control systemic signs of mixed cryoglobulinemia. With few exceptions, no consistent evidence of acute hepatic damage with the combination of these treatments have been reported, even though the potential unfavourable effect on viremia and hepatic disease has been hypothesized.

The current understanding of the association between cryoglobulinemic syndrome and HCV infection has changed the rationale for the treatment of the systemic disease and its renal complications. Since 1987, before the viral cause of essential mixed cryoglobulinemia had been proven, Bonomo et al. (53) had already reported a consistent improvement of clinical signs in cryoglobulinemic patients treated with interferon alfa, used for its known potential antiproliferative and immunoregulatory properties. Although now the most extensively used antiviral agent for HCV infection, the use of interferon alfa in mixed cryoglobulinemia has some drawbacks, as confirmed by the three therapeutic trials which have been performed at this point. The trial of Ferri et al. was a cross-over controlled trial on 26 patients with documented HCV infection and mixed cryoglobulinemia with systemic involvement but without renal complication (54). The trial used 6 months of interferon alfa therapy (2 million IU daily for a month, then every other day for 5 months) together with low-dose steroid therapy. A significant improvement of purpura, together with a reduction of cryoglobulins and transaminases, was reported during interferon alfa therapy, but a rebound phenomenon was observed after discontinuation of therapy and development of nephritis was also observed. The controlled trial of Misiani et al. (55) in 53 patients with HCV-associated type II mixed cryoglobulinemia showed that the clinical effect of interferon alfa, accompanied by a reduction of cryoglobulin concentration, was limited to 60% of patients in whom HCV RNA disappeared from the serum, and was therefore due to its antiviral action. The study also showed that the virus reappears in the majority of treated patients after discontinuation of the drug, suggesting the advisability of using high doses for long periods of time. Misiani proposed doses of 4.5 to 6 million IU interferon alfa thrice weekly for 6 months, and to continue at doses of 3 million IU thrice weekly for 6 additional months if there is a beneficial effect and HCV RNA disappears from the serum. In another trial of Dammacco *et al.* (56) in 65 patients with type II mixed cryoglobulinemia secondary to HCV infection, a reduction of cryocrit associated with improvement of systemic signs was achieved in about half of the patients given interferon alfa alone or interferon alfa plus oral steroids compared to patients who received only oral steroids or nothing at all. As in the previous trial the favourable effect was limited to patients in whom HCV RNA became negative and recurrence of clinical signs after discontinuation of the trial was a frequent phenomenon, but clinical relapse was delayed in patients who received the combined treatment interferon plus steroids, compared with those treated with interferon alfa alone.

All the controlled trials described above were performed in patients with clinically active mixed cryoglobulinemia but without clearly established renal involvement. However in the trial of Misiani (55) the renal involvement, that was present in 75% of patients, tended to improve, as demonstrated by a slight reduction in serum creatinine without a significant change in proteinuria. Johnson *et al.* performed an uncontrolled study in 14 patients with membranoproliferative glomerulonephritis associated with HCV infection and chronic active hepatitis; not all of them had clear evidence of concomitant mixed cryoglobulinemia. Interferon alfa reduced proteinuria by 60% without significantly changing serum creatinine levels (57).

The results of these trials and the review of other uncontrolled studies on interferon alfa treatment of patients with HCV infection, associated or not associated with mixed cryoglobulinemia, allows us to draw the following conclusions:

- Interferon alfa is an effective drug for the complications of HCV infection almost exclusively in patients whose viremia is eradicated. It is effective also against production of cryoglobulins, athough systemic signs of mixed cryoglobulinemia improve more than the renal signs.
- The effectiveness of interferon alfa to reduce viraemia is related to HCV genotype (genotype 1b is definitely less responsive than the other genotypes), the magnitude of the initial viraemia, duration of viral infection, age of the patient and severity of liver damage before treatment.
- The favourable effects usually last for only a short period of time after treatment is discontinued and is generally followed by a virologic rebound and clinical flare-up within a few months.
- In patients with renal and systemic manifestation of mixed cryoglobulinemia, interferon alfa is frequently administered in combination with variable doses of steroids, which seems to potentiate the beneficial effects of the antiviral agent. These include a faster and longer-lasting remission of the systemic manifestation of mixed cryoglobulinemia.

● In the presence of acute cryoglobulinemic glomerulonephritis, interferon alfa does not prevent progression of renal damage. Combination therapy with anti-inflammatory and cytotoxic drugs, and sometimes also plasma exchange, is still necessary.

Recently other antiviral agents were being tested in HCV infection and cryoglobulinemia. Ribavirin, a guanidine analogue with activity against RNA and DNA viruses has received special attention. This drug has the advantage of oral administration (600 to 1200 mg/day in two doses) and its combination with interferon alfa seems to be more effective on virus clearing than interferon alfa alone.

References

1. Brouet J.C., Clauvel J.P., Danon F., Klein M., and Seligman M. Biological and clinical significance of cryoglobulins. A report of 86 cases. *Am J Med* 1974, Vol. 57: 775–778.
2. Meltzer M., Franklin E.C., Elias K., McCluskey R.Y., and Cooper N. Cryoglobulinemia a clinical and laboratory study. II cryoglobulins with rheumatoid factor activity. *Am J Med* 1966, Vol. 40: 837–856.
3. Gorevic P.D., Kassab H.J., Levo Y., Kohn R., Meltzer M., Prose P., and Franklin E.C. Mixed cryoglobulinemia: Clinical aspects and long-term follow-up of 40 patients. *Am J Med* 1980, Vol. 69: 287–308.
4. Ferri C., Greco F., and Longobardo G. Antibodies to hepatitis C virus in patients with mixed cryoglobulinemia. *Arthritis Rheum* 1991, Vol. 34: 1606–1610.
5. Galli M., Monti G., and Monteverde A. Hepatitis C virus and mixed cryoglobulinemias. *Lancet* 1992, Vol. 1: 989.
6. Dammacco F. and Sansonno D. Antibodies to hepatitis C virus in essential mixed cryoglobulinemia. *Clin Exp Immunol* 1992, Vol. 87: 352–356.
7. Pechére-Bertschi A., Perrin L., De Sassure P., Widmann J.J., Giostra E., and Schifferli J.A. Hepatitis C: A possible etiology for cryoglobulinemia type II. *Clin Exp Immunol* 1992, Vol. 89: 419–422.
8. Misiani R., Bellavita P., and Fenili D. Hepatitis C virus infection in patients with essential mixed cryoglobulinemia. *Ann Intern Med* 1992, Vol. 117: 573–577.
9. Misiani R., Bellavita P., and Fenili D. Hepatitis C virus and cryoglobulinemia. *N Engl J Med* 1993, Vol. 328: 1121, (letter).
10. Agnello V., Chung R.T., and Kaplan L.M. A role for hepatitis C virus infection in type II cryoglobulinemia. *N Engl J Med* 1992, Vol. 327: 1490–1495.
11. Cacoub P., Lunel Fabiani F., Musset L., Perrin M., Franguel L., Leger J.M., Huraux J.M., Piette J.C., and Godeau P. Mixed cryoglobulinemia and hepatitis C virus. *Am J Med* 1994, Vol. 96: 124–132.
12. Pasquariello A., Ferri C., Moriconi L., La Civita L., Longobardo G., Lombardini F., Greco F., and Zignego A.L. Cryoglobulinemic membranoproliferative glomerulonephritis associated with hepatitis C virus. *Am J Nephrol* 1993, Vol. 13: 300–304, (letter).
13. Johnson R.J., Gretch D.R., Yamabe H., Hart J., Bacchi C.E., Hartwell P., Couser W.G., Corey L., Wener M.H., Alpers C.E., and Willson R. Membranoproliferative

44. Gumber C.S. and Chopra S. Hepatitis C. A multifaceted disease. *Ann Intern Med* 1995, Vol.123: 615–621.
45. Ferri C., Caracciolo F., Zignego A.L. *et al.* Hepatitis C virus infection in patients with non-Hodkin's lymphoma. *Br J Haematol* 1994, Vol. 88: 392–398.
46. Monga A., Mazzucco G., Barbiano di Belgioioso G., and Busnach G. The presence and possible role of monocyte infiltration in human chronic proliferative glomerulonephritis. *Am J Pathol* 1979, Vol. 94: 271–284.
47. Ferrario F., Castiglione A., Colasanti G., Barbiano di Belgioioso G., Bertoli S., and D'Amico G. The detection of monocytes in human glomerulonephritis. *Kidney Int* 1985, Vol. 28: 513–519.
48. Castiglione A., Bucci A., Fellin G, D'Amico G., and Atkins R.C. The relationship of infiltrating renal leucocytes to disease activity in lupus and cryoglobulinemic glomerulonephritis. *Nephron* 1988, Vol. 50: 14–23.
49. Mihatsch M.J. and Banfi G. Ultrastructural features in glomerulonephritis in essential mixed cryoglobulinemia. In: C. Ponticelli, L. Minetti and G. D'Amico (eds) *Antiglobulins, Cryoglobulins and Glomerulonephritis*, Dordrecht, M. Nijhoff, 1986, p. 211.
50. Cordonnier D., Martin H., Groslambert P., Micouin C., Chenais F., and Stoebner P. Mixed IgG-IgM cryoglobulinemia with glomerulonephritis. Immunochemical fluorescent and ultrastructural study of kidney and *in vitro* cryoprecipitate. *Am J Med* 1975, Vol. 59: 867–872.
51. Feiner H. and Gallo G. Ultrastructure in glomerulonephritis associated with cryoglobulinemia. *Am J Pathol* 1977, Vol. 88: 145–162.
52. Sinico A.R., Winearls C.G., Sabadini E., Fornasieri A., Castiglione A., and D'Amico G. Identification of glomerular immune deposits in cryoglobulinemia glomerulonephritis. *Kidney Int* 1988, Vol. 34: 1–8.
53. Bonomo L., Casato M., Afeltra A., and Caccavo D. Treatment of idiopathic mixed cryoglobulinemia with alpha interferon. *Am J Med* 1987, Vol. 83: 726–730.
54. Ferri C., Marzo E., and Longobardo G. Interferon-alfa in mixed cryoglobulinemia patients: a randomized, crossover-controlled trial. *Blood* 1993, Vol. 81: 1132–1136.
55. Misiani R., Bellavita P., Fenili D., Vicari O., Marchesi D., Sironi P.L., Zilio P., Vernocchi A., Massazza M., Vendramin G., Tanzi E., and Zanetti A. Interferon alfa-2a therapy in cryoglobulinemia associated with hepatitis C virus. *N Engl J Med* 1994, Vol. 330: 751–756.
56. Dammacco F., Sansonno D., Han J.H., Shyamaia V., Cornacchiulo V., Iacobelli A.R., Lauletta G., and Rizzi R. Natural Interferon-a versus its combination with 6-Methyl-Prednisolone in the therapy of type II mixed cryoglobulinemia: a long-term, randomized, controlled study. *Blood* 1994, Vol. 84: 3336–3343.
57. Johnson R.J., Gretch D.R., Couser W.G., Alpers C.E., Wilson J., Chung M., Hart J., and Willson R. Hepatitis C virus-associated glomerulonephritis, Effect of α-interferon therapy. *Kidney Int* 1994, Vol. 46: 1700–1704.

PART VII

24

Hepatitis B associated renal diseases

Kar Neng Lai

Introduction

Hepatitis B Virus (HBV) has been implicated in the pathogenesis of human glomerular disease. Persistent viral infections that could lead to immune complex-mediated nephritis have attracted a lot of interest.

The host range of hepatitis B virus (HBV) appears to be limited to humans and chimpanzees. In the chimpanzee, an acute experimental transmission results in a serological pattern that is similar to that of human HBV infection and cloned HBV DNA has been shown to be infective (1). HBV of humans and hepatitis B-like viruses found in woodchucks, ground squirrels, and Peking ducks share many common features and belong to a family of hepatotropic DNA viruses called hepadna-viruses. Human HBV has been classified as hepadnavirus type 1.

Each virus has a double-shelled virion 42–47 nm in diameter, a 27 nm internal core, and an excess of incomplete 22 nm spheres except for the duck HBV, tubular forms, and circular partially double-stranded and partially single-stranded DNA, with a length varying between 3000 and 3300 base pairs. All four viruses contain endogenous DNA polymerase and protein kinase, share some DNA and virion polypeptide homology, replicate within the liver, and may be associated with acute or persistent infection and immune complex-mediated extrahepatic disease (2).

Three antigens are clearly defined in HBV, namely hepatitis B surface antigen (HBsAg), hepatitis B core antigen (HBcAg), and hepatitis B e antigen (HBeAg). HBsAg has an estimated molecular weight of 2.4 to 4.6 million daltons and has the chemical characteristics of a lipoprotein with carbohydrate components. HBcAg reactivity does not circulate freely in infected patients and is not detected in sera unless HBV particles are present in a non-intact, disrupted form. It can be demonstrated by immunofluorescence or electron microscopy in the nucleus and cytoplasm of infected cells. HBeAg is a 22000 molecular weight polypeptide derived from denatured HBcAg.

Epidemiology and transmission of HBV infection

The prevalence of HBsAg carrier states varies widely from 0.3% to 1.0% in North America, 1% in Western Europe, 7% in Africa and 10% in Southeast Asia (3). Infection through blood transfusion is uncommon in developed countries; instead transmission associated with intravenous drug abuse and through the venereal route in promiscuous heterosexual and homosexual population is frequently encountered. Hence, the infected patients are usually adolescents or adults, not infrequently with clinical or subclinical manifestation of hepatitis. In Southeast Asia, vertical transmission from carrier mothers to their offspring may be important in maintaining the higher carrier rate (4). The patients are not uncommonly asymptomatic (without any previous history of liver disease) and the hepatitis B surface antigenaemia is only detected during routine serological screening. Furthermore, the affected subjects are not infrequently young children and the antigenaemia tends to persist.

Definition of hepatitis B virus-associated glomerulonephritis (GN)

The pathogenetic role of HBV in renal disease has attracted much attention, since Combes *et al.* (5) in 1971 reported glomerulonephritis with immune complexes of HBsAg and its antibody (anti-HBs) in a patient infected with HBV. Previous observations of a greater-than-expected incidence of chronic HBsAg carriers among the patients with various forms of glomerulonephritides compared with the general hospital population in different geographic areas tend to support the hypothesis of a pathogenetic association between chronic HBV infection and glomerulonephritis (6–8). Various morphological patterns including membranous nephropathy, mesangiocapillary glomerulonephritis, minimal change nephropathy, mesangial proliferative glomerulonephritis have since been described (6–9).

The only definitive means to prove that a particular glomerulonephritis is aetiologically associated with chronic HBV infection is to fulfill the following criteria:

(i) The pathology should be reproducible in experimental animals infected with the virus.
(ii) Demonstration of HBV-specific antigen(s) in the glomerulus.
(iii) Disappearance of the pathological lesion with eradication of the virus.

Unfortunately, solid research work reproducing the glomerulonephritis in infected experimental animals was lacking until recently. Gyorkey *et al.* (10) inoculated primates (10 baboons and 5 rhesus monkeys) with varying amounts of human plasma containing HBsAg. The lesions consisted of progressive focal glomerulonephritis with mesangial alterations that developed over a period of four to ten months after inoculation. The most likely explanation is immune complex deposition. The possibility that the immune complex deposition may have resulted from an antibody response to human plasma that was injected can be excluded since in rabbits injected with a single dose of bovine serum albumin any renal lesions were reversible and undetectable by the fourth week after injection. In the primates the renal lesions were progressive and a temporal progression of these lesions was observed which was similar to that reported in the chronic bovine serum albumin-rabbit model (11).

Recent observations from chronic woodchuck hepatitis virus infection in woodchucks revealed three types of glomerulonephritis, namely, membranous nephropathy with capillary HBcAg deposits, mesangial proliferative glomerulonephritis with mesangial deposits of HBsAg, and mixed membranous and mesangial proliferative glomerulonephritis with capillary deposits of HBcAg and mesangial deposits of HBsAg (12). The animal model of woodchuck hepatitis may be valuable for experimental study of the natural progression of renal lesion, as their pathological findings are similar to those of humans. Membranous nephropathy is the most common type of glomerulonephritis in humans and is particularly frequent in male children (7, 9, 13–15). Mesangial proliferative forms with IgA deposits appear to be more common in adults (8, 9, 16). Woodchucks with a membranous component appeared to be younger, whereas woodchucks with mesangial proliferative glomerulonephritis appeared to be older. The male/female ratio of the affected animals was significantly greater than that of the chronic carrier population. Thus, the pattern of occurrence of these types of glomerulonephritis was similar to that observed in human kidneys with the exception of HBeAg, as the woodchuck hepatitis antigen system has not been characterized.

Complete disappearance of the pathology with eradication of the virus in human beings is not easily demonstrated because of the ethical consideration of renal biopsy in patients in clinical remission. Hence, the diagnosis of HBV-associated GN, at present, depends on the demonstration of HBV specific antigen(s) in the glomeruli.

Pathology of HBV-related GN

Membranous nephropathy

This pathological entity was first described by Brzoko *et al.* (13) and subsequent reports from other countries reveal that membranous nephropathy remains the best recognized glomerulopathy associated with chronic HBV infection (6, 7, 9, 14–15).

Mesangial proliferative glomerulonephritis

Coexistence of mesangial proliferative glomerulonephritis with predominant mesangial IgA deposits and persistent hepatitis B surface antigenaemia was first reported in five patients by Nagy *et al.* (8) and later in two patients by Sluzarczk *et al.* (15). Mesangial IgA nephropathy associated with chronic HBV infection is supported by subsequent investigators from different geographic regions (9, 18, 19, 20).

Focal glomerulosclerosis

The association between chronic HBV infection and focal glomerulosclerosis remains unclear. Focal glomerulosclerosis in HBsAg carriers is likely to be secondary to progression of other types of HBV-associated GN or a sequel of hepatic cirrhosis (21).

Minimal change nephropathy

Although minimal change nephropathy has been reported in chronic HBV carriers (8, 12), the pathogenetic association is unlikely as glomerular deposition of immunoglobulin and HBV antigen is rarely observed. Furthermore, the prevalence of hepatitis B surface antigenaemia in nephrotic patients with minimal change nephropathy is not higher than that of the general population (22).

Lupus nephritis

An association between HBV infection and lupus nephritis had been reported with glomerular deposits of HBsAg in renal biopsy (23). This was not confirmed in subsequent studies using monospecific antibody for immunofluorescence examination (24).

Polyarteritis nodosa/microscopic polyangiitis

The association between polyarteritis nodosa (PAN) and hepatitis B was first reported in 1970 by two separate studies (25, 26). Subsequently, the presence of HBsAg in the serum amongst various series has been noted in 0 to 54% of cases of PAN (reviewed by Johnson and Couser (27)). Of interest is the observation that PAN associated with hepatitis B has been primarily reported in Europe and the United States where the prevalence of the HBsAg carrier state is greatest in adults, and infection is usually acquired via a parental routine (3). In contrast, PAN associated with hepatitis B is uncommon in endemic areas such as Southeast Asia and Africa where most infection occurs in childhood via transmission from parents or siblings. Furthermore, the variability in incidence of HBsAg in PAN within the United States may be partially explained by the underlying prevalence of intravenous drug abuse and the HBV carrier rate at the various reporting centres. Thus, in New York, up to 40% of PAN is HBV associated as opposed to Ann Arbor, Michigan and Rochester, Minnesota, where the rates are from 6 to 25% (27). A recent review of PAN and microscopic polyangiitis (MPA) failed to demonstrate any association between HBV and systemic vasculitides (28). Despite the earlier observation, the aetiological association between chronic HBV infection and PAN/MPA has not been substantiated.

Available data from human and animal studies (especially from the woodchucks) reveal, amongst HBV carriers, three distinct glomerulopathic entities (membranous nephropathy, mesangiocapillary glomerulonephritis and mesangial proliferative glomerulonephritis) are associated with a high prevalence of glomerular deposits of HBV antigens. This suggests that HBV antigens may have played a pathogenetic role in a proportion of these conditions. Therefore, our present review will focus mainly on these glomerulopathies.

Nature of HBV antigens in glomeruli

HBV-associated GN is generally considered to be an immune complex-mediated disease (29). Three distinct antigens, HBsAg, HBcAg, and HBeAg have been detected by immunofluorescent studies in renal biopsies from patients with HBV-associated GN. The nature of glomerular HBV antigen in different glomerulopathies remains controversial due to the different antibodies used in histopathological studies.

Both HBcAg and HBsAg have a molecular weight in excess of two million. HBeAg, which is a part of the viral nucleoprotein, is found in two forms with molecular weights of 19,000 and 300,000. HBeAg is expected to be capable of inducing membranous nephropathy by being preferentially deposited along capillary wall (29). Experiments with serum sickness induced by immunization with bovine serum albumin in rabbits showed that small immune complexes were deposited on the epithelial side of the glomerular basement membrane, whereas the larger immune complexes were deposited mainly in the mesangium (12). If HBV antigens with a lower molecular weight (i.e. HBeAg) induce membranous nephropathy, one would predict mesangial proliferative or mesangiocapillary glomerulonephritis associated with chronic HBV infection would show immune complexes with high molecular weight antigens (i.e. HBsAg). Furthermore, a mixed picture of mesangial IgA and membranous nephropathy should be seen in HBV-associated GN since immune complexes with different molecular weights may be present simultaneously in some of these patients. Such a glomerulopathic entity has been reported with mesangial HBsAg and capillary HBeAg deposits (17, 30, 31), thus confirming the above-mentioned hypothesis and also complying with the experimental findings of Germuth *et al.* (11).

HBV-associated membranous nephropathy

Glomerular capillary deposition of HBsAg (13, 14), HBcAg (9, 15), and HBeAg (32, 33) in HBV-associated membranous nephropathy have been observed by various investigators using different reagents. False-positive HBsAg staining may arise from IgM deposits with antiglobulin activity mainly in non-HBsAg carriers with either mixed cryoglobulinaemia or lupus nephritis (6). Hirose *et al.* [32] had used F(ab')$_2$ fragments of anti-HBsAg monoclonal antibody to demonstrate that capillary deposits were HBeAg in nature. Using the same F(ab')$_2$ fragment of anti-HBeAg monoclonal antibody and another monoclonal antibody against HBeAg, Lai *et al.* (34) demonstrated capillary HBeAg deposits in two-thirds of the biopsies, and the incidence is similar to that reported by Hirose *et al.* (32) However, identical capillary HBeAg immunostaining was demonstrated when polyclonal antibody was used (34). Further studies revealed that commercial polyclonal anti-HBeAg antiserum contains both anti-HBeAg and anti-HBcAg activities (34). This can be explained by the fact that the HBeAg is an integral component of HBcAg. Hence, the recent studies have confirmed that HBeAg is the HBV antigen deposited in HBV-associated GN.

HBV-associated mesangial proliferative glomerulonephritis with mesangial IgA deposits

Since the first description of IgA nephropathy associated with chronic hepatitis B surface antigenaemia (8), the possible pathogenetic association has attracted further attention since the same geographical area with highest endemicity of HBV infection has also the highest incidence of IgA nephropathy (9, 35). Lai *et al.* (9) had reported the detection of glomerular HBsAg in 30% of renal biopsies from patients with coexisting IgA nephropathy and persistent hepatitis B surface antigenaemia by polyclonal antisera. Contrary to the findings in membranous nephropathy, glomerular HBeAg deposits were not detected in the renal biopsy from IgA nephritic patients with coexisting chronic HBV carriers using both polyclonal and monoclonal antibodies. Mesangial deposits of HBsAg similar to the distribution of IgA immunostaining were detected in 40% and 21% of the renal biopsies by polyclonal and monoclonal antibodies respectively (19, 34), suggesting HBsAg rather than HBeAg may play a pathogenetic role in some of the patients with IgA nephropathy associated with chronic HBV infection.

HBV-associated mesangiocapillary glomerulonephritis

The nature of HBV antigen in mesangiocapillary glomerulonephritis related to chronic hepatitis B surface antigenaemia has not been conclusively defined. Three well documented reports of such glomerulopathic entities both demonstrated simultaneous glomerular deposition of HBeAg and HBsAg (17, 20, 36), supporting the hypothesis that immune complexes with HBV antigens of different molecular weights could induce a mixed pattern of glomerulonephritis as shown previously in cases of mixed IgA and membranous nephropathy (30, 37).

Immunopathology of HBV-associated GN

Animal experiments and observations on human subjects have demonstrated that HBV-containing immune complexes may be formed in the course of HBV-induced acute and chronic hepatitis (38). Immune complex-mediated glomerulonephritis requires a continuous supply of antigen and a maintained antibody response and, apparently, these requirements seem to be met in chronic HBV carriers. Circulating immune complexes have been reported in association with HBV and membranous nephropathy (38). Yet, HBV antigen(s) forming an integral part of the circulating immune complexes in these patients has not been unequivocally demonstrated. This raises the question of immune complex formation *in situ* (which occurs in primary membranous nephropathy) in HBV-associated membranous nephropathy.

Extrahepatic HBV replication occurs in human subjects but it is unclear whether viral replication occurs within the kidney in these patients with HBV-associated GN. Receptors for the small S protein of HBV is detected only in two cell lines derived from primates but is absent in other cell lines derived from liver (including hepatoma), lymphocyte, pancreas, spleen, and fibroblast (39). Spherical virus-like particles of 40–50 nm diameter have been demonstrated within the glomerular electron-dense deposits in renal biopsies from patients with HBV-associated GN (14, 19, 40). HBV viral replication in the kidneys of some of these HBV-associated GN is suggested by the localization of HBV DNA genome by *in situ* hybridization in glomeruli (41, 42). This mechanism is supported by the findings in woodchucks. *De novo* synthesis of viral antigens in viral infection has been demonstrated in renal tissues of woodchucks and small amounts of viral-specific mRNA, including full-length transcripts, have been demonstrated in the glomeruli of woodchuck hepatitis virus-infected woodchucks (43).

Lin (44) had detected HBV DNA in glomeruli and tubular epithelia by *in situ* hybridization in patients with early-onset HBV-MGN, but the glomerular HBV DNA was exclusively extracellularly located. Similarly, a study of Peking ducks infected with duck HBV revealed only cytoplasmic localization of HBcAg in the tubular epithelia of the kidney (45). It is plausible that such presence of HBcAg or HBV DNA results from endocytosis by proximal tubular epithelia when the HBV DNA in the urinary filtrate crosses their luminal borders. Alternatively, the presence of HBV DNA in the tubular epithelia could indicate HBV replication in the tubular epithelia, and these findings are in keeping with other transgenic mice studies revealing the expression of viral genome of HBcAg or HBeAg only in convoluted tubular epithelia (46, 47). Recently, using polymerase chain reaction and *in situ* hybridization, Lai *et al.* (48) demonstrated the frequent presence of HBV DNA within the cytoplasm of the renal proximal tubules in different HBV-associated glomerulonephritides of long duration. However, they detected HBV transcriptionally active genomes or mRNA in the glomeruli of these biopsies by *in situ* hybridization with a HBV-specific RNA probe (Fig. 24.1). The HBcAg mRNA was localized mainly in epithelial cells in HBV-associated membranous nephropathy and in both epithelial and mesangial cells in HBV-associated IgA nephropathy. These findings strongly suggest the notion that nephropathy may arise from immune complex formation *in situ*.

Clinical presentation

The clinical manifestations in paediatric and adult patients tend to be different. Paediatric chronic HBV carriers are frequently asymptomatic and HBV-associated GN is suspected by routine urine and serological screening (9, 22, 49). The other common clinical presentation in children is a nephrotic syndrome, not infrequently relapsing, which mimics minimal change nephropathy. The pathology

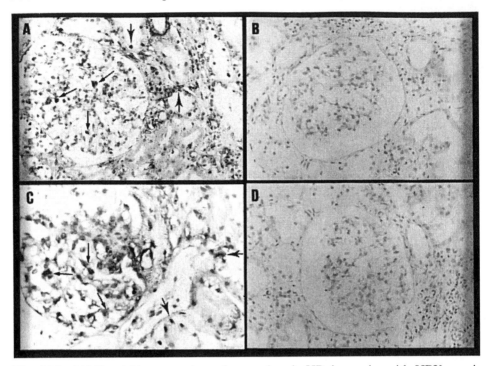

Fig. 24.1 [A] Renal biopsy specimen from a chronic HBsAg carrier with HBV–associated membranous nephropathy. Nuclear and cytoplasmic HBcAg RNA (purple colour) is detected with *in situ* hybridization in glomerular (small arrows) and tubular cells (large arrows) (anti-digoxigenin-alkaline phosphatase stain; ×366). [B] HBcAg RNA is not detected in the same kidney biopsy specimen by *in situ* hybridization if the specimen was pretreated with RNase (negative signals in nuclei were counterstained as pink by Nuclear Fast Red, ×274). [C] Renal biopsy specimen from a chronic HBsAg carrier with HBV-associated IgA nephropathy. Nuclear and cytoplasmic HBcAg RNA (purple colour) is detected with *in situ* hybridization in glomerular (small arrows) and tubular cells (large arrows) (anti-digoxigenin-alkaline phosphatase stain; ×366). [D] HBcAg RNA is not detected in the same kidney biopsy specimen by *in situ* hybridization if the specimen was pretreated with RNase (negative signals in nuclei were counterstained as pink by Nuclear Fast Red, ×274). Adopted from Lai K.N. *et al. Kidney Int* (1996), **50**: 1965–1977 with permission.

of HBV-associated GN in children tends to be exclusively membranous nephropathy with an obvious male predominance (14, 22, 30, 32). Other glomerulopathic entities are rarely encountered in HBV-associated GN amongst the paediatric population. Nephrotic syndrome and proteinuria are the commonest manifestations of HBV-associated membranous nephropathy and mesangiocapillary glomerulonephritis in adults. The male predominance of the nephritis in adults is less prominent than in children (22, 49). Microscopic haematuria is often present with asymptomatic proteinuria (9) and macroscopic haematuria could be the only presenting symptom in HBV-associated mesangial IgA nephropathy (8, 19).

Clinical course and prognosis

The natural history of HBV-associated GN is incompletely understood. No relationship of glomerulonephritis to preceding hepatitis A, hepatitis D, or non-A, non-B hepatitis has been recognized (9, 19, 49).

The rate of spontaneous regression of nephrotic syndrome varies between 23% and 92% of HBV-associated membranous nephropathy, and most patients usually remained symptomatic for 12 months or longer (9, 14, 33, 50–53). The remaining patients had persistent proteinuria with fluid retention (9, 14, 51). Reviews of 108 paediatric cases of HBV-associated membranous nephropathy revealed progression to renal insufficiency or end-stage renal failure in 17.6% and 4.6% respectively (14, 33, 38, 50, 52, 54, 55). In a recent study of adult HBV-associated membranous nephropathy, 29% of the patients had progressive renal failure and 10% required maintenance dialysis therapy after a mean follow-up period of 5 years (56).

Contrary to a 'favourable' benign course in children with HBV-associated membranous nephropathy, a definitive conclusion is difficult to draw in IgA nephropathy associated with HBV antigenaemia, as primary IgA nephropathy is characterized by a relentless, slowly progressive clinical course. Nevertheless, Lai *et al.* (41) reported that 19% of patients with HBV-associated IgA nephropathy had deterioration of renal function during a mean follow-up period of 40 months. One-quarter of these patients had progressed to end-stage renal failure requiring dialysis therapy. These observations suggest that these HBV-associated IgA nephropathies are progressive diseases that lead to renal insufficiency similar to cases of primary IgA nephropathy.

Treatment of HBV-associated GN

Attempts have been made to treat HBV-associated GN for the following reasons:

(i) Spontaneous resolution does not necessarily occur in all patients and 40–77% of patients remains symptomatic. Complications related to overt nephrotic syndrome such as hyperlipidaemia, edema, and venous thrombosis have been observed in these patients.
(ii) Anecdotal observations report the improvement of renal involvement as well as liver disease following clearance of HBsAg from blood (57).
(iii) The disease may progress and could result in chronic renal insufficiency (14, 56).

Corticosteroid therapy

Corticosteroid therapy used in primary membranous nephropathy has been administered to some patients as a therapeutic trial for symptomatic relief (49, 51, 58). Furthermore, it is not uncommon for corticosteroid to be given to nephrotic children suspected of having steroid-responsive minimal change nephropathy, and for subsequent serology and pathological examination to reveal the diagnosis of HBV-associated membranous nephropathy (7, 22). An isolated case report has suggested that short-term corticosteroid therapy, given at the onset of nephrotic syndrome, does not seem to interfere with the favourable course of the infection and related renal disorder (58).

A deleterious effect of corticosteroid with exacerbation of liver impairment following abrupt withdrawal has been reported in patients with chronic HBV hepatitis (59). In contrast to patients with chronic active hepatitis, most patients with HBV-associated membranous nephropathy may not have evidence of hepatic dysfunction and their liver biopsies may even be normal (9, 14). A prospective trial (compared with historic controls) of corticosteroid in nephrotic patients with HBV-associated membranous nephropathy has been conducted by Lai *et al.* (49). Serial serological measurements suggested that corticosteroid therapy was associated with active viral replication with increased serum concentrations of alanine aminotransferase, HBeAg and HBV DNA, although symptomatic liver dysfunction was not often detected. Histopathological examination of post-treatment renal biopsy in a single patient revealed histological progression that did not support a protective value of corticosteroid therapy (40). Furthermore, the appearance of virus-like particles in the glomeruli after corticosteroid therapy supported the serological evidence of active viral replication. Hence, these studies reveal corticosteroid should not be used in HBV-associated membranous nephropathy.

Anti-viral agents and thymic extract

Recently, Lin and Lo (60) have reported the administration of adenine arabinoside for two weeks and thymic extract (Thymostimulin) for 6 months in 24 children with HBV-associated membranous nephropathy. Proteinuria was reduced in 87% of patients with simultaneous reduction of HBV DNA in T cells, B cells, and macrophages. Four patients (17%) had seroconversion from HBeAg to anti-HBe. The exact mechanism of these therapeutic agents is not known although modulation of the immune response of T cells is suggested. Further studies are warranted to confirm these intriguing results.

Interferon therapy

If it could be shown that resolution of glomerulonephritis in a HBV carrier followed a response to interferon therapy, this would be strong presumptive evidence for a causal connection between HBV antigens and glomerulonephritis. No confirmative conclusion can be drawn from earlier anecdotal reports of resolution of proteinuria associated with interferon therapy (61, 62). Lisker-Melman *et al.* (63) reported a clinical, biochemical, and serological remission in four adult patients with HBV-associated membranous nephropathy who were treated with interferon-α for four months. Three of these four patients had acquired HBV infection during adulthood by either sexual or intravenous transmission. Immunofluorescence staining of glomerular deposits of HBeAg was not carried out in their renal biopsy specimens. On the contrary, Lai *et al.* (56) had examined the effect of interferon in five patients with HBV-associated membranous nephropathy who probably acquired chronic HBV infection in childhood and whose renal biopsy specimens contained evidence of the deposition of HBeAg. Reduction of proteinuria was observed in over 50% of the patients but disappearance of antibody to HBeAg occurred only in 20%, a figure similar to that observed in interferon treatment of chronic HBV hepatitis in children (64). In a separate study of using alfa-interferon in treating adult patients with HBV-associated mesangiocapillary glomerulonephritis, poor therapeutic response was also documented (65).

In contrast, two studies of long-term outcome of hepatitis B virus-associated glomerulonephritis following alfa-interferon with beneficial effect have been reported. Lin (66) studied 40 children with HBV-MN. After 12 months of alfa-interferon treatment, all patients were free of proteinuria and 80% had seroconversion of HBeAg to anti-HBe. For those receiving supportive treatment alone (i.e. no alfa-interferon), 10% were free of proteinuria and 60% had mild proteinuria, yet none had seroconversion of HBeAg.

In other studies by Conjeevaram *et al.* (67), 15 adult patients with HBV-associated glomerulonephritis were treated with alfa-interferon for 16 weeks. Most of these patients (86.7%) acquire HBV infection via sexual contact or needle injury. Eight responded with loss of HBV DNA and HBeAg. The remaining seven non-responders included the only Asian patient with maternal-infant spread. The responders tended to be younger and to have shorter known duration of liver and kidney disease, high initial liver enzymes, and lower levels of HBV DNA, DNA polymerase, and HBeAg than non-responders do. In both studies, a higher incidence of side effects was observed with the higher dose of alfa-interferon.

These findings tend to suggest a satisfactory response rate to interferon amongst children or adults infected with the virus with short duration. For adults with early infection through maternal-infant spread, the poor result of interferon therapy is not unexpected. Integration of HBV DNA into host cell chromosomal DNA may occur, and in some instances fragments of HBV DNA are integrated, thus rendering the interferon therapy less effective.

New anti-viral agents

With the failure of alfa-interferon to achieve a satisfactory therapeutic effect on chronic HBV infection in endemic areas, newer anti-viral agents have emerged for clinical studies. These consist of immunomodulators and nucleoside analogues. The former group include HBV/MF59 vaccine (phases I and II studies) and pegylated alfa-interferon (phase III study) whereas the latter comprises of β-L-2′-deoxythymidine (phases I and II studies), β-L-2′-deoxycytidine (phases I and II studies), entacavir (phase III study), emtoicitabine (phase III study), FMAU (phases II and III study) and adefovir dipivoxil (phase III study).

Lamivudine, an oral nucleoside analogue, has recently been shown promise for treatment of chronic hepatitis B. In a one-year study, lamivudine given at a dose of 100 mg daily was associated with substantial histologic improvement (liver biopsy) in 56% of patients with chronic hepatitis B (68). A 98% reduction of serum HBV DNA and 16% disappearance of serum HBV DNA at week 52 was reported. The major concerns of new nucleoside analogues are the uncertain length of treatment and the emergence of drug resistant mutants and break-through of hepatitis following prolonged treatment. Example of mutants includes the YMDD motif of domain C at polymerase region of the HBV genome.

The experience of using lamivudine to treat HBV-associated membranous nephropathy is limited. In a preliminary report of 4-month lamivudine treatment in eight HBsAg carriers with nephrotic syndrome, the proteinuria fell from 12 g/day to 4.7 gm/day with simultaneous reduction of serum HBV DNA (69). Figure 24.2 depicts the clinical course of our two HBsAg carriers with symptomatic HBV-associated membranous nephropathy. Treatment with lamivudine was associated with a rapid disappearance of serum HBV DNA (within 6 months). Both patients had partial remission of nephrotic syndrome. Despite the reduction of proteinuria by more than two-thirds, completion disappearance of proteinuria was not observed even after 12 months of treatment.

Symptomatic treatment of HBV-related IgA nephropathy

HBV-associated IgA nephropathy is a slowly progressive disease and supportive treatment such as normalization of blood pressure (preferably using agents blocking the renin-angiotensin system) and low protein diet (in case of renal impairment) should be the mainstay of treatment.

Conclusion

There is strong evidence that chronic HBV infection is associated with the development of glomerulonephritis. Membranous nephropathy, mesangiocapillary nephropathy and mesangial proliferative glomerulonephritis (with IgA deposits) are the best documented HBV-associated GN. Although the natural history of these glomerulonephritides is now better known, complete cure may not always be possible. Alfa-interferon therapy should only be considered in HBV-associated glomerulonephritis in children or adult with short duration of infection. The role of nucleoside analogues is uncertain and a controlled trial should be conducted. Prevention by vaccinating all newborns with HBV vaccine should be practised in endemic areas. Vaccination of all newborns over the last decade in some endemic regions such as Hong Kong has dramatically reduced the incidence of chronic hepatitis B and HBV-associated glomerulonephritis in children and adolescents. This practice will provide the best and most cost-effective means to combat hepatitis B infection and its complications.

Acknowledgment

Part of the work was supported by the Jardine Charity Fund and the Croucher Foundation (Hong Kong).

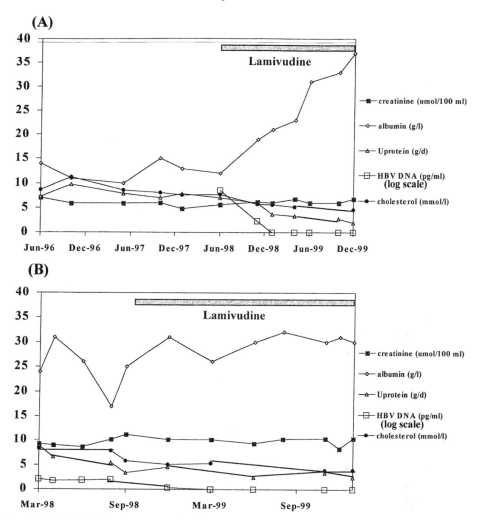

Fig. 24.2 [A] Clinical course of a 21-year old female HBsAg carrier presented with ankle edema and renal biopsy showed membranous nephropathy. [B] Clinical course of a 61-year old male HBsAg carrier with mildly elevated liver enzymes for 6 years and presented with nephrotic syndrome. Renal biopsy showed membranous nephropathy. In both cases, the serum HBV DNA disappeared within 6 months after commencing lamivudine treatment. The proteinuria was greatly reduced but both patients did not go into complete remission after treatment for 12 months.

References

1. Will H., Cattaneo R., Koch H.G., *et al.* Cloned HBV DNA causes hepatitis B in chimpanzees. *Nature* 1982, 299: 740–2.
2. Robinson W.S., Marion P.L., and Miller R.H. The hepadna viruses of animals. *Semin Liver Dis* 1984, 4: 347–60.
3. Szmuness W., Harley E.J., Ikram H., and Stevens C.E. Sociodemographic aspects of the epidemiology of hepatitis B. In: G.N. Vyas, S.N. Cohen and R. Schmid (eds) *Viral Hepatitis*. Philadelphia, Franklin Institute, 1978, 297–320.

4. Wong V., Ip H., Reesink H., *et al.* Prevention of the HBsAg carrier state in newborn infants of mothers who are chronic carriers of HBsAg and HBeAg by administration of hepatitis B vaccine and hepatitis B immunoglobulin. *Lancet* 1984, 1: 921–6.

5. Combes B., Stastny P., Shorey J., *et al.* Glomerulonephritis with deposition of Australia antigen-antibody complexes in glomerular basement membrane. *Lancet* 1971, 2: 234–7.

6. Maggiore Q., Bartolomeo F., L'Abbate A., and Misefari V. HBsAg glomerular deposits in glomerulonephritis: Fact or artifacts? *Kidney Int* 1981, 19: 579–86.

7. Takekoshi Y., Tanaka M., Shida N., *et al.* Strong association between membranous nephropathy and hepatitis-B surface antigenemia in Japanese children. *Lancet* 1978, 2: 1065–8.

8. Nagy J., Bajtai G., Brasch H., *et al.* The role of hepatitis B surface antigen in the pathogenesis of glomerulonephritis. *Clin Nephrol* 1979, 12: 109–16.

9. Lai K.N., Lai F.M., Chan K.W., *et al.* The clinico-pathological features of hepatitis B virus associated glomerulonephritis. *Q J Med* 1987, 63: 323–33.

10. Gyorkey F., Hollinger F., Eknoyan G., *et al.* Immune-complex glomerulonephritis, intra-nuclear particles in hepatocytes, and *in vivo* clearance rates in sub-human primates inoculated with HBsAg-containing plasma. *Exp Mol Pathol* 1975, 22: 350–65.

11. Germuth F.G., Senterfit L.B., and Dreesman G.R. Immune complex disease V. The nature of the chronic HSA-rabbit system. *Johns Hopkins Med J* 1972, 130: 814–19.

12. Peters D.N., Steinberg H., Anderson W.I., Hornbuckle W.E., Cote P.J., Gerin J.L., Lewis R.M., and Tennant B.C. Immunopathology of glomerulonephritis associated with chronic woodchuck hepatitis virus infection in woodchucks. *Am J Pathol* 1992, 141: 143–52.

13. Brzoko W., Krawczynski K., Nazarewicz T., *et al.* Glomerulonephritis associated with hepatitis B surface antigen immune complexes in children. *Lancet* 1974, 2: 476–82.

14. Hsu H.C., Lin G.H., Chang M.H., *et al.* Association of hepatitis B surface antigenemia and membranous nephropathy in children in Taiwan. *Clin Nephrol* 1983, 20: 121–9.

15. Sluzarczk J., Michalak T., Nazarewicz-de Mezer T., *et al.* Membranous glomerulopathy associated with hepatitis B core antigen immune complexes in children. *Am J Pathol* 1980, 98: 29–39.

16. Venkatasseshan V.S., Lieberman K., Kim D.U., *et al.* Hepatitis-B-associated glomerulonephritis: Pathology, pathogenesis, and clinical course. *Medicine* 1990, 69: 200–16.

17. Amemiya S., Ito H., Kato K., *et al.* A case of membranous proliferative glomerulonephritis type III (Burkholder) with the deposition of both HBsAg and HBeAg. *Int J Pediatr Nephrol* 1983, 4: 267–73.

18. Lai K.N., Lai F.M., Lo S., *et al.* IgA nephropathy associated with hepatitis B virus antigenemia. *Nephron* 1987, 47: 341–3.

19. Lai K.N., Lai F.M., and Tam J.S. IgA nephropathy associated with chronic hepatitis B virus infection in adults: The pathogenetic role of HBsAg. *J Pathol* 1989, 157: 321–7.

20. Tadokoro M. The clinico-pathological studies of hepatitis B virus nephropathy in adults. *Nippon Jinzo Gakkai Shi* 1991, 33: 257–266.

21. Takeda S., Kida H., Katagiri M., *et al.* Characteristics of glomerular lesions in hepatitis B virus infection. *Am J Kidney Dis* 1988, 11: 57–62.
22. Lai K.N., Lai F.M., Tam J.S., *et al.* High prevalence of hepatitis B surface antigenemia in nephrotic syndrome in Hong Kong. *Ann Trop Paediatr* 1989, 9: 45–8.
23. Looi L.M. and Prathap K. Hepatitis B virus surface antigen in glomerular immune complex deposits of patients with systemic lupus erythematosus. *Histopathology* 1982, 6: 141–7.
24. Lai K.N., Lai F.M., Leung A., and Lo S. Is there a pathogenetic role of hepatitis B virus in lupus nephritis? *Arch Pathol Lab Med* 1987, 111: 185–8.
25. Gocke D.J., Morgan C., Lockshin N., Hsu H., Bombardieri S., and Christian C.L. Association between polyarteritis and Australia antigen. *Lancet* 1970, 2: 1149–1153.
26. Trepo C. and Thivolet J. Hepatitis associated antigen and periarteritis nodosa. *Vox Sang* 1970, 19: 410–411.
27. Johnson R.J. and Couser W.G. Hepatitis B infection and renal disease: Clinical, immunopathogenetic and therapeutic considerations. *Kidney Int* 1990, 37: 663–676.
28. Lhote F., Cohen P., Genereau T., Gayraud M., and Gillevin L. Microscopic polyangiitis: clinical aspects and treatment. *Ann Med Interne (Paris)* 1996: 147: 165–177.
29. Editorial. HBV and glomerulonephritis. *Lancet* 1987, 2: 252–3.
30. Lai K.N., Lai F.M., Lo S., and Lam C.W.K. IgA nephropathy and membranous nephropathy associated with hepatitis B surface antigenemia. *Hum Pathol* 1987, 18: 411–14.
31. Ohba S., Kimura K., Mise N., *et al.* Differential localization of s and e antigens in hepatitis B virus-associated glomerulonephritis. *Clin Nephrol* 1997, 48: 44–47.
32. Hirose H., Udo K., Kojima M., *et al.* Deposition of hepatitis B e antigen in membranous glomerulonephritis. *Kidney Int* 1984, 26: 338–41.
33. Ito H., Hattori S., Matusda I., *et al.* Hepatitis B e antigen-mediated membranous glomerulonephritis. *Lab Invest* 1981, 44: 214–20.
34. Lai K.N., Lai F.M., and Tam J.S. Comparison of polyclonal and monoclonal antibodies in determination of glomerular deposits of hepatitis B virus antigens in hepatitis B virus-associated glomerulonephritis. *Am J Clin Pathol* 1989, 92: 159–65.
35. Sham M.K., Pun K.K., Yeung C.K., *et al.* hepatitis B induced glomerulonephritis, fact or fiction. *Aust NZ J Med* 1985, 15: 256–8.
36. Collins A.B., Bhan A.K., Dienstag J.L., *et al.* Hepatitis B immune complex glomerulonephritis: Simultaneous glomerular deposition of hepatitis B surface and e antigens. *Clin Immunol Immunopathol* 1983, 26: 137–53.
37. Magil A., Webber D., and Chan V. Glomerulonephritis associated with hepatitis B surface antigenemia: Report of a case with features of both membranous and IgA nephropathy. *Nephron* 1986, 42: 335–9.
38. Furuse A., Hattori S., Terashima T., *et al.* Circulating immune complexes in glomerulopathy associated with hepatitis B virus infection. *Nephron* 1982, 31: 212–18.
39. Peeples M.E., Komai K., Radek R., and Bankowski M.J. A cultured cell receptor for the small S protein of hepatitis B virus. *Virology* 1987, 160: 135–42.
40. Lai F.M., Tam J.S., Li P., and Lai K.N. Replication of hepatitis B virus with corticosteroid therapy in hepatitis B virus related membranous nephropathy. *Virchows Arch Pathol Anat* 1989, 414: 279–98.

41. Lai K.N., Lai F.M., Tam J.S., and Vallance-Owen J. Strong association between IgA nephropathy and hepatitis B surface antigenemia in endemic area. *Clin Nephrol* 1988, 29: 229–34.

42. He X.Y., Fang L.J., Zhang Y.E., Sheng F.Y., Zhang X.R., and Guo M.Y. *In situ* hybridization of hepatitis B DNA in hepatitis B-associated glomerulonephritis. *Pediatr Nephrol* 1998, 12: 117–120.

43. Korba B.E., Brown J.L., Wells R.V., *et al.* Natural history of experimental WHV infection: Molecular virologic features of the pancreas, kidney, ovary and testis. *J Virol* 1990, 60: 4499–506.

44. Lin C.Y. Hepatitis B virus DNA in kidney cells probably leading to viral pathogenesis among hepatitis B virus associated membranous nephropathy patients. *Nephron* 1993, 63: 58–64.

45. Halpern M.S., England J.M., Deery D.T., Peteu D.J., Mason W.S., and Molnar-Kimber K.L. Viral nucleic acid synthesis and antigen accumulation in pancreas and kidney of Peking ducks infected with duck hepatitis B virus. *Proc Natl Acad Sci USA* 1983, 80: 4865–4869.

46. Farza H., Hadchouel M., Scotto J., Tiollais P., Babinet C., and Pourcel C. Replication and gene expression of hepatitis B virus in a transgenic mouse that contains the complete viral genome. *J Virol* 1988, 62: 4144–4152.

47. Araki K., Miyazaki J.I., Hino O., Tomita N., Chisaka O., Matsubara K., and Yamamura K. Expression and replication of hepatitis B virus genome in transgenic mice. *Proc Natl Acad Sci USA* 1989, 86: 207–211.

48. Lai K.N., Ho R.T.H., Tam J.S., and Lai F.M. Detection of hepatitis B virus DNA and RNA in kidneys of HBV-related glomerulonephritis. *Kidney Int* 1996, 50: 1965–1977.

49. Lai K.N., Tam J.S., Lin H.J., and Lai F.M. The therapeutic dilemma of usage of corticosteroid in patients with membranous nephropathy and persistent hepatitis B virus surface antigenemia. *Nephron* 1990, 54: 12–17.

50. Kleinknecht C., Levy M., Peix A., *et al.* Membranous glomerulonephritis and hepatitis B surface antigen in children. *J Pediatr* 1979, 95: 946–52.

51. Kohler P.F., Chromin R.E., Hammond W.S., *et al.* Chronic membranous glomerulonephritis caused by hepatitis antigen-antibody immune complexes. *Ann Intern Med* 1974, 81: 448–51.

52. Van Buuren A.J., Bates W.D., and Muller N. Nephrotic syndrome in Namibian children. *S Afr Med J* 1999, 89: 1088–1091.

53. Hsu H.C., Wu C.Y., Lin C.Y., Lin G.J., Chen C.H., and Huang F.Y. Membranous nephropathy in 52 hepatitis B surface antigen carrier children in Taiwan. *Kidney Int* 1989, 36: 1103–1107.

54. Seggie J., Nathoo K., and Davies P.G. Association of hepatitis B antigenaemia and membranous glomerulonephritis in Zimbabwean children. *Nephron* 1984, 38: 115–119.

55. Lin C.Y. Hepatitis B virus-associated membranous nephropathy: clinical features, immunological profiles and outcome. *Nephron* 1990, 55: 37–44.

56. Lai K.N., Li P.K.T., Lui S.F., *et al.* Membranous nephropathy related to hepatitis B virus in adults. *N Engl J Med* 1991, 324: 1457–63.

57. Knecht G.L. and Chisari F.V. Reversibility of hepatitis B virus-induced glomerulonephritis and chronic active hepatitis after spontaneous clearance of serum hepatitis B surface antigen. *Gastroenterology* 1978, 75: 1152–6.

58. Cadrobbi P., Bortolotti F., Zacchello G., *et al.* Hepatitis B virus replication in acute glomerulonephritis with chronic active hepatitis. *Arch Dis Child* 1985, 60: 583–5.
59. Hoofnagle J.H., Davis M.D., Pappas C., *et al.* A short course of prednisolone in chronic type B hepatitis. *Ann Intern Med* 1986, 104: 12–17.
60. Lin C.Y. and Lo S. Treatment of hepatitis B virus-associated membranous nephropathy with adenine arabinoside and thymic extract. *Kidney Int* 1991, 39: 301–6.
61. Garcia G., Scullard G., Smith C., *et al.* Preliminary observation of hepatitis B-associated membranous glomerulonephritis treated with leukocyte interferon. *Hepatology* 1985, 5: 317–20.
62. Mizushima N., Kanai K., Matsuda H., *et al.* Improvement of proteinuria in a case of hepatitis B-associated glomerulonephritis after treatment with interferon. *Gastroenterology* 1987, 92: 524–6.
63. Lisker-Melman M., Webb D., Di Bisceglie, A.M., *et al.* Glomerulonephritis caused by hepatitis B virus infection: Treatment with recombinant human a-interferon. *Ann Intern Med* 1989, 111: 479–83.
64. Lai C.L., Lok A.S., Lin H.J., *et al.* Placebo-controlled trial of recombinant a 2-interferon in Chinese HBsAg carrier children. *Lancet* 1987, 2: 877–80.
65. Chung D.R., Yang W.S., Kim S.B., Yu E., Chung Y.H., Lee Y., and Park J.S. Treatment of hepatitis B virus associated glomerulonephritis with recombinant human alpha interferon. *Am J Nephrol* 1997, 17: 112–117.
66. Lin C.Y. Treatment of hepatitis B virus-associated membranous nephropathy with recombinant alpha-interferon. *Kidney Int* 1995, 47: 225–230.
67. Conjeevarum H.S., Hoofnagle J.H., Austin H.A., Park Y., Fried M.W., and Di Bisceglie A.M. Long-term outcome of hepatitis B virus-related glomerulonephritis after therapy with Interferon Alfa. *Gastroenterology* 1995, 109: 540–546.
68. Lai C.L., Chien R.N., Leung N.W., *et al.* A one-year trial of lamivudine for chronic hepatitis B. Asia Hepatitis Lamivudine study group. *N Engl J Med* 1998, 339: 61–68.
69. Lee H.Y., Shin S.K., Lee R.T., *et al.* Usefulness of lamivudine in high dose steroid taking in nephrotic syndrome patients with hepatitis B. *J Am Soc Nephrol* 1998, 9: 93A (abstract).

PART VIII

25

The nephrotoxicity of calcineurin inhibitors

Ihab M. Wahba and William M. Bennett

Introduction

Short-term survival of solid organ grafts has reached unprecedented levels over the last two decades, mainly because of calcineurin inhibitor (CI)-based immuno-suppressive regimens, namely cyclosporin A (CsA) and tacrolimus (FK-506) (1). Because of their 'incomplete' immunosuppressive effects, CI have also been successfully used in the treatment of a variety of primary glomerular and auto-immune diseases. Although generally well tolerated, the long-term use of such agents has been hampered by chronic nephrotoxicity. This chapter will address the mechanism of immunosuppression with CI, and the clinical aspects, types, pathogenesis and prevention of nephrotoxicity.

Immunosuppressive mechanisms of calcineurin inhibitors

CI reversibly inhibit early T cell signal transduction pathways which are import-ant for the activation of lymphokine genes (2). This effect is the result of binding of CsA and FK-506 to cyclophilin and FK-binding protein (FKBP), re-spectively, a family of cytosolic proteins called immunophilins (3, 4). The CI-cyclophilin or FKBP complex then binds to and inhibits calcineurin, a calcium calmodulin-dependent phosphatase whose normal function is to dephosphorylate a nuclear regulatory protein, the nuclear factor of activated T cells (NF-AT) (5). By inhibiting this dephosphorylation step, CI prevent NF-AT from translocating to the nucleus (6), thereby preventing the transcription of T cell activating genes, including IL-2, IL-3, IL-4, and gamma interferon (7). In addition, CsA upregulates transforming growth factor-β (TGF-β) which decreases T cell acti-vation (8, 9). The net result is reduced lymphokine formation. In addition to their effects on T lymphocytes, CI can directly inhibit B lymphocyte and poly-morphoneuclear leukocyte function (10, 11).

Classification of CI-induced nephrotoxicity

The adverse effects of CsA and FK-506 are very similar with few exceptions (12, 13). The clinical manifestations of nephrotoxicity are hypertension, acute haemo-dynamic renal dysfunction and chronic nephropathy. Thrombotic microangiopathy is rare. Electrolyte disorders are common but only rarely cause patient morbidity.

Hypertension

Clinical aspects

Hypertension commonly complicates CI therapy. The incidence of hypertension varies between 40% and 85% in renal, liver, lung, bone marrow and stem cell transplant recipients, and approaches 95% in cardiac transplant recipients (14–18). Even with low-dose CsA treatment, the rate of *de novo* hypertension may exceed 30% in non-transplant patients (19). Dosage reduction usually results in reduction of blood pressure, but rarely returns it to normal levels (14, 20). Characteristically, patients lose the normal nocturnal blood pressure decline (21). There is no preference as to the type of antihypertensive medication to use for therapy, but non-dihydropyridine calcium channel blockers have traditionally been preferred because of their safe renal profile and their renal vasodilatory properties (1, 22).

Pathogenesis

The pathogenesis of CI-induced hypertension is uncertain. It may be the result of (a) enhanced proximal tubular reabsorption of sodium (23), (b) renal vasoconstriction and reduced GFR (24), (c) a direct vasoconstrictive effect (24), (d) increased sympathetic neural stimulation via calcineurin inhibition in the central nervous system (25, 26), (e) inhibition of nitric oxide synthase (27) , (f) increased production of endothelin (28), or a combination of such factors. The latter two mechanisms deserve emphasis since both nitric oxide precursors and endothelin receptor antagonists attenuate CsA-induced hypertension in animals (29, 30). Furthermore, the circulating levels of endothelin-1 are usually elevated in CsA-treated patients with solid organ transplants as compared to controls (28).

Acute nephrotoxicity

Clinicopathologic aspects

CI induce afferent arteriolar vasoconstriction (Fig. 25.1), which may result in marked reduction of the glomerular filtration rate (GFR) (20, 31). Clinically, this results in an acute rise of the serum creatinine. This effect is dose-dependent and is largely reversible by dose reduction (20).

Pathogenesis

The mechanism by which CI increase afferent arteriolar tone is not well understood. A few studies suggested that CsA may stimulate the production of vaso-

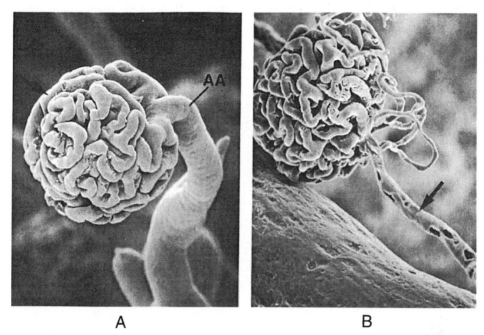

A   B

Fig. 25.1 (A) Scanning electron micrograph of a normal rat afferent arteriole (AA) and glomerular tuft (arrow) (×390). (B) Rat afferent arteriolar constriction (arrow) after 14 days of CsA treatment (×390). Reproduced by permission of Lippincott, Williams & Wilkins from: English J, Evan A, Houghton D.C, Bennett W.M. Cyclosporin-induced acute renal dysfunction. Evidence of arteriolar vasoconstriction with preservation of tubular function. *Transplantation* 1987;44:135–41 (31).

constrictor substances such as thromboxane A_2 and angiotensin II or may directly increase sympathetic nerve traffic to the kidney (25, 32, 33). Stronger evidence indicates that CI can stimulate the production and the intrarenal binding of endothelin (24, 28, 34, 35), and inhibit nitric oxide synthesis (36). In support of this hypothesis, administration of endothelin antagonists or of the nitric oxide precursor, L-arginine, reverses CsA-induced vasoconstriction in rats (37, 38).

Chronic nephropathy

Clinicopathologic aspects

Chronic CI-induced nephropathy is a clinicopathologic entity which results from exposure to CI for a period of 6–12 months (1, 39, 40). It was first described in heart transplant recipients who received relatively large doses of CsA (41). The lesion is characterized by tubulointerstitial fibrosis in a striped pattern, beginning in the renal medulla and progressing to the medullary rays of the cortex (1, 39, 42) (Fig. 25.2). This is usually associated with afferent arteriolar thickening and

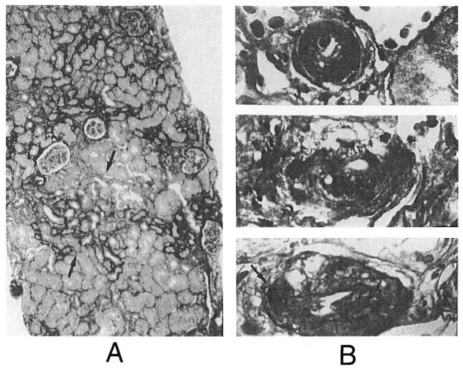

A   **B**

Fig. 25.2   (A) Renal biopsy specimen showing typical lesions of chronic CsA nephropathy. (A) Areas of striped tubulointerstitial fibrosis and tubular atrophy (arrows) (van Gieson's stain ×55). (B) Three examples of CsA-induced arteriolopathy with smooth muscle cell-necrosis and replacement by protein deposits (arrows). (acid fuchsin–orange G stain, ×267). Reproduced by permission of the Massachusetts Medical Society from: Feutren G., Mihatsch MJ. Risk factors for cyclosporin-induced nephropathy in patients with autoimmune diseases. *N Engl J Med* 1984;11:699–705 (42).

hyalinosis, which is due to the deposition of an eosinophilic protein material replacing the pericytes and the smooth muscle cells of the arterioles (Fig 25.2). Glomerular sclerosis and obsolescence may occur (1, 39). As opposed to acute nephrotoxicity, these chronic changes are usually irreversible even with dosage reduction (40, 43) and may lead to progressive renal failure and end-stage renal disease (ESRD) (1, 44).

Clinically, serum creatinine elevation is usually but not invariably present. Advanced structural changes may indeed be present in the absence of significant serum creatinine elevation (45, 46). This is due to the relative insensitivity of the serum creatinine as a marker of the true GFR, making the renal biopsy a gold standard for the diagnosis of structural chronic CI nephropathy. It may be difficult, however, to distinguish the structural changes of CI nephropathy from chronic renal allograft rejection in renal transplant recipients since they share similar histologic changes (47).

Risk factors

Although there usually is no correlation between CI blood levels and chronic nephropathy, the risk increases in relation to the duration of exposure and to the total dosage (42, 45). A CsA dosage above 5 mg/kg/d increases the risk of nephropathy (42). Chronic nephropathy can still occur, however, in patients receiving low-dose CsA (48). Other risk factors for chronic nephropathy include older age, the number of CI-induced episodes of acute renal toxicity, pre-existing renal dysfunction, number of rejection episodes in renal transplants and the number of nephrotoxic drugs used (42, 49).

Pathogenesis

The pathogenesis of chronic CI nephropathy is not well understood. Chronic low-grade ischaemia from afferent arteriolar constriction and thickening may certainly be contributing to the tubulointerstitial fibrosis and the glomerulosclerosis (46). However, this logical cause and effect relationship has not been proven in humans. Both human and animal data provide evidence that other factors independent of ischaemia may be contributing to the fibrotic process (1, 50). Because salt-depletion is necessary for the development of the characteristic structural lesions in the rat, angiotensin II has been implicated in the pathogenesis of chronic CsA nephropathy (51, 52). In support of this hypothesis, both angiotensin converting enzyme (ACE) inhibitors and angiotensin II receptor type 1 (AT1R) blockers and not other antihypertensive agents strikingly reduce the tubulointerstitial fibrosis and arteriolopathy in this animal model (53). There is also evidence that CsA promotes apoptosis of the renal tubular cells (54), and increases TGF-β and osteopontin production (50, 55) leading to the deposition of type IV collagen (56) in the renal interstitium. All of such effects are attenuated by AT1R blockade, suggesting that angiotensin II at least partially mediates the fibrotic process, perhaps via the AT1R (50, 57). Recently, endothelin-1, the inflammatory chemokine monocyte chemoattractant protein-1 (MCP-1) and RANTES (regulated upon activation, normal T cell expressed and secreted) were found to be preferentially upregulated in renal allografts of patients with histologic evidence of CsA nephropathy and not in those with chronic rejection (58). A suggested mechanism integrating all such factors is depicted in Figure 25.3.

The role of angiotensin II in human CsA nephropathy is debated due to the fact that plasma renin activity is reduced in CsA-treated patients (39). However, this finding is not uniform, and plasma total renin and prorenin are usually elevated in such patients (39, 59). Furthermore, juxtaglomerular apparatus hyperplasia is almost uniformly present and intrarenal renin is upregulated in CsA-treated animals and humans, implicating a role for intrarenal renin-angiotensin system activation, similar to patients with diabetic nephropathy (39, 52). Additionally, ACE inhibitors are at least as equally effective as calcium antagonists in the treatment of hypertension in transplant recipients (60). Their effect on chronic CI nephropathy in humans, however, has not been tested in long-term studies.

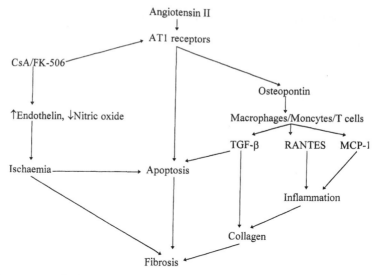

Fig. 25.3   Factors contributing to chronic CsA-induced tubulointerstitial fibrosis.

Thrombotic microangiopathy

A rare complication of CsA therapy is a microangiopathic haemolytic anaemia causing an obliterative arteriolopathy due to microthrombi. This has been reported in 3–5% of all types of solid organ transplants (61–64) and is especially important in bone marrow transplant recipients (65, 66). It usually occurs a few weeks after transplantation, but its onset may be delayed for more than 12 months (66, 67) . Apparently this syndrome is not invariably dose-related (68, 69) but has been associated with elevated CsA blood levels (64). The most common presentation of thrombotic microangiopathy is acute rapidly progressive renal failure. Evidence of haemolysis is not always present and renal biopsy is often the only clue to the diagnosis (63). Renal histopathology consists of glomerular endothelial cell swelling, mesangial hypercellularity, and fibrin and platelet thrombi (64). The pathogenesis is poorly understood and may be related to renal endothelial injury with increased thromboxane A_2, endothelin release, reduced prostacyclin production and increased platelet aggregation.

Switching to FK-506 may be safe as rescue therapy (70); however a few cases of FK-506-induced microangiopathy have also been reported (71, 72). The therapeutic efficacy of plasmapheresis, intravenous immunoglobulins, antiplatelet agents and corticosteroids has not been firmly established (64, 66). Dosage reduction or discontinuation of CsA is necessary, but permanent renal damage may persist.

Other adverse effects

A detailed discussion of other renal and extrarenal adverse effects of CI is beyond the scope of this chapter and will be mentioned briefly. Hyperkalaemia is not an uncommon complication, and may be the result of increased sodium reabsorption and reduced distal tubular flow rate (73), inhibition of distal basolateral Na^+/K^+ ATPase and apical potassium secretory channels (74, 75), extracellular migration of potassium (76), or a type IV-like renal tubular acidosis (77). Hypomagnesaemia (78) and hyperuricaemia leading to clinical gout (79, 80) may also occur as a result of renal magnesium wasting (81) and reduced tubular secretion of urate (82), respectively.

Non-renal adverse effects of CI include gingival hyperplasia (83), hirsutism (84), hepatotoxicity (85), tremors, seizures, headache (12, 86, 87), bone pain (88), hyperlipidaemia (89), glucose intolerance (90), and predisposition to infection and malignancy especially lymphoma (91, 92).

Adverse effects profile of CsA versus FK-506

CsA and FK-506 have a similar adverse profile with a few differences. Gingival hyperplasia and hirsutism are less frequent with FK-506, which makes it more favourable to use in women (12, 93). The incidence and severity of hypertension is less (13), whereas glucose intolerance and neurotoxicity are more pronounced with FK-506 than CsA (94). The risk of long-term nephrotoxicity and the histopathology appear to be similar with both agents (13, 87, 95, 96).

Clinical aspects of CI use and nephrotoxicity

In autoimmune diseases

As opposed to CsA, FK-506 is still considered an investigational drug in the treatment of most autoimmune diseases. CsA use was best studied in rheumatoid arthritis. CsA alone or in combination with non-steroidal anti-inflammatory drugs or methotrexate is indicated in patients with advanced, refractory and long-standing rheumatoid arthritis. High doses (5–10 mg/kg/d) invariably cause a significant rise of the serum creatinine by 20–40% above baseline after a 4–12 month-therapy (97–99). Lower doses (2.5–5 mg/kg/d) are less nephrotoxic with comparable efficacy (100–102).

The use of CsA in other autoimmune diseases has not been rigorously studied. Some benefits have been reported in patients with non-renal systemic lupus erythematosus (103), scleroderma (104), refractory dermatomyositis (105), Sjögren's syndrome (106), Behçet's syndrome with uveitis (107), psoriasis (108), type 1 diabetes mellitus (109), primary biliary cirrhosis (110), myasthenia gravis (111) and others, but not without the risk of causing chronic interstitial nephropathy (48, 104, 112).

In glomerular diseases

CsA has been successfully used in the primary glomerulopathies. The main indications for its use are steroid-dependent or steroid-resistant minimal-change disease, steroid-resistant focal segmental glomerulosclerosis (113–115), and progressive membranous nephropathy (116). It may also be used in resistant diffuse proliferative or membranous lupus nephritis (117, 118). A high rate of relapse has been documented after CsA discontinuation (114, 115). It is unclear if the antiproteinuric effect of CsA is due to its immunologic effects or a mere reduction of the GFR and glomerular permeability, since renal histologic indices of inflammation often remain unchanged or even worsen after therapy (119). Chronic tubulointerstitial nephropathy may occur after prolonged treatment, even if serum creatinine remains stable (120, 121).

In transplant recipients

Renal dysfunction is well document in transplant recipients receiving CI. Significant GFR decline occurs in 30–50% of cardiac and lung allograft recipients and about 6–8% may develop ESRD by 3–4 years following transplantation (15, 39, 122). Renal dysfunction and chronic nephropathy also occur in a substantial number of liver (123, 124), pancreas (43), bone marrow (125), and renal transplant patients (126). Further, CI nephrotoxicity cannot be excluded as one of the causes of chronic renal allograft nephropathy (127).

Contraindications to CsA use in autoimmune diseases

According to two evidence-based reviews on CsA use in rheumatoid arthritis, the following precautions should be undertaken (128, 129). CsA should not be used in patients who have malignancy other than non-melanomatous skin cancer (130), uncontrolled hypertension, renal dysfunction, serious infections, or hypersensitivity to CsA (129). It should be used with caution in patients older than 65 years and in those with immunodeficiency. Careful consideration of therapeutic drug levels and dosage adjustment is necessary in patients concomitantly using drugs that induce or inhibit the cytochrome P450 3A4 enzyme which is responsible for CsA hepatic and intestinal metabolism (Table 25.1). There are insufficient data available on CI use during pregnancy (129).

Table 25.1

Inhibitors of P450 3A4 (Increase CI levels)	Inducers of P450 3A4 (Reduce CI levels)
Calcium channel blockers: verapamil, diltiazem, nicardipine	Antituberculous drugs: rifampin, isoniazide
Antifungal agents: ketoconazole, fluconazole, itraconazole	Anticonvulsants: barbiturates, phenytoin, carbamazepine
Antibiotics: erythromycin	Antibiotics: nafcillin, imipenem

Prevention of CsA nephrotoxicity in autoimmune and glomerular diseases

Since the risk of chronic CsA nephropathy is dose-dependent, CsA should be started at a dosage between 2.5–3 mg/kg/d of the microemulsion form in two divided doses, and continued at the lowest effective dose if optimal efficacy is achieved. If the response is not satisfactory, the dose can be escalated gradually to a maximum of 4 mg/kg/d. If still ineffective, CsA should be discontinued (128, 129). If serum creatinine rises by 30% above baseline on two occasions one week apart, the dosage should be reduced by 25%. If renal function does not improve despite dosage reduction, CsA should be discontinued and restarted if serum creatinine returns near the patient's baseline value (128, 129). These guidelines should be followed in patients with primary glomerular diseases as well.

It should be noted that the combination of CsA and non-steroidal anti-inflammatory drugs may cause a significant reduction of the GFR (131). A recent study, however, showed that this combination is safe provided that careful monitoring of renal function is followed (132). If renal dysfunction occurs despite precautious measures, it may be prudent to withdraw the non-steroidal agent. The safety of one particular anti-inflammatory agent over the others has not been firmly established (132).

Prevention of CI nephrotoxicity in transplant recipients

The use of strong mono and polyclonal antibodies for induction therapy in transplant recipients allows for avoiding CI in the immediate post-transplant period (133, 134). This may reduce the incidence of acute renal dysfunction or delayed graft function in renal transplants. Monitoring CI blood levels is useful especially in the early post-transplant period and whenever a new medication affecting CI metabolism is introduced (Table 25.1) (22). However, current protocols for measuring the total CsA blood levels may not be optimal due to the complex kinetics of CsA following oral administration, and because the unmeasured drug metabolites may be nephrotoxic (22, 87, 135).

In the long term, unfortunately, the risk of chronic rejection may be increased if very low doses of CI in combination with conventional antirejection therapy such as azathioprine are used, due to inadequate immunosuppression (136). Combining CI with stronger immunosuppressives such as mycophenolate mofetil may allow safer reduction of their dosage or even their withdrawal (137, 138). It is unclear if the administration of calcium antagonists to counteract the vasoconstrictive effects of CI is beneficial. Recently, ACE inhibitors and AT1R blockers were safely used in hypertensive renal transplant recipients without causing renal dysfunction (139), but their long-term effects have not been studied. Ultimately, if studies aiming at induction of immune tolerance in humans prove to be successful (140), the need for CI to prevent allograft rejection may be mitigated.

References

1. Bennett W.M., DeMattos A., Meyers M.M., Andoh T., and Barry J.M. Chronic cyclosporin nephropathy. The Achille's heel of immmunosuppressive therapy. *Kidney Int* 1996, 50: 1089–100.
2. Bierer B.E., Holländer G., Fruman D., and Burakoff S.J. Molecular mechanisms of immunosuppression and probes for transplantation biology. *Curr Opin Immunol* 1993, 5: 763–73.
3. Wiederrecht G., Lam E., Hung S., Martin M., and Sigal N. The mechanism of action of FK-506 and cyclosporin A. *Ann NY Acad Sci USA* 1993, 696: 9–19
4. Clipstone N.A. and Crabtree G.R. Identification of calcineurin as a key signaling enzyme in T Lymphocyte activation. *Nature* 1992, 357, 695–7.
5. Park J., Yaseen N.R., Hogan P.G., Rao A., and Sharma S. Phosphorylation of the transcription factor NFATp inhibits its DNA binding activity in cyclosporin A-treated human B and T cells. *J Biol Chem* 1995, 270: 20653–9.
6. Flanagan W.M., Corthésy B., Bram R.J., and Crabtree G.R. Nuclear association of a T cell transcription factor blocked by FK-506 and cyclosporin A. *Nature* 1991, 352: 803–7.
7. Andersson J., Nagy S., Groth C.G., and Andersson U. Effects of FK-506 and cyclosporin A on cytokine production studied *in vitro* at a single-cell level. *Immunology* 1992, 75: 136–42.
8. Khanna A., Li B., Stenzel K.H., and Suthanthiran M. Regulation of new DNA synthesis in mammalian cells by cyclosporin. Demonstration of a transforming growth factor β-dependent mechanism of inhibition of cell growth. *Transplantation* 1994, 57: 577–82.
9. Brabletz T., Pfeuffer I., Schorr E., Siebelt F., Wirth T., and Serfling E. Transforming growth factor β and cyclosporin A inhibit the inducible activity of the interlukin-2 gene in T cells through a noncanonical octamer-binding site. *Mol Cell Biol* 1992, 13: 1155–62.
10. Thomson A.W. The effects of cyclosporin A on non-T cell components of the immune system. *J Autoimmun* 1992, 5: 167–76.
11. Forrest M.J., Jewell M.E., Koo C.G., and Sigal N.H. FK-506 and cyclosporin A: Selective inhibition of calcium ionophore-induced polymorphonuclear leukocyte degranulation. *Biochem Pharmacol* 1991, 42: 1221–8.
12. The U.S. Multicentre FK-506 Liver Study Group. A comparison of tacrolimus (FK-506) and cyclosporin in liver transplantation. *N Engl J Med* 1994, 331: 1110–5.
13. Textor S.C., Wiesner R., Wilson D.J., Porayko M., Romero J.C., Burnett J.C. Jr, Gores G., Hay E., Dickson E.R., and Krom R.A. Systemic and renal haemodynamic differences between FK-506 and cyclosprin in liver transplant recipients. *Transplantation* 1993, 55: 1332–9.
14. Textor S.C., Canzanello V.J., Taler S.J., Wilson D.J., Schwartz L.L., Augustine J.E., Raymer J.M., Romero J.C., Wiesner R.H., Krom R.A., and Burnett J.C. Cyclosporin-induced hypertension after transplantation. *Mayo Clin Proc* 1994, 69: 1182–93.
15. Zaltzman J.S., Pei Y., Mauer J., Patterson A., and Cattran D.C. Cyclosporin nephrotoxicity in lung transplant recipients. *Transplantation* 1992, 54: 875–8.
16. Loughran T.P., Deeg H.J., Dahlberg S., Kennedy M.S., Storb R., and Thomas, E.D. Incidence of hypertension after bone marrow transplantation among 112

patients randomized to either cyclosporin or methotrexate as graft versus host disease prophylaxis. *Br J Haematol* 1985, 59: 547–53.

17. Woo M., Przepiorka D., Ippoliti C., Warkentin D., Khouri I., Fritsche H., and Korbling M. Toxicities of tacrolimus and cyclosporin A after allogeneic blood stem cell transplantation. *Bone Marrow Transplant* 1997, 20: 1095–8.

18. Ventura H.O., Mehra M.R., Stapleton D.D., and Smart F.W. Cyclosporin-induced hypertension in cardiac transplantation. *Med Clin North Am* 1997, 81: 1347–57.

19. Quereda C., Soria C., Sabater J., Orte L., Lucas M.F., Gonzalo A., and Ortuño J. Low-dose cyclosporin A nephrotoxicity in non-renal patients. *Transplant Proc* 1994, 26: 2693–4.

20. Curtis J.J., Luke R.G., Dubovsky E., Diethelm A.G., Whelchel J.D., and Jones P. Cyclosporin in therapeutic doses increases renal allograft vascular resistance. *Lancet* 1986, 2: 477–9.

21. Van de Borne P., Gelin M., Van de Sadt J., and Degaute J.P. Circadian rhythms of blood pressure after liver transplantation. *Hypertension* 1993, 21: 398–405.

22. de Mattos A.M., Olyaei A.J., and Bennett W.M. Nephrotoxicity of immunosuppressive drugs: Long-term consequences and challenges for the future. *Am J Kidney Dis* 2000, 35: 333–46.

23. Cusi D., Barlassina C., Niutta E., Elli A., Quarto di Palo F., and Bianchi G. Mechanisms of cyclosporin-induced hypertension. *Clin Invest Med* 1991, 14: 607–13.

24. Textor S.C., Burnett Jr J.C., Romero J.C., Canzanello V.J., Taler S.J., Wiesner R., Porayko M., Krom R., Gores G., and Hay E. Urinary endothelin and renal vasoconstriction with cyclosporin or FK-506 after liver transplantation. *Kidney Int* 1994, 47: 1426–33.

25. Sherrer U., Vissing S.F., Morgan B.J., Rollins J.A., Tindall R.S.A., Ring S., Hanson P., Mohanty P.K., and Victor R.G. Cyclosporin-induced sympathetic activation and hypertension after heart transplantation. *N Engl J Med* 1990, 323: 693–9.

26. Sander M., Lyson T., Thomas G.D., and Victor R.G. Sympathetic neural mechanisms of cyclosporin-induced hypertension. *Am J Hypertens* 1996, 9: 121S–38S.

27. Vaziri N.D., Ni Z., Zhang Y.P., Ruzics E.P., Maleki P., and Ding Y. Depressed renal vascular nitric oxide synthase expression in cyclosporin-induced hypertension. *Kidney Int* 1998, 54: 482–91.

28. Grieff M., Loertscher R., Shohaib S.L., and Stewart, D.J. Cyclosporin-induced elevation in circulating endothelin-1 in patients with solid-organ transplants. *Transplantation* 1993, 56: 880–4.

29. Bartholomeusz B., Hardy K.J., Nelson A.S., and Phillips P.A. Modulation of nitric oxide improves cyclosporin A-induced hypertension in rats and primates. *J Human Hypertens* 1998, 12: 839–44.

30. Oriji G.K. and Keiser H.R. Role of nitric oxide in cyclosporin A-induced hypertension. *Hypertension* 1998, 32: 849–55.

31. English J., Evan A., Houghton D.C., and Bennett, W.M. Cyclosporin-induced acute renal dysfunction. Evidence of arteriolar vasoconstriction with preservation of tubular function. *Transplantation* 1987, 44: 135–41.

32. Elzinga L., Kelley V.E., Houghton D.C., and Bennett W.M. Fish oil vehicle for cyclosporin lowers renal thromboxanes and reduces experimental nephrotoxicity. *Transplant Proc* 1987, 19: 1403–6.

67. Lucca L.J., Ressurreiçao F.A.M.S., Ferraz A.S., Costa R.S., Costa J.A.C., Pisi T.M., and Alves M.R. De novo haemolytic uraemic syndrome: A rare adverse effect in renal transplant recipients immunosuppressed with cyclosporin. *Transplant Proc* 1992, 24, 3098–9.

68. Van Buren D., Van Buren C.T., Flechner S.M., Maddox A.M., Verani R., and Kahan B.D. De novo haemolytic uraemic syndrome in renal transplant recipients immunosuppressed with cyclosporin. *Surgery* 1995, 98: 54–62.

69. Zent R., Katz A., Quaggin S., Cattran D., Wade J., Cardella C., Zaltzman J., Fenton S., and Cole E. Thrombotic microangiopathy in renal transplant recipients treated with cyclosporin A. *Clin Nephrol* 1997, 47: 181–6.

70. Franz M., Regele H., Schmaldienst S., Stummvol H.K., Horl W.H., and Pohanka E. Post-transplant haemolytic uraemic syndrome in adult retransplanted kidney graft recipients: advantage of FK-506 therapy? *Transplantation* 1998, 66: 1258–62.

71. Walder B., Ricou B., and Suter P.M. Tacrolimus (FK-506)-induced haemolytic uraemic syndrome after heart transplantation. *J Heart Lung Transplant* 1998, 17: 1004–6.

72. Schmidt R.H., Lenz T., Grone H.J., Geiger H., and Scheuermann, E.H. Haemolytic uraemic syndrome after tacrolimus rescue therapy for cortisone-resistant rejection. *Nephrol Dial Transplant* 1999, 14: 979–83.

73. Laine J. and Holmberg C. Renal and adrenal mechanisms in cyclosporin-induced hyperkalaemia after renal transplantation. *Eur J Clin Invest* 1995, 25: 670–6.

74. Tumlin J.A. and Sands J.M. Nephron segment-specific inhibtion of Na^+/K^+-ATPase activity by cyclosporin A. *Kidney Int* 1993, 43: 246–51.

75. Ling B.N. and Eaton D.C. Cyclosporin A inhibits apical secretory K^+ channels in rabbit cortical collecting tubule principal cells. *Kidney Int* 1993, 44: 974–84.

76. Pei Y., Richardson R., Greenwood C., Math M., Wong P.Y. and Baines A. Extrarenal effect of cyclosporin A on potassium homeostasis in renal transplant recipients. *Am J Kidney Dis* 1993, 22: 314–9.

77. Jones J.W., Gruessner R.W., Gores P.F., and Matas A.J. Hypoaldosteronaemic hyporeninaemic hyperkalaemia after renal transplantation. *Transplantation* 1993, 56: 1013–5.

78. Thompson C.B., June C.H., Sullivan K.M., and Thomas E.D. Association between cyclosporin neurotoxicity and hypomagnesaemia. *Lancet* 1984, 2: 116–20.

79. Burack D.A., Griffith B.P., Thompson M.E., and Kahl L.E. Hyperuricaemia and gout among heart transplant recipients receiving cyclosporin. *Am J Med* 1992, 92: 141–6.

80. Delaney V., Sumrani N., Daskalakis P., Hong J.H., and Sommer B.G. Hyperuricaemia and gout in renal allograft recipients. *Transplant Proc* 1992, 24: 1773–4.

81. Nozue T., Kobayashi A., Sako A., Satoh T., Kodama T., Yamazaki H., Kurosawa M., Uemasu F., Endoh H., and Takagi Y. Evidence that cyclosporin causes both intracellular migration and inappropriate urinay excretion of magnesium in rats. *Transplantation* 1993, 55: 346–9.

82. Colussi G., Rombola G., De Ferrari M.E., Rolando P., Surian M., Malberti F., and Minetti L. Pharmacologic evaluation of urate renal handling in humans: pyrazinamide test vs combined pyrazinamide and probenecid administration. *Nephrol Dial Transplant* 1987, 2: 10–6.

83. Pan W.L., Chan C.P., Huang C.C., and Lai M.K. Cyclosporin-induced gingival overgrowth. *Transplant Proc* 1992, 4: 1393–4.

84. Fernando O.N., Sweny P., and Varghese Z. Elective conversion of patients from cyclosporin to tacrolimus for hypertrichosis. *Transplant Proc* 1998, 30: 1243–4.

85. Klintmalm C.B.G., Iwatsuki S., and Starzl T.E. Cyclosporin A hepatotoxicity in 66 renal allograft recipients. *Transplantation* 1981, 32: 488–9.

86. Shah, A.K. Cyclosporin A neurotoxicity among bone marrow transplant recipients. *Clin Neuropharmacol* 1999: 22: 67–73.

87. de Mattos A.M., Olyaei A.J., and Bennett W.M. Pharmacology of immunosuppressive medications used in renal diseases and transplantation. *Am J Kidney Dis* 1996, 28: 631–60.

88. Lucas V.P., Ponge T.D., Plougastel-Lucas M.C., Glemain P, Hourmant M., and Soulillou J.P. Musculoskeletal pain in renal transplant recipients (Letter). *N Engl J Med* 1991, 325: 1449–50.

89. Massy A.Z. and Kasiske B.L. Post-transplant hyperlipidaemia: Mechanisms and management. *J Am Soc Nephrol* 1996, 7: 971–7.

90. Jindal R.M. Post-transplant diabetes mellitus – a review. *Transplantation* 1994, 58: 1289–98.

91. Penn I. Tumors after renal and cardiac transplantation. *Haematol Oncol Clin North Am* 1993, 7: 431–45.

92. Rubin R.H. Infectious disease complications of renal transplantation. *Kidney Int* 1993, 44: 221–36.

93. Fung J.J., Alessiani M., Abu-Elmagd K., Todo S., Shapiro R., Tzakis A., Van Thiel D., Armitage J., Jain A., McCauley J., Selby R., and Starzl T.E. Adverse effects associated with the use of FK-506. *Transplant Proc* 1991, 23: 3105–8.

94. Pirsch J.D., Miller J., Deierhoi M.H., Vincenti F., and Filo R.S. A comparison of tacrolimus (FK-506) and cyclosporin for immunosuppression after cadaveric renal transplantation. FK-506 Kidney Transplant Study Group. *Transplantation* 1998, 65: 142–5.

95. Randhawa P.S, Shapiro R., Jordan M.L., Starzl T.E., and Demetris A.J. The histopathological changes associated with allograft rejection and drug toxicity in renal transplant recipients maintained on FK-506. *Am J Surg Path* 1993, 17: 60–8.

96. Mayer A.D., Dmitrewski J., Squifflet J.P., Besse T., Grabensee B., Klein B., Eigler F.W., Heeman U., Pichlmayr R., Behrend M., Vanrenterghem Y., Donck J., van Hooff J., Christiaans M., Morales J.M., Andres A., Johnson R.W., Short C., Buchholz B., Rehmert N., Land W., Schleibner S., Forsythe J.L., Talbot D, and Pohanka E. Multicentre randomized trial comparing tacrolimus (FK-506) and cyclosporin in the prevention of renal allograft rejection: A report of the European Tacrolimus Multicentre Renal Study Group. *Transplantation* 1997, 64: 436–43.

97. Van Rijthoven A.W.A.M., Dijkmans B.A.C., Goei The H.S., Hermans J., Montnor-Beckers Z.L.M.B., Jacobs P.C.J., and Cats A. Cyclosporin treatment for rheumatoid arthritis: a placebo-controlled, double-blind, multicentre study. *Ann Rheum Dis* 1986, 45: 726–31.

98. Dougados M., Awada H., and Amor B. Cyclosporin in rheumatoid arthritis: A double blind, placebo controlled study in 52 patients. *Ann Rheum Dis* 1988, 47: 127–33.

99. Yocum D.E., Klippel J.H., Wilder R.L., Gerber N.L., Austin H.A., Wahl S.M., Lesko L., Minor J., Preuss H.G., Yarboro C., Berkebile C., and Dougherty B.S. Cyclosporin A in severe, treatment-refractory rheumatoid arthritis. *Ann Intern Med* 1988, 109: 863–9.

100. Tugwell P., Bombardier C., Gent M., Bennett K.J., Bensen W.G., Carette S., Chalmers A., Esdaile J.M., Klinkhoff A.V., Kraag G.R., Ludwin D., and Roberts R.S. Low-dose cyclosporin versus placebo in patients with rheumatoid arthritis. *Lancet* 1990, 335: 1051–5.

101. Tugwell P., Pincus T., Yocum D., Stein M., Gluck O., Kraag G., McKendry R., Tesser J., Baker P., and Wells G. For the methotrexate-cyclosporin combination study group. Combination therapy with cyclosporin and methotrexate in severe rheumatoid arthritis. *N Engl J Med* 1995, 333: 137–41.

102. Landewé R.B.M., Goei The H.S., Van Rijthoven A.W.A.M., Breedveld F.C., and Dijkmans B.A.C. A randomized, double-blind, 24-week controlled study of low-dose cyclosporin versus chloroquine for early rheumatoid arthritis. *Arthritis Rheum* 1994, 37: 637–43.

103. Caccavo D., Lagana B., Mittehofer A.P., Ferri G.M., Alfeltra A., Amoroso A., and Bonomo L. Long-term treatment of systemic lupus erythematosus with cyclosporin A. *Arthritis Rheum* 1997, 40: 27–35.

104. Ippoliti G., Miori L., Negri B., Rovati F., Lorenzutti F., Zerbinati N., and Rabbiosi G. Cyclosporin in the treatment of progressive systemic sclerosis: Clinical and immunologic findings. *Transplant Proc* 1994, 26: 3117–18.

105. Lueck C.J., Trend P., and Swash M. Cyclosporin in the management of polymyositis and dermatomyositis. *J Neurol Neurosurg Psych* 1991, 54: 1007–8.

106. Droros A.A., Skopouli F.N., and Costopoulos J.S. Cyclosporin A in primary Sjögren's syndrome: A double blind study. *Ann Rheum Dis* 1986, 45: 732–5.

107. Binder A.I., Graham E.M., Sanders M.D., Dinning W., James D.G., and Denman A.M. Cyclosporin A in the treatment of severe Behçet's uveitis. *Br J Rheumatol* 1987, 26: 285–91.

108. Berth-Jones J., Henderson C.A., Munro C.S., Rogers S., Chalmers R.J.G., Boffa M.J., Norris P.G., Friedmann P.S., Graham-Brown R.A.C., Dowd P.M., Marks R., and Sumner M.J. Treatment of psoriasis with intermittent short course cyclosporin (Neoral). A multicentre study. *Br J Dermatol* 1997, 136: 527–30.

109. Feutren G., Papoz L., Assan R., Vialettes B., Karsenty G., Vexiau P., Du Rostu H., Rodier M., Sirmai J., and Lallemand A. Cyclosporin increases the rate and length of remissions in insulin-dependent diabetes of recent onset. Results of a multicentre double-blind trial. *Lancet* 1986, 2: 119–24.

110. Wiesner R.H., Ludwig J., Lindor K.D., Jorgensen R.A., Baldus W.P., Homburger H.A., and Dickson E.R. A controlled trial of cyclosporin in the treatment of primary biliary cirhosis. *N Engl J Med* 1990, 322: 1419–24.

111. Tindall R.S., Rollins J.A., Phillips J.T., Greenlee R.G., Wells L., and Belendijk G. Preliminary results of a double-blind, randomized, placebo-controlled trial of cyclosporin in myasthenia gravis. *N Engl J Med* 1987, 316: 719–24.

112. Palestine A.G., Austin H.A., Balow J.E., Antonovych T.T., Sabnis S.G., Preuss H.G., and Nussenblatt R.B. Renal histopathologic alterations in patients treated with cyclosporin for uveitis. *N Engl J Med* 1986, 14: 1293–8.

113. Ponticelli C., Rizzoni G., Edefonti A., Altieri P., Rivolta E., Rinaldi S., Ghio L., Lusvarghi E., Gusmano R., Locatelli F., Pasquali S., Castellani A., and Casa-Alberighi O.D. A randomized trial of cyclosporin in steroid-resitant idiopathic nephrotic syndrome. *Kidney Int* 1993, 43: 1377–84.

114. Niaudet P. Comparison of cyclosporin and chlorambucil in the treatment of steroid-dependent idiopathic nephrotic syndrome: A multicentre randomized controlled trial. *Paediatr Nephrol* 1992, 6: 1–3.

115. Niaudet P. Treatment of childhood steroid-resistant idiopathic nephrosis with a combination of cyclosporin and prednisone. French Society of Paediatric Nephrology. *J Paediatr* 1994, 125: 981–6.

116. Cattran D.C., Greenwood C., Ritchie S., Bernstein K., Churchill D.N., Clark W.F., Morrin P.A., and Lavoie S. A controlled trial of cyclosporin in patients with progressive membranous nephropathy. Canadian Glomerulonephritis Study Group. *Kidney Int* 1995, 47: 1130–5.

117. Tam L.S., Li E.K., Leung C.B., Wong K.C., Lai F.M., Wang A., Szeto C.C., and Lui S.F. Long-term treatment of lupus nephritis with cyclosporin A. *Q J Med* 1998, 91: 573–80.

118. Radhakrishnan J., Kunis C.L., D'Agati V., and Appel G.B. Cyclosporin A treatment of lupus membranous nephropathy. *Clin Nephrol* 1994, 42: 147–54.

119. Ambalavanan S., Fauvel J.P., Sibley R.K., and Myers B.D. Mechanism of the antiproteinuric effect of cyclosporin in membranous nephropathy. *J Am Soc of Nephrol* 1996, 7: 290–8.

120. Melocoton T.L., Kamil E.S., Cohen A.H., and Fine R.N. Long-term cyclosporin A treatment of steroid-resistant and steroid-dependent nephrotic syndrome. *Am J Kidney Dis* 1991, 18: 583–8.

121. Niaudet P., Broyer M., and Habib R. Serial biopsies in children with idiopathic nephrosis receiving cyclosporin. In: A. Tejani (ed.) *Cyclosporin in the Therapy of Renal Disease*. Krager, Basel 1995, pp. 78–83.

122. Goldstein D.J., Zeuch N., Seghal V., Weinberg A.D., Drusin R., and Cohen D. Cyclosporin-associated end-stage nephropathy after cardiac transplantion: Incidence and progression. *Transplantation* 1997, 63: 664–8.

123. Gonwa T.A., Morris C.A., Goldstein R.M., Husberg B.S., and Klintmalm G.B. Long-term survival and renal function following liver transplantation in patients with and without hepatorenal syndrome-experience in 300 patients. *Transplantation* 1991, 51: 428–30.

124. Porayko M.K., Textor S.C., Krom R.A.F., Hay J.E., Gores G.J., Richards T.M., Crotty P.H., Beaver S.J., Steers J.L., and Wiesner R.H. (1994). Nephrotoxic effects of primary immunosuppression with FK-506 and cyclosporin regimens after liver transplantation. *Mayo Clin Proc* 1994, 69: 105–11.

125. Dieterle A., Gratwohl A., Nizze H., Huser B., Mihatsch M.J., Thiel G., Tichelli A., Singer E., Nissen C., and Speck B. Chronic cyclosporin-associated nephrotoxicity in bone marrow transplant patients. *Transplantation* 1990, 49: 1093–100.

126. Mourad G., Vela C., Ribstein J., and Mimran A. Long-term improvement in renal function after cyclosporin reduction in renal transplant recipients with histologically proven chronic cyclosporin nephropathy. *Transplantation* 1998, 65: 661–7.

127. Halloran P.F., Melk A., and Barth C. Rethinking chronic allograft nephropathy: The concept of accelerated scenescence. *J Am Soc Nephrol* 1999, 10: 167–81.

128. Payani G.S. and Tugwell P. The use of cyclosporin A microemulsion in rheumatoid arthritis: Conclusions of an international review. *Br J Rheumatol* 1997, 36: 808–11.

129. Cush J.J., Tugwell P., Weinblatt M., and Yocum D. US consensus guidelines for the use of cyclosporin A in rheumatoid arthritis. *J Rheumatol* 1999, 26: 1176–86.

130. Arellano F. and Krupp P. Malignancies in rheumatoid arthritis patients treated with cyclosporin A. *Br J of Rheumatol* 1993, 32(Suppl. 1): 72–5.

131. Altman R.D., Perez G.O., and Sfakianakis G.N. Interaction of cyclosporin A and nonsteroidal anti-inflammatory drugs on renal function in patients with rheumatoid arthritis. *Am J Med* 1992, 93: 396–402.

132. Tugwell P., Ludwin D., Gent M., Roberts R., Bensen W., Grace E., and Baker P. Interaction between cyclosporin A and nonsteroidal anti-inflammatory drugs. *J Rhemuatol* 1997, 24: 1122–5.

133. Norman D.J., Kimball J.A., Bennett W.M., Shihab F., Batiuk T.D., Meyer M.M., and Barry J.M. A prospective, double-blind randomized study of low-dose OKT3 induction immunosuppression in cadaveric renal transplantation. *Transpl Int* 1994, 7: 356–61.

134. Norman D.J. Rationale for OKT3 monoclonal antiobody treatment in transplant patients. *Transplant Proc* 1993, 25: 2(Suppl. 1): 1–3.

135. Christians U. and Sewing K.-F. Cyclosporin metabolism in transplant patients. *Pharmacol Ther* 1993, 57: 291–345.

136. Almond P.S., Matas A., Gillingham K., Dunn D.L., Payne W.D., Gores P., Gruessner R., and Najarian J.S. Risk factors for chronic rejection in renal allograft recipients. *Transplantation* 1993, 55: 752–6.

137. Hueso M., Bover J., Seron D., Gil-Vernet S., Sabate I., Fulladosa X., Ramos R., Coll O., Alsina J., and Grinyo J.M. Low-dose cyclosporin and mycophenolate mofetil in renal allograft recipients with suboptimal renal function. *Transplantation* 1998, 66: 1727–31.

138. Abramowicz D., Manas D., Lao M., Vanrenterghem Y., del Castillo D., and Barker D. Preliminary results of a randomized, controlled study investigating the withdrawal of Neoral in stable renal transplant recipients receiving mycophenolate mofetil in addition to Neoral and steroids. *Transplantation* 1999, 67(Suppl. 1, Abstract 934): S240A

139. Stigant C.E., Cohen J., Vivera M., and Zaltzman J.S. ACE inhibitors and angiotensin II antagonists in renal transplantation: An analysis of safety and efficacy. *Am J Kidney Dis* 2000, 35: 58–63.

140. Sayegh M.H. and Turka L. The role of T cell costimulatory activation pathways in transplant recipients. *N Engl J Med* 1998, 338: 1813–21.

26

Non-steroidal anti-inflammatory drugs and the kidney

Wai Y. Tse and Dwomoa Adu

Introduction

Many patients with rheumatic diseases and joint pains take non-steroidal anti-inflammatory drugs (NSAIDs) for symptom control. Despite their recognized efficacy, their safe use requires an awareness of their well-recognized side-effects, the most significant of which are gastric and renal toxicity. Although the renal side effects of these drugs are uncommon, the widespread use of NSAIDs and the availability of some NSAIDs as 'over-the-counter' drugs make it likely that renal side effects will be seen more frequently. These include salt and water retention, acute deterioration of renal function, acute tubular necrosis, acute interstitial nephritis with or without heavy proteinuria, hyperkalaemia, renal papillary necrosis and chronic renal failure (1–3). The incidence of these renal side-effects is unknown. A large hospital-based study of 41,000 inpatients, including 1222 who were taking NSAIDs, demonstrated no increase in renal disease attributable to NSAIDs. Furthermore long-term follow up of 50,000 outpatient users of NSAIDs disclosed that none required hospital admission for acute kidney disease (4). However, more recent case control studies have shown that the use of NSAIDs is associated with a two fold to four fold increase in the risk of hospitalization with acute renal failure (5), (6). Many of the renal abnormalities encountered as a result of NSAID use can be attributed to the action of these drugs on prostaglandins (PGs) through cyclooxygenase-1 (COX-1) and COX-2 inhibition. Questions still remain as to whether some NSAIDs might spare effects on renal function and, in particular, whether COX-2 selective inhibitors might differ in their effects on the kidney.

Prostaglandin biochemistry

Pharmocodynamics

The NSAIDs are a chemically heterogeneous group of compounds that were first reported to inhibit PGs synthesis in 1971 (7). Most of the therapeutic and adverse effects of NSAIDS are mediated through inhibition of PGs synthesis. PGs are unsaturated fatty acid compounds synthesized from cell membrane

Renin release

PGE$_2$, PGI$_2$ and arachidonic acid are potent stimuli of renin release (19). NSAIDs inhibit renin secretion although this can still occur through baroreceptor and adrenergic stimuli if these are sufficiently activated. In some circumstances NSAIDs can lead to hyporeninaemia and hypoaldosteronism. The most common manifestation of this complication is hyperkalaemia, especially in patients with pre-existing renal impairment (27), (28). The renin inhibitory effects of NSAIDs have been used in the management of Bartter's syndrome where hypokalaemia is associated with increased levels of prostaglandins (29), (30).

Potassium homeostasis

In addition to their effects on renin and aldosterone secretion described above, PGs synthesis inhibition can also lead to hyperkalaemia through decreased distal tubular flow rate and sodium delivery, both of which can limit potassium secretion (31), (32). Moreover, the increased action of anti-diuretic hormone that results from inhibition of PGs synthesis can further decreases flow rate and lowers the patient's ability to secrete potassium (33).

Natriuresis and diuresis

There is good experimental evidence that renal PGs have a natriuretic tubular effect through inhibition of sodium and chloride reabsorption in the proximal and distal nephron and the loop of Henle (34), (35). They also reduce renal cortico-medullary solute gradient and antagonize the action of vasopressin *in vivo* (36) leading to a diuresis. Whilst PGs acutely influence salt and water excretion they do not regulate this under normal conditions. Inhibition of renal PG synthesis can cause salt and water retention but this is transitory unless there are circumstances such as heart failure, cirrhosis or the nephrotic syndrome that are associated with sodium retention (2).

Conditions in which renal prostaglandins are important

Under normal euvolaemic conditions, PGs play a negligible role in the maintenance of renal and glomerular blood flow, and the administration of NSAIDs under such circumstances produce negligible effects on renal haemodynamics (37), (38). However, in the presence of salt depletion, or conditions where there is ineffective circulating plasma volume or conditions characterized by high circulating levels of vasoconstrictor hormones, NSAIDs use can lead to nephrotoxicity. Examples of these conditions include cirrhosis, hypovolaemia, cardiac disease, chronic renal failure, septic shock, advanced age, diuretic use and diabetes mellitus (39) (Table 26.2). Elderly people, particularly those with arterial disease or gout, rely on renal PGs to maintain renal function and are therefore susceptible to NSAID-induced renal side-effects. The majority of patients reported to have developed acute renal failure on NSAIDs have been over the age of 60 years (2).

Table 26.2 Conditions that predispose to NSAIDs-induced renal failure

Hypovolaemia
Haemorrhage
Septic shock
Congestive cardiac failure/Heart disease
Nephrotic syndrome
Cirrhosis with ascites
Anaesthesia/Surgery
Pre-eclampsia
Sodium depletion: Diuretics
                    Gastrointestinal losses
Renal artery stenosis
Glomerulonephritis
Urinary tract obstruction
Toxic injury: Cyclosporin A
            Tacrolimus
            Gentamicin
Urinary tract infection
Hypercalcaemia
Advancing age
Chronic renal failure

Clinical syndromes associated with NSAIDs

Acute renal impairment/acute tubular necrosis

The risk for these adverse renal effects is largely dose-dependent, and is negligible for healthy individuals, whose renal haemodynamics is minimally dependent upon intact PG synthesis. In high renin states the kidney is dependent on PGs to maintain blood flow and renal function (discussed above). Inhibition of PGs synthesis by NSAIDs under these conditions can lead to a fall in glomerular filtration rate and acute renal failure. This complication has been reported with most of the NSAIDs but only rarely with aspirin. Predisposing causes of acute renal failure include previous diuretic therapy, sodium depletion, congestive heart failure, underlying chronic renal failure, diabetes and hepatocellular insufficiency. Renal function usually improves on stopping the drug although in some cases the development of acute renal failure may necessitate dialysis.

Acute tubulo-interstitial nephritis

Most NSAIDs of different chemical classes have been associated with acute renal failure caused by an acute tubulo-interstitial nephritis. The original description of this association was reported by Brezin *et al.* (1979) (42) and since that time, there have been many further reports (40), (41), (1). Acute allergic tubulo-interstitial nephritis due to NSAIDs is much less common than the haemodynamic form of renal failure. The patients are often elderly and the drug may have been taken for months or years before the development of acute interstitial nephritis. There is often little clinical evidence of an allergic reaction; fever, rash, arthralgia, eosinophilia and eosinophiluria are uncommon. An unusual feature of NSAID-induced tubulo-interstitial nephritis is the development of proteinuria that is often in the nephrotic range. This is a particular feature of fenoprofen-induced tubulo-interstitial nephritis (42–44). The histologic picture is unusual in combining minimal-change glomerulonephropathy with acute interstitial nephritis. These combined histological findings have also been reported in patients who had ingested other NSAIDs, including piroxicam, indomethacin, tolmetin, ibuprofen and zomepirac (41). Many of these features differ from that seen in tubulo-interstitial nephritis caused by other drugs in which the onset is earlier, there is often evidence of an allergic reaction and in which, apart from occasional reports with ampicillin, heavy proteinuria is not seen. The insidious nature of onset of NSAID-induced tubulo-interstitial nephritis and the wide use of NSAIDs makes it important to obtain a careful drug history in patients with unexplained acute renal failure.

Diagnosis of NSAID-induced acute tubulo-interstitial nephritis is by renal biopsy (Fig. 26.1). Renal histology shows patchy acute tubular damage and a tubulo-interstitial infiltrate that consists predominantly of T lymphocytes and to

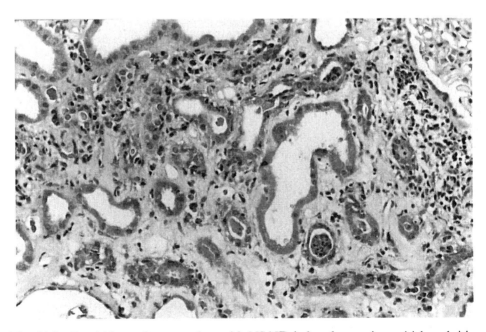

Fig. 26.1 Renal biopsy from a patient with NSAID-induced acute interstitial nephritis. Cortex in a renal biopsy specimen showing an infiltrate of mixed inflammatory cells in acute interstitial nephritis. Haematoxylin and eosin ×170. (By courtesy of Dr A.J. Howie.)

a lesser extent monocytes/macrophages, B lymphocytes, plasma cells and eosinophils (44), (45). Rarely a granulomatous interstitial nephritis is seen (46). Immunofluorescent microscopy is usually negative or non-specific. The predominance of T lymphocytes in the interstitial infiltrate has led to speculation that T lymphocyte activation may be the immunologic process that mediates this syndrome rather than a humoral mechanism as in other forms of acute interstitial nephritis due to drugs (43), (44). Likewise, suggestions that the heavy proteinuria might be due to an increased glomerular permeability caused by lymphokines released by activated T cells remains speculative. The observation that NSAIDs of different chemical structures can cause an acute tubulo-interstitial nephritis has led to the suggestion that this lesion is a consequence of inhibition of renal COX. This can lead to stimulation of the lipoxygenase pathway of arachidonic acid metabolism with the production of leukotrienes which are potent chemotactic factors for lymphocytes. Furthermore, PGs have immunomodulatory functions and it is possible that inhibition of their secretion may lead to an escape from immunological control (47). There is evidence that inhibition of PGs can lead to sustained or enhanced expression of proinflammatory and profibrogenic mediators, resulting in tubulo-interstitial damage and fibrosis (48).

The main functional derangements relates to uraemia, but a consistent hyperchloraemic acidosis has been noted (49), together with impaired concentrating ability which may persist for many months after the acute episode in those cases which recover renal function (50). Renal failure in these patients may be severe enough to necessitate dialysis. Withdrawal of the drug leads in most cases to resolution of the renal failure and proteinuria although this may take up to a year. Recovery of renal function may be only partial (45) and progression to chronic interstitial fibrosis and chronic renal failure has been reported (40,51). There is no conclusive evidence that corticosteroids hasten the resolution of the renal lesion (1) and the use of prednisolone is based on anecdotal reports. Experimental acute interstitial nephritis typically precedes fibrogenesis by as short a time as 7 to 14 days (52). The potential for incomplete resolution leads us to advocate a one month course of prednisolone starting at a dose of 30 mg daily that is rapidly reduced as renal function improves. Whether cross-reactivity among NSAIDs occurs in this syndrome is unknown. If a patient develops this syndrome, further administration of any NSAIDs should be avoided. If this is not possible, a compound of a different structural class should be selected and the patient should be monitored closely.

Vasculitis/glomerulonephritis

Membranous nephropathy with nephrotic syndrome may occur as idiosyncratic reaction to various classes of NSAIDs (53), (54). The temporal association with the intake of modest doses of NSAIDs, the prompt and complete recovery after drug discontinuation, and the absence of recurrent disease may help to clinically distinguish NSAID-associated membranous nephropathy from the idiopathic form (55). There are also anecdotal reports of generalized vasculitis and glomerulitis in patients taking NSAIDs. It is difficult to be certain of a causal relationship with NSAIDs in many of these cases. However in one case of generalized vasculitis associated with piroxicam the same clinical picture developed on re-challenge with the drug (56).

Renal papillary necrosis

Renal papillary necrosis is a well-recognized complication of chronic and excessive ingestion of compound analgesic drugs particularly those containing phenacetin, and this was an important cause of chronic renal failure (57–59) (see Chapter 27). There are also infrequent reports of renal papillary necrosis occurring in patients treated with ibuprofen, indomethacin, phenylbutazone, fenoprofen and mefenamic acid (60), (61), (41), (51), (62) and with paracetamol (63), (64).

Chronic renal failure

Sandler *et al.* (1991) evaluated the risk for chronic renal disease associated with regular use of non-aspirin NSAIDs in 554 patients with newly diagnosed chronic renal dysfunction (65). They found a twofold risk for chronic renal disease was associated with previous daily use of NSAIDs. The increased risk was predominantly limited to men older than 65 years, for whom the odds ratio was 10 after adjusting for use of other analgesics. These observations were confirmed in a case control study of 716 patients with end-stage renal failure and 361 controls (66). In this study a high cumulative intake of NSAIDs (>5000 tablets) was associated with a 4.5 fold excess risk of end-stage renal failure although the confidence interval was wide (1.0–19.5) and curiously this excess risk was not seen when average annual intake of NSAIDs was examined. Other studies of NSAID usage in hospitalized patients, however, did not confirm this association (4), (67). Adams *et al.* (1986) reported six patients who presented with chronic renal failure associated with the use of NSAIDs (51). One patient had renal papillary necrosis and five the histological findings of chronic tubulo-interstitial fibrosis. In other reports of NSAID-induced acute tubulo-interstitial nephritis, a proportion of patients showed moderate impairment of renal function after recovery (45). On balance it seems likely that chronic usage of NSAIDs may be associated with a slightly increased risk for the development of chronic renal failure.

Salt and water retention

Sodium retention is the most common renal side-effect associated with NSAIDs therapy (68). This occurs more commonly in conditions where there is renal hypoperfusion and sodium retention, such as heart failure, cirrhosis or the nephrotic syndrome (2). The administration of NSAIDs in such circumstances may lead to salt and water retention and the development of oedema.

Hyponatraemia may occur if water retention is disproportionate to sodium retention (69) and this may be worsened by the concomitant administration of diuretics, particularly thiazides (1).

Hypertension

Two large meta-analyses encompassing more than 90 studies demonstrated that NSAIDs can indeed perturb blood pressure, especially in those who were already hypertensive (3), (70). In the meta-analysis by Johnson *et al.* (1994), NSAIDs were found to elevate supine mean blood pressure by 5 mmHg (70).

Hyperkalaemia and hyporeninaemic hypoaldosteronism

NSAIDs may lead to the development of hyperkalaemia and this occurs more commonly in patients with chronic renal failure, diabetes mellitus and Type IV tubular acidosis (71) (72), (28). In addition, NSAIDs must be used with caution in patients taking other drugs known to decrease renal potassium excretion, such as potassium sparing diuretics and angiotensin converting enzyme inhibitors and beta-blockers. The hyperkalaemia in these patients may be accompanied by a mild metabolic acidosis and a deterioration in renal function.

Drug interactions with NSAIDs

NSAIDs and diuretics

In addition to sodium retention caused by NSAIDs, these agents may blunt the natriuretic action of thiazides, aldosterone antagonists and frusemide in patients with heart failure, nephrotic syndrome, renal impairment, cirrhosis and hypertension (39). Notably, the combination of diuretics and NSAIDs in patients with impaired renal function, especially in the elderly, may result in an appreciable deterioration in renal function, as well as precipitating congestive cardiac failure (73).

NSAIDs and anti-hypertensive drugs

NSAIDs have been reported to impair the effectiveness of diuretics (74) and beta-blocking agents (70) in the treatment of hypertension.

NSAIDs and cyclosporin A

Cyclosporin A is now established as a disease modifying drug in rheumatoid arthritis and has also been used in systemic lupus erythematosis. The nephrotoxicity of cyclosporin A is well established (see Chapter 25). It reduces the formation of vasodilatory PGs (75), but increases the formation of the vasoconstrictor thromboxane (76). Furthermore, cyclosporin A induces tubulo-interstitial fibrosis in renal transplants, possibly through increased transforming growth factor β-mediated collagen deposition (77). Recent studies show that NSAIDs significantly worsen cyclosporin nephrotoxicity (78), (79). Patients being treated with cyclosporin A should not also be given NSAIDs, unless there is no alternative. If NSAIDs are to be given, they should only be used with close monitoring of renal function.

NSAIDs and tacrolimus

Tacrolimus is now widely used as an immunosuppressant in liver and renal allograft recipients. Like cyclosporin A, it is potentially nephrotoxic. Acute renal failure has been reported in liver allograft recipients associated with the use of ibuprofen (80).

Renal sparing NSAIDs

Selective inhibitors of COX-2

Attention has therefore been focused on the development of NSAIDs which are selective toward PGHS-2, in the hope that they would reduce renal inflammation without altering renal haemodynamics (81), (82). A number of studies have been conducted with COX-2-selective inhibitors in an attempt to define the roles of the different COX isoenzymes in renal function. Meloxicam has modest selectivity toward COX-2. One study showed that meloxicam had no effect on the pharmacokinetics or the diuretic response to frusemide (83). However, this study did not control for dietary sodium, and this precludes valid conclusions regarding the effects of meloxicam on renal function. A randomized crossover comparisons of meloxicam and indomethacin showed that both NSAIDs inhibited frusemide-stimulated plasma renin activity and PGE_2 (84). This study suggests that COX-2 is important for PGE_2 synthesis and renin release, and implies that COX-2 selective inhibitors would have the same effects on renal function as conventional NSAIDs.

Celecoxib and rofecoxib are two newer COX-2 selective inhibitors. Both have greater COX-2 selectivity than meloxicam. Data presented at the Food and Drug Administration Advisory committee of December 1998, showed that celecoxib had similar effects on blood pressure and sodium excretion reduction, compared with naproxen. Further, excretion of urinary 6-keto-$PGF_{1\alpha}$ was comparable in response to celecoxib and traditional NSAIDs (85). In salt-depleted subjects, selective inhibition with celecoxib, compared with naproxen, resulted in sodium and potassium retention, and transient decreases in glomerular filtration rate and renal blood flow (86). In another study, both indomethacin and rofecoxib resulted in decreases in sodium excretion, but rofecoxib had little impact on the glomerular filtration rate (87). Thus COX-1 may be important in maintaining renal haemodynamics, and COX-2 is preferentially involved in sodium reabsorption. Since COX-2 expression is intertwined with dietary sodium intake and renin release (13), (88), inhibition of COX-2 may lead to undesirable renal side effects. Similar considerations may pertain to maintenance of renal medullary blood flow by PGs produced by COX-2 in medulla interstitial cells (14). There is a recent report of acute renal failure in two patients with chronic renal insufficiency treated with celecoxib (89).

Conclusion

The increasing use of NSAIDs both from prescription and from over-counter sales will result in increased prevalence of nephrotoxicity. A history of NSAID use should be sought in all patients presenting with unexplained impairment of renal function and or proteinuria. In patients with an increased risk of developing NSAID-induced renal insufficiency, the use of NSAIDs should be avoided. Patients with chronic renal impairment, or with a functioning renal transplant, also should not be prescribed NSAIDs. Patients with a NSAID-induced glomerulonephritis, interstitial nephritis or papillary necrosis should not be given NSAIDs again. It may be possible in some individuals who had developed NSAID-induced acute renal failure and who have recovered renal function, to re-introduce a NSAID; provided that the at risk circumstances that led to the enhanced susceptibility have been corrected. NSAIDs should only be given if absolutely indicated, and renal function must be closely monitored in these patients. Preliminary data from COX-2-selective inhibitors suggest that they also affect renal prostaglandins. Therefore, the same cautions should be exercised with their use as with traditional NSAIDs.

References

1. Clive D.M. and Stoff J.S. Renal syndromes associated with anti-inflammatory drugs. *New Engl J Med* 1984, 310: 563–72.
2. Blackshear J.L., Napier J.S., Davidman M. and Stillman M.T. Renal complications of non-steroidal anti-inflammatory drugs: identification and monitoring of those at risk. *Sem Arthritis Rheum* 1985, 14: 163–75.
3. Whelton A. Nephrotoxicity of nonsteroidal anti-inflammatory drugs: Physiologic foundations and clinical implications. *American Journal of Medicine* 1999, 106(5B): 13S–24S.
4. Fox D.A. and Jick H. Non-steroidal anti-inflammatory drugs and renal disease. *J Am Med Association* 1984, 151: 1299–1300.
5. Perez Gutthann S., Garcia Rodriguez L., Raiford D. and Ris Romeu J. Nonsteroidal anti-inflammatory drugs and the risk of hospitalization for acute renal failure. *Archives of Internal Medicine* 1996, 156(21): 2433–9.
6. Evans J., McGregor E., McMahon A. *et al*. Non-steroidal anti-inflammatory drugs and hospitalization for acute renal failure. *Quarterly Journal of Medicine* 1995, 88(8): 551–7.
7. Ferreira S.H., Moncada S. and Vane J.R. Indomethacin and aspirin abolish prostaglandin release from the spleen. *Nature* 1971, 231: 237–9.

8. Aiken J.W. and Vane J.R. Intrarenal prostaglandin release attenuates the renal vasoconstrictor activity of angiotensin. *J Pharmacol Exp Therapeutics* 1973, 184: 678–87.

9. DeWitt D.L. and Smith W.L. PGH synthase isoenzyme selectivity: the potential for safer nonsteroidal antiinflammatory drugs. *Am J Med* 1993, 95(suppl 2A):40S–44S.

10. Jones D.A., P C.D., M M.T., Zimmerman G.A. and Prescott S.M. Molecular cloning of human prostaglandin endoperoxide synthase type II and demonstration of expression in response to cytokines. *J Biological Chemistry* 1993, 268: 9049–54.

11. Siebert K., Masferrer J.L. and Needleman Salvemini D. Pharmacological manipulation of cyclo-oxygenase-2 in the inflamed hydronephrotic kidney. *Br J Pharmacol* 1996, 117: 1016–20.

12. O'Neill G.P. and Ford-Hutchinson A.W. Expression of mRNA for cyclooxygenase-1 and cyclooxygenase-2 in human tissues. *FEBS Lett* 1993, 330: 156–60.

13. Harris R.C., McKanna J.A., Alcai Y., Jacobson H.R., Dubois R.N. and Breyer M.D. Cyclo-oxygenase-2 is associated with the macula densa of rat kidney and increases with salt restriction. *J Clin Invest* 1994, 94: 2504–10.

14. Guan Y., Chang M., Cho W. *et al.* Cloning, expression, and regulation of rabbit cyclooxygenase-2 in renal medullary interstitial cells. *Am J Physiol* 1997, 283: F18–F26.

15. Hartner A., Goppelt-Struebe M. and Hilgers K.F. Coordinate expression of cyclooxygenase-2 and renin in the rat kidney in renovascular hypertension. *Hypertension* 1998, 31(part 2): 201–5.

16. Komhoff M., Grone H.J., Klein T. *et al.* Localization of cyclooxygenase-1 and -2 in adult and fetal human kidney: implication for renal function. *Am J Physiol* 1997, 272: F460–F68.

17. Zhang M.Z., Wang J.L., Cheng H.F. *et al.* Cyclooxygenase-2 in rat nephron development. *Am J Physiol* 1997, 273: F994–F1002.

18. Morham S.G., Langenbach R., Loftin C.D. *et al.* Prostaglandin synthase 2 gene disruption causes severe renal pathology in the mouse. *Cell* 1995, 83: 473–82.

19. Henrich W.L. Role of the prostaglandins in renin secretion. *Kid Inter* 1981, 19: 822–30.

20. Lifschitz M.D. Prostaglandins and renal blood flow: *in vivo* studies. *Kid Inter* 1981, 19: 781–5.

21. Dunn M.J. Nonsteroidal anti-inflammatory drugs and renal function. *Annual Rev Medicine* 1984, 35: 411–28.

22. Patrono C., Ciabattoni G., Remuzzi G. *et al.* Functional significance of renal prostacyclin and thromboxane A2 production in patients with systemic lupus erythematosus. *J Clin Invest* 1985, 76: 1011–8.

23. Dibona G.F. Prostaglandins and non-steroidal anti-inflammatory drugs: effects on renal haemodynamics. *Am J Med* 1986, 80(suppl 1A): 12–21.

24. Pelayo J.C. Renal adrenergic effector mechanisms: glomerular sites for prostaglandin interaction. *Am J Physiol* 1988, 254(23): F184–F90.

25. Scharschmidt L.A., Simonson M.S. and Dunn M.J. Glomerular prostaglandins, angiotensin II, and nonsteroidal antiinflammatory drugs. *Am J Med* 1986, 81(2B): 30–42.

26. Takahashi K., Nammour T.M., Fukunaga M. *et al.* Glomerular action of a free radical-generated novel prostaglandin, 8-epi-prostaglandin F2 alpha in the rat. *J Clin Invest* 1992, 90: 136–41.

27. Goldzer R.C., Coodley E.L., Rosner M.J., Simons W.M. and Schwartz A.M. Hyperkalaemia associated with indomethacin. *Archives Int Med* 1980, 141: 802–4.

28. Galler M., Folkert V.W. and Schlondorff D. Reversible acute renal insufficiency and hyperkalemia following indomethacin therapy. *J Am Med Association* 1981, 246: 154–5.

29. Donker A.J.M., de Jong P.E., Statius van Eps L.W., Brentjens J.R., Bakker K. and Doorenbos H. Indomethacin in Bartter's syndrome. *Nephron* 1977, 19: 200–13.

30. Verberckmoes R., van Damme B., Clement J., Amery A. and Michielsen P. Bartter's syndrome with hyperplasia of renomedullary cells: successful treatment with indomethacin. *Kid Inter* 1976, 9: 200–13.

31. Tannen R.L. Potassium in cardiovascular and renal medicine, arrhythmias, myocardial infarction and hypertension. In: Whelton P.K., Whelton A. and Walker W.G., eds. *Drug interactions causing hyperkalaemia*. New York: Marcel Dekker, 1986.

32. Field M.J. and Giebisch G. Mechanisms of segmental potassium reabsorption and secretion. In: Seldin D.W., Giebisch G., eds. *The regulation of potassium balance.* New York: Raven, 1989.

33. Berl T., Raz A. and Wald H. Protsglandin synthesis inhibition and the action of vasopressin: studies in man and rat. *Am J Physiol* 1977, 232: 529–37.

34. Stokes J.B. Effect of prostaglandin E2 on chloride transport across the rabbit thick ascending limb of Henle. Selective inhibition of the medullary portion. *J Clin Invest* 1979, 64: 495–502.

35. Kinoshita Y., Romero J.C. and Knox F. Effect of renal interstitial infusion of arachidonic acid on proximal sodium reabsorption. *Am J Physiol* 1989, 26: F237–F42.

36. Lum G.M., Aisenberg G.A., Dunn M.J., Berl T., Schrier R.W. and McDonald K.M. *In vivo* effect of indomethacin to potentiate the renal medullary cyclic AMP response to vasopressin. *J Clin Invest* 1977, 59: 8–13.

37. Muther R.S. and Bennett W.M. Effect of aspirin on glomerular filtration rate in normal humans. *Annals Int Med* 1980, 92: 386–7.

38. Donker A.J.M., Arisz L., Brentjens J.R.H., van der Hem G.K. and Hollemans H.J.G. The effect of indomethacin on kidney function and plasma renin activity in man. *Nephron* 1976, 17: 288–96.

39. Garella S. and Matarese R.A. Renal effects of prostaglandins and clinical adverse effects of non-steroidal anti-inflammatory drugs. *Medicine* 1984, 63: 165–81.

40. Abraham P.A. and Keane W.F. Glomerular and interstiti disease induced by nonsteroidal anti-inflammatory drugs. *Am J Nephrol* 1984, 4: 1–6.

41. Carmichael T. and Shankel S.W. Effects of non-steroidal anti-inflammatory drugs on prostaglandins and renal function. *Am J Med* 1985, 78: 992–1000.

42. Brezin J.H., Katz S.M., Schwartz A.B. and Chinitz J.L. Reversible renal failure and nephrotic syndrome associated with nonsteroidal anti-inflammatory drugs. *New Engl J Med* 1979, 310: 1271–3.

43. Finkelstein A., Fraley D.S., Stachura I., Feldman H.A., Grandy D.R. and Bourke E. Fenoprofen nephropathy: lipoid nephrosis and interstitial nephritis: a possible T lymphocyte disorder. *Am J Med* 1982, 72: 81–7.

44. Bender W.L., Whelton A., Beschorner W.E., Darwish M.O., Hall-Craggs M. and Solez K. Interstitial nephritis, proteinuria and renal failure caused by non-steroidal anti-inflammatory drugs. Immunological characterisation of the infiltrate. *Am J Med* 1984, 1006–12.

45. Cameron J.S. Allergic interstitial nephritis: clinical features and pathogenesis. *Quarterly J Med* 1988, 66(250): 97–115.

46. Schwartz A., Krause P.H., Keller T., Offerman G. and Mihatsch M.J. Granulomatous interstitial nephritis after non-steroidal anti-inflammatory drugs. *Am J Nep* 1988, 8: 410–6.

47. Torres V.E. Present and future of non-steroidal anti-inflammatory drugs in nephrology. *Majo Clin Proceedings* 1982, 57: 390–3.

48. Schneider A., Jocks T., Wenzel U., Reszka M. and Stahl R.A.K. Prostaglandin G/H synthase (PGHS) inhibitors modulate glomerular MCP-1 mRNA expression in anti-Thy-1 antiserum (ATS) induced glomerulonephritis in rats. *J Am Soc Nephrol* 1996, 7: 1720.

49. Baldwin D.S., Levine B.B., McCluskey R.T. and Gallo G.R. Renal failure and interstitial nephritis due to penicillin and methicillin. *N Engl J Med* 1968, 279: 1245–52.

50. Woodroffe A.J., Thomson N.M., Meadows R. and Lawrence J.R. Nephropathy associated with methicillin administration. *Aust N Z J Med* 1974, 4: 256–61.

51. Adams D.H., Howie A.J., Micheal J., McConkey B., Bacon P.A. and Adu D. Nonsteroidal anti-inflammatory drugs and renal failure. *Lancet* 1986, i: 57–60.

52. Neilson E.G. Pathogenesis and therapy of interstitial nephritis (clinical conference). *Kidney Int* 1989, 35: 1251–70.

53. Campistol J.M., Galofre J., Botey A., Torras A. and Revert L.I. Reversible membranous nephropathy associated with diclofenac. *Nephrol Dialysis Transplantation* 1989, 4: 393–5.

54. Tattersall J., Greenwood R. and Farrington K. Membranous nephropathy associated with diclofenac (letter). *Postgraduate Med J* 1992, 68(799): 392–3.

55. Radford M.G., Holley K.E., Grande J.P. *et al.* Reversible membranous nephropathy associated with the use of nonsteroidal antinflammatory drugs. *JAMA* 1996, 276: 466–9.

56. Goebal K.M. and Muellar-Brodmann W. Reversible overt nephropathy with Henoch-Schönlein purpura due to piroxicam. *Br Med J* 1982, 284: 311.

57. McCredie M., Stewart J.H. and Mahony J.F. Is phenacetin responsible for analgesic nephropathy in New South Wales? *Clin Nephrol* 1982, 17(3): 134–40.

58. Morlans M., Laporte J.-R., Vidal X., Cabeza D. and Stolley P.D. End-stage renal disease and non-narcotic analgesics: A case-control study. *Br J Clin Pharmacol* 1990, 30: 717–23.

59. Sandler D.P. Analgesic use and chronic renal disease. *New Engl J Med* 1989, 320: 1238–43.

60. Munn E., Lynn K.L. and R B.R. Renal papillary necrosis following regular consumption of NSAIDs. *New Zealand J Med* 1976, 95: 213–4.

61. Shah G.M., Muhalwas K.K. and Winer R.L. Renal papillary necrosis due to ibuprofen. 1981, 24: 1208–10.

62. Segasothy M., Thyaparan A., Kamal A. and Sivalingam S. Mefanamic acid nephropathy. 45 1987: 156–7.

63. Krikler D.M. Paracetamol and the kidney. *Br J Med* 1967, 2: 615.

64. Master D.R. and Krikler D.M. Analgesic nephropathy associated with paracetamol. *Proceedings of Royal Society of Medicine* 1973, 66: 904.

65. Sandler D.P., Burr F.R. and Weinberg C.R. Nonsteroidal anti-inflammatory drugs and the risk for chronic renal disease. *Annals Int Med* 1991, 115: 165–72.

66. Perneger T.V., Whelton P.K. and J. K.M. Risk of kidney failure associated with the use of acetaminophen, aspirin, and nonsteroidal antiinflammatory drugs. *New Engl J Med* 1994, 331: 1675–9.

67. Beard K., Perera D.R. and Jick H. Drug-induced parenchymal renal disease in outpatients. *J Clin Pharmacol* 1988, 28(5): 431–5.

68. Coles S.L., Fries J.F., Kraines R.G. and Roth S.H. From experiment to experience: side effects of nonsteroidal anti-inflammatory drugs. *Am J Med* 1983, 74: 820–8.

69. Blum M. and Aviram A. Ibuprofen-induced hyponatraemia. *Rheumatology Rehabilatation* 1980, 19: 258–9.

70. Johnson A.G., Nguyen T.V. and Day R.O. Do nonsteroidal anti-inflammatory drugs affect blood pressure? *Annals of Internal Medicine* 1994, 121: 289–300.

71. Kutyrina I.M., Androsova S.O. and Tareyeva I.E. Indomethacin-induced hyporeninaemic hypoaldosteronism. *Lancet* 1979, 1: 785.

72. Findling J.W., Beckstrom D., Rawsthorne L., Kozin F. and Itskovitz H. Indomethacin-induced hyperkalaemia in three patients with gouty arthritis. *J Am Med Association* 1980, 244: 1127–8.

73. Kleinknecht D., Landais P. and Goldfarb B. Analgesic and non-steroidal anti-inflammatory drug-associated acute renal failure: a prospective collaborative study. *Clin Nephrol* 1986, 25: 275–81.

74. Brater D. Diuretic therapy. *New England Journal of Medicine* 1998, 339: 387–95.

75. Stahl R.A.K., Kanz L. and Kudelka S. Cyclosporine and renal prostaglandin E2 production. *Ann Int Med* 1985, 103: 474.

76. Perico N., Benigni A. and Zoja C. Functional significance of exaggerated thromboxane A2 synthesis induced by cyclopsorine A. *Am J Physiol* 1986, 251: F581–F7.

77. Wolf G., Zahner G., Ziyadeh F.N. and Stahl R.A.K. Concise Report: Cyclosporine A Induces transcription of transforming growth factor beta in a cultured murine tubular cell line. *Exp Nephrol* 1996, 4: 304–08.

78. Berg K.J., Forre O., Djoselanel O., Mikkelsen M., Marnervol J. and Rugstad J.E. Renal side-effects of high and low cyclosporin A doses in patients with rheumatoid arthritis. *Clin Nephrol* 1989, 31: 225–31.

79. Altman R.D., Perez G.O. and Sfakianakis G.N. Interaction of cyclosporin A and nonsteroidal anti-inflammatory drugs on renal function in patients with rheumatoid arthritis. *Am J Med* 1992, 93: 396–402.

80. Sheiner P.A., Mor E., Chodoff L. *et al.* Acute renal failure associated with the use of ibuprofen in two liver transplant recipients on FK506. *Transplantation* 1994, 57: 1132–3.

81. Meade E.A., Smith W.L. and Dewitt D.L. Differential inhibition of prostaglandin endoperoxide synthase (cyclooxygenase) isozymes by aspirin and other non-steroidal anti-inflammatory drugs. *J Biol Chem* 1993, 268: 6610–4.

82. Smith W.L. and Dewitt D.L. Biochemistry of prostaglandin endoperoxide H synthase-1 and synthase-2 and their differential susceptibility to nonsteroidal anti-inflammatory drugs. *Semin Nephrol* 1995, 15: 179–94.

83. Müller F.O., Middle M.V., Schall R., Terblanché J., Hundt H.K.L. and Groenewoud G. An evaluation of the interaction of meloxicam with furosemide in patients with compensated chronic cardiac failure. *Br J Clin Pharmacol* 1997, 44: 393–8.

84. Stichtenoth D.O., Wagner B. and Frölich J.C. Effect of selective inhibition of the inducible cyclooxygenase on renin release in healthy individuals. *J Invest Med* 1984, 46: 290–6.

85. McAdam B.F., Catella-Lawson F., Mardini I.A., Kapoor S., Lawson J.A. and FitzGerald G.A. Systemic biosynthesis of prostacyclin by cyclooxygenase (COX)-2: the human pharmacology of a selective inhibitor of COX-2. *Proc Natl Acad Sci USA* 1999, 96: 272–7.

86. Rossat J., Maillard M., Nussberger J., Brunner H.R. and Burnier M. Renal effects of selective cyclooxygenase-2 inhibition in normotensive salt-depleted subjects. *Clin Pharmacol Ther* 1999, 66: 76–84.

87. Catella-Lawson F., McAdam B., Morrison B.W. *et al.* Effects of specific inhibition of cyclooxygenase-2 on sodium balance, hemodynamics and vasoactive eicosanoids. *J Pharmacol Exp Ther* 1999, 289: 735–41.

88. Harding P., Sigmon D.H., Alfie M.E. *et al.* Cyclooxygenase-2 mediates increased renal renin content induced by low-sodium diet. *Hypertension* 1997, 29: 297–302.

89. Parazella M. and Eras J. Are selective COX-2 inhibitors nephrotoxic. *American Journal of Kidney Diseases* 2000, 35(5): 937–40.

27

Nephrotoxicity of drugs used in rheumatology: Analgesic nephropathy

Marc E. De Broe

Introduction

Patients having long-lasting systemic diseases involving the muscular-skeletal system suffer intermittently from pain for which they take several types of pain killing medicine over prolonged periods of time. Since several of these drugs may have a nephrotoxic effect, renal damage failure may occur after some time in a not well-identified number of these patients.

Chronic analgesic nephropathy (AN) is a form of renal disease characterized by renal papillary necrosis and chronic interstitial nephritis caused by prolonged and excessive consumption of analgesic mixtures. It is invariably caused by compound analgesic mixtures containing aspirin or antipyrin in combination with phenacetin, paracetamol, or salicylamide and caffeine or codeine in popular 'over the counter' proprietary mixtures (1).

Diagnosis

The renal manifestations of analgesic nephropathy are usually non-specific: slowly progressive chronic renal failure, with urea analysis that may be normal or may reveal sterile pyuria and a mild proteinuria (less than 1.5 g/day) (2, 3). Hypertension and anaemia are commonly seen with moderate to advanced disease; more prominent proteinuria that can exceed 3.5 g/day can also occur at this time, a probable reflection of secondary haemodynamically mediated glomerular injury.

Most patients have no symptoms referable to the urinary tract, although flank pain or macroscopic/microscopic haematuria from a sloughed or obstructing papilla may occur or as a result of transectional cell carcinoma. Urinary tract infection is also somewhat more common in women with this disorder.

Despite the non-specific nature of the renal presentation, there are frequently other findings that point toward the presence of analgesic nephropathy (2, 3). Most patients are between the ages of 30 to 70. Careful questioning often reveals a history of chronic headaches or low back pain that leads to the analgesic use. Also common are other somatic complaints (such as malaise and weakness), and ulcer-like symptoms or a history of peptic ulcer disease due in part to chronic aspirin ingestion.

Table 27.1 Sensitive and specificity of CT imaging criteria used to diagnose analgesic nephropathy in 40 patients with end-stage renal disease (ESRD) and 53 patients with incipient, mild, or moderate renal failure (RF)*

Finding on renal imaging	Sensitivity %	Specificity %
Decrease in length		
patients with ESRD	95	10
patients with RF	77	86
Bumpy contours		
patients with ESRD	50	90
patients with RF	62	93
Papillary calcifications		
patients with ESRF	87	97
patients with RF	92	100
Decrease in length and either		
bumpy contours or papillary		
calcifications		
patients with ESRD	90	90
patients with RF	77	100

* CT was performed without contrast medium. In patients with incipient, mild, or moderate renal failure, serum creatinine concentration ranged from 1.5 to 4 mg per decilitre (133 to 354 μmol per litre).

consumption and renal functional impairment (14, 15). Because of the small number of patients with analgesic abuse who had signs of renal impairment, the nephrotoxicity of particular types of analgesic mixtures could not be analysed. In contrast, the case–control design of several other studies did allow such an analysis (Table 27.2). For analgesic mixtures, particularly those containing phenacetin and acetaminophen, nephrotoxicity was demonstrated. No consistent results were obtained with respect to single analgesics.

Additional evidence of the nephrotoxicity of various analgesic mixtures came from a cohort of 226 patients with documented abuse of analgesics and a clear diagnosis of analgesic nephropathy. All but seven patients admitted abusing analgesic mixtures containing caffeine, codeine, or both (16). In 46 patients with no previous phenacetin consumption, classic analgesic nephropathy was associated with the following combinations: aspirin and acetaminophen, aspirin and a pyrazolone, acetaminophen and a pyrazolone, and two pyrazolones, all of which were combined with caffeine, codeine, or both (17). The pyrazolones included antipyrine, salipyrine, aminopyrine, and dipyrone.

Acetaminophen

An important question that remains incompletely resolved is the renal risk of monotherapy with acetaminophen (paracetamol), which is the primary metabolite of phenacetin and which is now widely used as a minor analgesic. Three recent studies suggest that acetaminophen alone is nephrotoxic (10, 13, 18), although the risk is probably less than that of phenacetin-aspirin combinations (10). This difference in risk could be due to acetaminophen having less intrinsic nephrotoxicity than phenacetin. Alternatively, if acetaminophen and phenacetin had the same risk when used in combination with other analgesics, but less risk when used alone, case-control studies would show a lower risk for acetaminophen relative to phenacetin. This would occur because acetaminophen is used both alone and in combinations whereas phenacetin was always used in combinations, never as a single agent (19). This hypothesis is supported by one study (11) showing that risk of acetaminophen and phenacetin combinations was similar.

That acetaminophen alone is nephrotoxic is described in one case-control study of patients with end-stage renal failure (13). There were, however, important methodological problems with this study. In particular, it could not be excluded that patients with renal disease were more likely to have symptoms requiring analgesics and confounding by indication may have occurred whereby patients with renal disease are taking acetaminophen because they were told to avoid aspirin and nonsteroidal anti-inflammatory drugs.

The latter issues may have been less important in another study that looked at analgesic use in 554 adults presenting with new renal insufficiency (plasma creatinine concentration $\geq$ 1.5 mg/dl (13 µmol/L)), rather than end-stage renal disease (10). This study estimated that the adjusted odds ratio for renal disease was 3.21 in patients taking daily acetaminophen. There was no increase in risk with weekly or less frequent use.

The greater frequency with which acetaminophen is taken alone rather than in combination with aspirin may explain the apparently greater risk seen with phenacetin.

In summary, the withdrawal of phenacetin from the market did not completely eradicate analgesic nephropathy. There is experimental, pharmacological, and epidemiological evidence that other analgesic mixtures that do not contain phenacetin can also become nephrotoxic and may produce the classic renal lesions of the disease (20). There is suggestive but not definitive evidence that chronic, especially daily acetaminophen use may have dose dependent long-term nephrotoxicity.

Chronic renal failure and analgesic use

A small number of epidemiological studies (10–13) generated the hypothesis that habitual analgesic use influences the progression of chronic renal disease. Given the study designs, however, it is impossible to determine whether exposure to analgesics is the initial cause of renal failure or a factor contributing to the progression of the renal disease, whether there is an interplay between the two possibilities, or whether the association is noncausal (21). Furthermore, the only clearly increased odds ratios for chronic renal failure were found in the groups of patients with interstitial nephritis and end-stage renal disease from unclear

Table 27.2 Epidemiological studies demonstrating the nephrotoxicity of different kind of analgesics

Study design	Cases	Controls	Definition of minimal abuse
Case-control studies			
McCredie et al. Australia, 1982 (8)	80 women with RPN	80 healthy women	3 units/week for one year
Murray et al. USA, 1983 (9)	527 p. with ESRD	1047 hospitalized p.	almost daily for 30 days
Sandler et al. USA, 1989 (10)	554 p. with newly diagnosed CRF	516 population based	daily for one year
Pommer et al. West Berlin, 1989 (11)	517 p. with ESRD	517 outpatient clinic p.	15 units/month for one year
Morlans et al. Barcelona, 1990 (12)	340 p. with ESRD	673 hospitalized p.	15 units/month for 30 days
Perneger et al. USA 1994 (13)	716 p. with ESRD	361 population based	daily for one year
Prospective studies			
Dubach et al. Switzerland, 1983 (14)	623 healthy women followed during 10 years	621 healthy women	NAPAP in urine positive
Elseviers and De Broe, Belgium, 1995 (15)	200 healthy subjects followed during 7 years	200 population based	daily for one year overall at least 1000 units

Table 27.2 Epidemiological studies demonstrating the nephrotoxicity of different kind of analgesics *continued*

Results

Case control studies (1)	Any analgesic	Single analgesics			Analgesic mixtures		
		Any	Aspirin	Acetaminophen	Any	Phenacetin	Acetaminophen
McCredie et al. (8)	17.2	–	–	–	–	18.1	ns
Murray et al. (9)	ns	–	–	–	–	–	–
Sandler et al. (10)	2.79	–	ns	3.21	–	7.59	6.9
Pommer et al. (11)	2.44	ns	–	–	2.69	4.76	4.06
Morlans et al. (12)	2.89	–	2.54	–	–	19.05	–
Perneger et al. (13)	–	–	ns (3)	–	–	–	2.1 (4)
Prospective studies (2)							
Dubach et al. (14)	–	–	–	–	–	8.10	–
Elseviers and De Broe (15)	6.10	–	–	–	–	–	–

(1) Results are odds ratios showing significant differences between cases and controls.
(2) Results are relative risks for the development of renal failure during the study period.
(3) Results are obtained after adjustment for the use of other analgesics.
(4) Analgesic component either or not taken in mixture.
Abbreviations: NAPAP = N-acetyl-p-aminophenol (the main metabolite of phenacetin); ns = not significant.

causes, a finding that corroborates the well-documented clinicopathological entity of classic analgesic nephropathy.

The association between chronic renal failure from any cause and excess analgesic use reported by these three case-control studies does not establish cause and effect. In any analysis of these studies, flaws in the study design, inaccurate renal diagnoses, and confounding by indication have to be considered (22). Further investigation is needed to determine whether habitual analgesic use influences the progression of chronic renal disease.

While the collective evidence suggests that habitual analgesic use abuse may be associated with the development of chronic renal failure, it does not conclusively establish a casual link between use/abuse of specific analgesics, particularly acetaminophen, and chronic renal failure. Whether habitual analgesic use influences the progression of chronic renal disease also needs more solid scientific data. Improvements in study design could include the following:

- patients with early stage disease should be included, avoiding the possibility that renal disease provoked analgesic use/abuse;
- explicit knowledge of both the time in which the drug was started and stopped, and the amount of drug ingested should be obtained;
- personal, not telephone, interviews should be performed, and must include visual (book with colour photographs) aids to obtain accurate information concerning the type of drug ingested;
- patients and control individuals should be drawn from the same population source, and should be of adequate number to determine statistical significance.

Pathogenesis

The nephrotoxicity of analgesics is dose-dependent (2, 13). Decreased concentrating ability or a mild reduction in glomerular function rate can be seen after cumulative phenacetin, part of analgesic mixtures, intake of as little as 1 kg. In comparison, clinically evident renal disease requires a minimum intake of 2 to 3 kg each of phenacetin and aspirin. This will take 6 to 8 years in a patient ingesting 6 to 8 tablets (or about 1 gram) of phenacetin-containing compounds per day.

The renal damage induced by analgesics is most prominent in the medulla. The earliest changes consist of prominent thickening of the vasa recta capillaris (capillary sclerosis) and patchy areas of tubular necrosis; similar vascular lesions can be found in the renal pelvis and ureter, suggesting that the primary effect is damage to the vascular endothelial cells (23). Later changes include areas of papillary necrosis and secondary cortical injury with focal and segmental glomerulosclerosis and interstitial infiltration and fibrosis.

The mechanisms responsible for the renal injury are incompletely understood. Phenacetin is metabolized to acetaminophen and the reactive intermediates that can injure cells, in part by lipid peroxidation (24). These metabolites tend to accumulate in the medulla along the medullary osmotic gradient (created by the countercurrent system). As a result, the highest concentrations are seen at the papillary tip, the site of the initial vascular lesions (25).

The potentiating effect of aspirin with both phenacetin and acetaminophen may be related to two factors. First, acetaminophen undergoes oxidative metabolism by prostaglandin H synthase to reactive quinoneimine that is conjugated to glutathione. If acetaminophen is present alone, there is sufficient glutathione generated in the papillae to detoxify the reactive intermediate. If the acetaminophen is ingested with aspirin, the aspirin is converted to salicylate and salicylate becomes highly concentrated in both the cortex and papillae of the kidney. Salicylate is a potent depletor of glutathione. With the cellular glutathione depleted, the reactive metabolite of acetaminophen then produces lipid peroxides and arylation of tissue proteins, ultimately resulting in necrosis of the papillae (26, 27) (Fig. 27.2). Second, aspirin inhibit prostaglandin production by inhibition of cyclooxygenase enzymes. Renal blood flow is very dependent on systemic as well as local production of vasodilatory prostaglandins. This is especially true for renal medulla, which normally lives at the edge of hypoxia and therefore is more prone to ischaemic damage.

Course and complications

The course of the renal disease depends both upon the severity of the renal damage at the time of presentation and upon whether drug therapy is discontinued (3, 29, 30). The decline in renal function can be expected to progress if analgesics are continued. Even aspirin, which is generally not nephrotoxic when given alone (10), could promote further renal damage in analgesic nephropathy (29, 30).

On the other hand, renal function stabilizes or mildly improves in most patients if analgesic consumption is discontinued (29, 30). If, however, the renal disease is already advanced, then progression may occur in the absence of drug intake, presumably due to secondary haemodynamic and metabolic changes associated with nephron loss (31).

The late course of analgesic nephropathy also may be complicated by two additional problems: malignancy and atherosclerotic disease.

Transitional cell carcinomas of the renal pelvis, ureter, and bladder (which may be multiple and bilateral) all occur with increased frequency in this setting (32–34). The incidence of renal cell carcinoma also may be enhanced, but this remains controversial (35).

It is estimated that a urinary tract malignancy will develop in as many as 8 to 10% of patients with analgesic nephropathy (32–34), but in well under 1% of phenacetin-containing analgesic users without kidney disease (36). In women under the age of 50, for example, analgesic abuse is the most common cause of bladder cancer, an otherwise unusual disorder in young women (34). The potential magnitude of this problem has also been illustrated by histological examina-

Analgesic Nephropathy is a form of renal disease characterized by renal papillary necrosis and chronic interstitial nephritis caused by prolonged and excessive consumption of analgesic mixtures.

It is invariably caused by compound analgesic mixtures containing aspirin or antipyrine in combination with phenacetin, paracetamol, or salicylamide and caffeine or codeine in popular "over-the-counter" proprietary mixtures.*

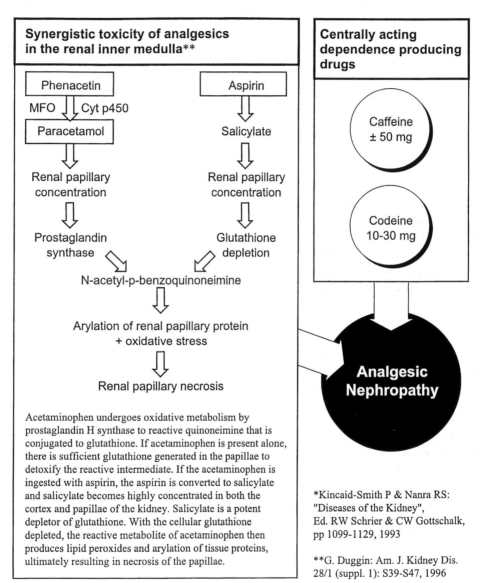

Synergistic toxicity of analgesics in the renal inner medulla**

Phenacetin

MFO ⇓ Cyt p450

Paracetamol

⇓

Renal papillary concentration

⇓

Prostaglandin synthase

Aspirin

⇓

Salicylate

⇓

Renal papillary concentration

⇓

Glutathione depletion

N-acetyl-p-benzoquinoneimine

⇓

Arylation of renal papillary protein + oxidative stress

⇓

Renal papillary necrosis

Acetaminophen undergoes oxidative metabolism by prostaglandin H synthase to reactive quinoneimine that is conjugated to glutathione. If acetaminophen is present alone, there is sufficient glutathione generated in the papillae to detoxify the reactive intermediate. If the acetaminophen is ingested with aspirin, the aspirin is converted to salicylate and salicylate becomes highly concentrated in both the cortex and papillae of the kidney. Salicylate is a potent depletor of glutathione. With the cellular glutathione depleted, the reactive metabolite of acetaminophen then produces lipid peroxides and arylation of tissue proteins, ultimately resulting in necrosis of the papillae.

Centrally acting dependence producing drugs

Caffeine ± 50 mg

Codeine 10-30 mg

Analgesic Nephropathy

*Kincaid-Smith P & Nanra RS: "Diseases of the Kidney", Ed. RW Schrier & CW Gottschalk, pp 1099-1129, 1993

**G. Duggin: Am. J. Kidney Dis. 28/1 (suppl. 1): S39-S47, 1996

Fig. 27.2   Adapted from [27] and [28].

tion of nephrectomy specimens obtained prior to renal transplantation; the incidence of urothelial atypia in this setting approaches 50% (32).

The tumours generally become apparent after 15 to 25 years of analgesic abuse (32), usually but not always in patients with clinically evident analgesic nephropathy (33). Most patients are still taking the drug at the time of diagnosis, but clinically evident disease can first become apparent several years after cessation of analgesic intake and even after renal transplantation has been performed (32). In Australia, for example, the incidence of analgesic nephropathy declined progressively in the first 10 years after phenacetin-containing compounds were removed from over-the-counter analgesic combinations and 5 years after over-the-counter sales of analgesic mixtures were banned (37). In comparison, the incidence of urinary tract malignancy continued to rise (at a greater rate than other malignancies), a possible reflection of late phenacetin-induced injury (37).

It is presumed that the induction of malignancy results from the intrarenal accumulation of N-hydroxylated phenacetin metabolites that have potent alkylating action (33). Because of urinary concentration, the highest concentration of these metabolites will be in the renal medulla, ureters, and bladder, possibly explaining the predisposition to carcinogenesis at these sites. The pathogenetic importance of phenacetin metabolites is suggested indirectly from the observation that there appears to be no association with tumour formation with the prolonged ingestion of other analgesics that can cause papillary necrosis but do not form these metabolites, such as acetaminophen and the nonsteroidal anti-inflammatory drugs (38–40).

The major presenting symptom of urinary tract malignancy in analgesic nephropathy is microscopic or gross haematuria. Thus, continued monitoring is essential, and new haematuria should be evaluated with urinary cytology, and, if indicated, cystoscopy with retrograde pyelography (32). It may also be prudent to obtain yearly urine cytology for the first several years if analgesics are discontinued or indefinitely if drug intake persists. The incidence of urothelial carcinoma after renal transplantation in patients with analgesic nephropathy is comparable to the general incidence of up to 10% of urothelial carcinomas in end-stage renal failure patients with analgesic nephropathy. Removal of the native kidneys prior to renal transplantation has also been suggested, but the efficacy of this regimen has not been proven (32).

Patients with analgesic nephropathy are more likely to develop premature aging and greying and *atherosclerotic vascular disease* (including myocardial infarction and thrombotic stroke) (2, 36). As examples, chronic ingestion of phenacetin containing analgesic mixtures in women aged 30 to 49 is, after 20 years, associated with a twofold increase risk of myocardial infarction and a threefold increase in risk of all cardiovascular diseases (36). It is possible that the analgesic microangiopathy that is the earliest sign of renal injury (23) may play an important role in this problem; the incidence of other risk factors (such as hypercholesterolemia, smoking, and hypertension) does not appear to be enhanced when compared to patients with other forms of chronic renal failure.

Conclusion

Classic analgesic nephropathy is a specific renal disease characterized by renal papillary necrosis and chronic interstitial nephritis caused by prolonged and excessive consumption of analgesic mixtures. Analgesic nephropathy can be accurately diagnosed at any stage by CT scanning without contrast medium, even in the absence of reliable information on previous analgesic use. The effects of habitual use of analgesics alone or in combination on the progression of other forms of renal disease remain unclear. Well-designed studies are needed to define the nephrotoxicity of analgesics in patients with renal disease. In the meantime it is prudent to continue to advise these patients that acetaminophen should be the nonnarcotic analgesic of choice for intermittent use.

References

1. De Broe M.E. and Elseviers M.M. Analgesic nephropathy. *N Engl J Med* 338: 446–452, 1998.
2. Nanra R.S., Stuart-Taylor J.M., deLeon A.H., and White K.H. Analgesic nephropathy: etiology, clinical syndrome, and clinicopathologic correlations in Australia. *Kidney Int* 13: 79–92, 1978.
3. Murray T.G. and Goldberg M. Analgesic-associated nephropathy in the USA: epidemiologic, clinical and pathogenetic features. *Kidney Int* 13: 64–71, 1978.
4. Elseviers M.M., Bosteels V., Cambier P., De Paepe M., Godon J.P., Lins R., Lornoy W., Matthys E., Moeremans C., Roose R., Theelen B., Van Caesbroeck D., Verbanck J., and De Broe M.E. Diagnostic criteria of analgesic nephropathy in patients with end-stage renal failure – results of the Belgian study. *Nephrol Dial Transplant* 7: 479–486, 1992.
5. Elseviers M.M., Waller I., Nenov D., Levora J., Matousovic K., Tanquerel T., Pommer W., Schwarz A., Keller E., Thieler H., Köhler H., Lemoniatou H., Cresseri D., Bonnucchi D., and De Broe M.E. Evaluation of diagnostic criteria for analgesic nephropathy in patients with end-stage renal failure: results of the ANNE study. *Nephrol Dial Transplant* 10: 808–814, 1995.
6. Elseviers M.M., De Schepper A., Corthouts B., Bosmans J.L., Cosyn L., Lins R.L., Lornoy W., Matthys E., Roose R., Van Caesbroeck D., Waller I., Horackova M., Schwarz A., and De Broe M.E. High diagnostic performance of CT scan for analgesic nephropathy in patients with incipient to severe renal failure. *Kidney Int* 48: 1316–1323, 1995.
7. Prescott L.F. Analgesic nephropathy: a reassessment of the role of phenacetin and other analgesics. *Drugs* 23: 75–149, 1982.
8. McCredie M., Ford J.M., Taylor J.S., and Stewart J.H. Analgesics and cancer of the renal pelvis in New South Wales. *Cancer* 49, 2617–2625, 1982.
9. Murray T.G., Stolley P.D., Anthony J.C., Schinnar R, Hepler-Smith E, and Jeffreys J.L. Epidemiologic study of regular analgesic use and end-stage renal disease. *Arch Intern Med* 143: 1687–1693, 1983.
10. Sandler D.P., Smith J.C., Weinberg C.R., Buckalew V.M. Jr, Dennis V.W., Blythe W.B., and Burgess W.P. Analgesic use and chronic renal disease. *N Engl J Med* 320: 1238–1243, 1989.
11. Pommer W., Bronder E., Greiser E., Helmert U., Jesdinsky H.J., Klimpel A., Borner K., and Molzahn M. Regular analgesic intake and the risk of end-stage renal failure. *Am J Nephrol* 9(5): 403–412, 1989.

12. Morlans M. Laporte J.R., Vidal X., Cabeza D., and Stolley P.D. End-stage renal disease and nonnarcotic analgesics: a case-control study. *Br J Clin Pharmacol* 30: 717–723, 1990.

13. Perneger T.V., Whelton P.K., and Klag M.J. Risk of kidney failure associated with the use of acetaminophen, aspirin, and nonsteroidal antiinflammatory drugs. *N Engl J Med* 331: 1675–1679, 1994.

14. Dubach U.C., Rosner B., and Pfister E. Epidemiologic study of abuse of analgesics containing phenacetin: renal morbidity and mortality (1968–1979). *N Engl J Med* 308: 357–362, 1983.

15. Elseviers M.M. and De Broe M.E. A long-term prospective controlled study of analgesic abuse in Belgium. *Kidney Int* 48: 1912–1919, 1995.

16. Murray R.M. Genesis of analgesic nephropathy in the United Kingdom. *Kidney Int* 13: 50–57, 1978.

17. Elseviers M.M. and De Broe M.E. Combination analgesic involvement in the pathogenesis of analgesic nephropathy: the European perspective. *Am J Kidney Dis* 28 (Suppl. 1): S48-S55, 1996.

18. Segasothy M., Suleiman A.B., Puvaneswary M., and Rohana A. Paracetamol: a cause for analgesic nephropathy and end-stage renal disease. *Nephron* 50(1): 50–54, 1988.

19. Buckalew V.M. Jr. Habitual use of acetaminophen as a risk factor for chronic renal failure: a comparison with phenacetin. *Am J Kidney Dis* 28(Suppl. 1): S7-S13, 1996.

20. Spühler O. and Zollinger H.U. Die Chronisch-Interstitiëlle Nephritis. *Z Klin Med* 151: 1–50, 1953.

21. Barrett B.J. Acetaminophen and adverse chronic renal outcomes: an appraisal of the epidemiologic evidence. *Am J Kidney Dis* 28 (Suppl. 1): S14-S19, 1996.

22. Delzell E. and Shapiro S. Commentary on the National Kidney Foundation position paper on analgesics and the kidney. *Am J Kidney Dis* 28: 783–785, 1996.

23. Mihatsch M.J., Hofer H.O., Gudat F., Knusli C., Torhorst J., and Zollinger H.U. Capillary sclerosis of the urinary tract and analgesic nephropathy. *Clin Nephrol* 20(6): 285–301, 1983.

24. Bennett W.M. and Porter G.A. Analgesic nephropathy and the use of nonsteroidal antiinflammatory drugs in renal patients: new insights. *J Nephrol* 11: 70–75, 1998.

25. Bach P.H. and Hardy T.L. Relevance of animal models to analgesic-associated renal papillary necrosis in humans. *Kidney Int* 28(4): 605–613, 1985.

26. Bennett W.M. and De Broe M.E. Analgesic nephropathy – a preventable renal disease. *N Engl J Med* 320(19): 1269–1271, 1989.

27. Duggin G.G. Combination analgesic-induced kidney disease: the Australian experience. *Am J Kidney Dis* 28 (Suppl. 1): S39–S47, 1996.

28. Kincaid-Smith P. and Nanra R.S. In: R.W. Schrier and C.W. Gottschalk (eds) *Diseases of the Kidney*, pp. 1099–1129, 1993.

29. Buckalew V.M. Jr and Schey H.M. Renal disease from habitual antipyretic analgesic consumption: an assessment of the epidemiologic evidence. *Medicine (Baltimore)* 65(5): 291–303, 1986.

30. Gault M.H. and Barrett B.J. Analgesic nephropathy. *Am J Kidney Dis* 32: 351–360, 1998.

31. Garber S.L., Mirochnik Y., Arruda J.A., and Dunea G. Evolution of experimentally induced papillary necrosis to focal segmental glomerulosclerosis and nephrotic proteinuria. *Am J Kidney Dis* 33(6): 1033–1039, 1999.

32. Blohme I. and Johansson S. Renal pelvic neoplasms and atypical urothelium in patients with end-stage analgesic nephropathy. *Kidney Int* 20: 671–675, 1981.

33. McCredie M., Stewart J.H., Carter J.J., Turner J., and Mahony J.F. Phenacetin and papillary necrosis: Independent risk factors for renal pelvic cancer. *Kidney Int* 30: 81–84, 1986.
34. Piper J.M., Tonascia J., and Matanoski G.M. Heavy phenacetin use and bladder cancer in women aged 20 to 49 years. *N Engl J Med* 313: 292–295, 1985.
35. Chow W.H., McLaughlin J.K., Linet M.S., Niwa S., and Mandel J.S. Use of analgesics and risk of renal cell cancer. *Int J Cancer* 59: 467–470, 1994.
36. Dubach U.C., Rosner B., and Sturmer T. An epidemiologic study of abuse of analgesic drugs. Effects of phenacetin and salicylate on mortality and cardiovascular morbidity. *N Engl J Med* 324: 155–160, 1991.
37. McCredie M., Stewart J.H., Mathew T.H., Disney A.P., and Ford J.M. The effect of withdrawal of phenacetin-containing compounds on the incidence of kidney and urothelial cancer and renal failure. *Clin Nephrol* 31: 35–39, 1989.
38. McCredie M. and Stewart J.H. Does paracetamol alone cause urothelial cancer or renal papillary necrosis? *Nephron* 49: 296–300, 1988.
39. Nanra R.S. Analgesic nephropathy in the 1990s – An Australian perspective. *Kidney Int* Suppl. 42: S86–S92, 1993.
40. Jensen O.M., Knudsen J.B., Tomasson H., and Sørensen B.L. The Copenhagen case-control study of renal pelvis and ureter cancer, role of analgesics. *Int J Cancer* 44: 965–968, 1989.

28

Renal toxicity of anti-rheumatic drugs

Sarah Bingham and Paul Emery

Many anti-rheumatic medications are nephrotoxic; this has implications both for patient selection and monitoring (Table 28.1 and 28.2). Some therapies are contraindicated in patients with renal impairment while others are allowed after dose reduction. Several drugs can induce renal impairment in previously normal kidneys necessitating vigilant monitoring of all patients. In this chapter the renal side effects of common anti-rheumatic medications will be outlined along with implications for patients with renal impairment. Guidance regarding routine monitoring will be given. The effects of cyclosporin and non-steroidal anti-inflammatory drugs are covered in separate sections of this book (Chapters 25 and 26).

Slow-acting antirheumatic drugs

Sulphasalazine

Sulphasalazine is used as the first line disease modifying anti-rheumatic drug (DMARD) in rheumatoid arthritis (in Europe), spondyloarthropathy and other rheumatic conditions as well as gastroenterological conditions. Via an unknown mechanism, the number of activated lymphocytes is reduced and the titres of IgM and rheumatoid factor both fall following 12 weeks therapy (1). Sulphasalazine is insoluble and little absorption occurs (10–20%). Sulphapyridine and 5-aminosalicylic acid are liberated from sulphasalazine in the colon following bacterial activation of the azo bond. Virtually no sulphasalazine is found in the stools. Sulphapyridine appears in the plasma 4–6 hours postdose and is metabolized by N^4-acetylation, ring hydroxylation and subsequent gluconuration. Individual differences in the rate of acetylation and oxidation leads to variations in steady state plasma concentrations of sulphapyridine. However, no relationship between the plasma level of sulphapyridine and response or toxicity has so far been ascertained (2). Both sulphasalazine and sulphapyridine are responsible for the anti rheumatic properties of sulphasalazine. Sulphasalazine is generally well tolerated and long-term toxic effects are rare (3). Serious side effects are most common in the first 12 weeks of therapy and include leukopenia and hepatotoxicity; these necessitate cessation of therapy. Gastrointestinal upset is common but can usually be improved by dose reduction. Patients should be warned to expect orange discoloration of the urine. Although serious renal side effects are rare, a

Table 28.1 Anti-rheumatic medications; effects, mechanism of action, indications and use

Class	Drug	Effects	Mechanism of action	Indications	Route
Non-steroidal anti-inflammatory drugs	Eg. Diclofenac (non-selective), rofecoxib, celecoxib (COX II selective)	Analgesic and anti-inflammatory effects	Inhibition of cyclo-oxygenase	Inflammatory arthritis, connective tissue disease, gout	Oral, topical, PR
Cortico-steroids	Depomedrone, triamcinolone	Anti-inflammatory	Changes in DNA transcription	Inflammatory arthritis, connective tissue disease, gout	Oral, IV, IA
Slow-acting anti-rheumatic drugs	Sulphasalazine	Disease modifying	Reduction in activated lymphocytes	RA, SPA, inflammatory bowel disease	Oral
	Antimalarials	Disease modifying	Lymphocyte antigen processing	RA, SLE	Oral
	Gold	Disease modifying	May regulate gene expression	RA	Oral, IM
	Penicillamine	Disease modifying	Sulphydryl exchange reactions	RA, systemic sclerosis	Oral
Immuno-suppressant drugs	Methotrexate	Disease modifying	Inhibition of dihydrofolate reductase, Increased adenosine	RA, SPA, CTD, vasculitis	Oral, IM, IV
	Leflunomide	Disease modifying	Inhibition of dihydroorate dehydrogenase	RA	Oral
	Azathioprine	Disease modifying	Suppression of inosinic acid synthesis	RA, SLE, vasculitis	Oral
	Cyclophosphamide	Disease modifying	DNA crosslinks	SLE, SSc, vasculitis	Oral, IV
	Chlorambucil	Disease modifying	DNA crosslinks	RA, vasculitis	Oral

Table 28.1 Anti-rheumatic medications; effects, mechanism of action, indications and use *continued*

Class	Drug	Effects	Mechanism of action	Indications	Route
	Mycophenolate Mofetil	Disease modifying	Inhibition of IMPDH	RA, SLE, JIA	Oral
	Antibiotics Eg minocycline	Disease modifying	See text	RA	Oral
Biological therapy	Infliximab	Anti-inflammatory, disease modifying	Chimeric human-mouse monoclonal antibody, inhibition of TNFα effects	RA	IV
	Etanercept	Anti-inflammatory, disease modifying	Fc-TNF receptor fusion molecule, inhibition of TNFα effects	RA, JIA	SC
	D2E7	Anti-inflammatory, disease modifying	Fully humanized monoclonal antibody, inhibition of TNFα effects	RA	SC
	Interleukin-1 receptor antagonist	Anti-inflammatory, disease modifying	Inhibition of IL1 effects	RA	SC
Drugs used in the treatment of gout	Colchicine	Anti-inflammatory, anti-function prophylaxis	Effects on neutrophils	Gout	Oral, IV
	Allopurinol	Prophylaxis	Xanthine-oxidase inhibitor	Gout	Oral
	Probenecid and sulphinpyrazone	Prophylaxis	Uricosuric	Gout	Oral

RA — rheumatoid arthritis, SPA — spondyloarthropathy, CTD — connective tissue disease, SLE — systemic lupus erythematosis, SSc — systemic sclerosis, JIA — juvenile inflammatory arthritis, IMPDH — inosine monophosphate dehydrogenase
PR — per rectum, IV — intravenous, IA — intra-articular, IM — intramuscular, SC — subcutaneous

Table 28.2 Renal side effects of anti-rheumatic medication

Drug	Use in renal impairment	Renal toxicity	Monitoring for renal toxicity	Comments
Sulphasalazine	Caution	Rare: Proteinuria Nephrotic	Blood U and Serum Cr test urine for protein	
Antimalerials	None	None	None	
Gold	Caution in mild impairment Contra-indicated in severe renal disease	Proteinuria Nephrotic Haematuria	Test urine with each injection or monthly with oral gold Blood U and Serum Cr	
Penicillamine	Caution in renal impairment	Proteinuria Nephrotic Haematuria Goodpastures syndrome	Test urine biweekly then monthly Blood U and Serum Cr	
Methotrexate	Reduce dose in renal impairment Contra-indicated in severe renal disease	Rare Blood U and Serum Cr	Creatinine clearance if indicated	Interaction with NSAIDs
Leflunomide	Not in moderate/severe renal impairment	None	None	
Azathioprine	Reduce dose in severe renal impairment	Rare: Interstitial nephritis Multiple-organ failure	Blood U and Serum Cr Increase frequency of blood count monitoring in presence of renal impairment	Interaction with allopurinol
Cyclophosphamide	Reduce dose in renal impairment	Haemorrhagic cystitis Bladder Carcinoma	Dip urine for blood during treatment, long-term monitoring if haemorrhagic cystitis occurs	Interaction with allopurinol and cimetidine

Table 28.2 Renal side effects of anti-rheumatic medication *continued*

Drug	Use in renal impairment	Renal toxicity	Monitoring for renal toxicity	Comments
Chlorambucil	Caution in renal impairment	None	None	
Mycophenolate	Caution in renal impairment	None	Can measure MPA levels	
Tetracyclines	Tetracycline contraindicated in renal disease	None	None	
TNFα-blocking Agents	None	None	None	
IL1 ra	None	None	None	
Colchicine	Caution	Rare	None	
	Reduce dose in severe renal disease			
Allopurinol	Caution	Rare	None	
	Reduce dose in severe renal disease			
Probenecid and Sulphinpyrazone	Not in severe renal disease or urate stones	Rare	None	

few cases of sulphasalazine induced renal failure have been reported (4) and therefore monitoring of renal function and caution when prescribing for patients with renal impairment is recommended (5). Sulphasalazine has also been reported to cause proteinuria and nephrotic syndrome; regular testing for proteinuria may therefore be beneficial (6).

Antimalarials

Chloroquine and hydroxychloroquine are used to treat rheumatoid arthritis and systemic lupus erythematosus. In recent years, hydroxychloroquine is commonly used in combination with sulphasalazine and/or methotrexate for RA as it has a lower efficacy when used as monotherapy. The mechanism of action is unclear, but the accumulation in liposomes of leucocyte and fibroblasts may interfere with antigen processing and hence lymphocyte response. In addition, interleukin-1 production by macrophages and monocytes is reduced. Apart from the rare cumulative side effect of retinopathy (more commonly seen with chloroquine), the majority of adverse events are transient and not serious. In general hydroxychloroquine is less toxic than chloroquine. Antimalarials are not reported to cause any renal toxicity either alone or in combination (7).

Gold therapy

Injectable gold (sodium aurothiomalate) and oral gold (Auranofin) are both used for the treatment of patients with rheumatoid arthritis. They are normally used in patients who have failed to adequately respond to methotrexate and sulphasalazine. The mechanism of action is not definitely known, but recently aurothiomalate has been found to inhibit the binding of transcription factors to DNA and hence may regulate gene expression. Toxicity is more common with injectable gold than the oral preparation and can be divided into two groups. Mucocutaneous reactions and anorexia tend to occur early during therapy and are likely to be a direct toxic effect of the drug. The second group consists of reactions that may involve an immunological mechanism and include renal toxicity, blood dyscrasias and hypersensitivity pneumonitis. Gold induced toxicity does not appear to be dose related probably due to therapy being given in standard regimes that involves intermittent administration.

Gold therapy should be avoided renal impairment and is contra-indicated in severe renal disease (5). Transient and minor proteinuria occurs commonly (10%) and urine should be tested with each injection or monthly if receiving oral gold. Minor proteinuria (< 300 mg/L) usually responds to suspension of gold therapy and exclusion of urinary tract infection. Gold therapy should be discontinued in the presence of persistent proteinuria at greater than 300 mg/L. Deterioration of renal function due to gold is unusual. Rarely nephrotic syndrome develops which always resolves, but may take months or years (8). Occasionally membranous glomerulonephritis associated with immune complex deposition occurs with more severe proteinuria and haematuria. Epimembranous spikes and a mild increase in mesangial cells are unusually seen, and the diagnosis can be confirmed with immunofluorescence/immunoperoxidase microscopy, which shows granular subepithelial deposits of predominately IgG. On electron-microscopy, electron dense deposits are seen. Mesangial glomerulonephritis is found in patients with RA irrespective of therapy, but in patients receiving gold therapy there is an increased association between this histological appearance and haematuria. Immunofluorescence may reveal either granular deposits of immunoglobulin (predominantly IgG) and complement, or may be negative. Patients with proteinuria and haematuria following gold therapy have been found to have thinner glomerular basement membranes when compared to controls (9). Gold may induce a disease of immune-complex type in which circulating immune complexes are either deposited in glomeruli or formed *in situ*. Tubular proteinuria and abnormal tubular function have also been described with gold therapy (10) and gold deposits have been demonstrated in proximal tubular cells (11). In those patients without renal abnormalities before treatment, renal biopsy should be confined to those who have deteriorating renal function, or who fail to improve after withdrawal of drug. Rechallenge with further gold therapy usually results in repeated toxicity. This may in part be due to an association between renal toxicity and the HLA alleles DR3/B8. Poor sulphoxidation ability has been shown to be a risk factor for increased toxicity with gold therapy although the mechanism is unknown (12). Shared risk factors may be involved in the observation that patients who develop proteinuria on gold are more likely to do so on penicillamine and vice versa (13).

D-penicillamine

D-penicillamine (DPA) is used in the treatment of rheumatoid arthritis and also to treat the skin manifestations of systemic sclerosis. The use in both these conditions is declining, as more efficacious therapies are now available. The mechanism of action is not known, but may involve modulation of the immune system via sulphydryl exchange reactions. In addition, DPA inhibits binding of the transcription factor AP-1 to DNA and therefore may influence gene transcription. DPA is cleared largely through oxidation to form disulphides with plasma albumin, L-cystine, homocysteine and itself. Patients with impaired sulphoxidation status have been shown to have an increased risk of side effects (14). In addition, increased risk of renal toxicity has been found to be associated with the presence of HLA allele DR3 (15). Although the two risk factors are not additive, the possession of either DR3 or poor sulphoxidation produces a relative risk of toxicity of 25.0 (14). Patients who develop proteinuria with penicillamine are more likely to do so with gold and vice versa (13).

Toxicity is common (50%), with mucocutaneous reactions, gastrointestinal upset, renal toxicity, blood dyscrasias and autoimmune phenomenon seen. The incidence of side effects with DPN is related to drug dose (16). Proteinuria is common and urine should be checked biweekly for 8 weeks then monthly after commencement of therapy. Mild proteinuria associated with immune complex nephritis occurs in up to 30% of patients (17), but may resolve despite continuation of treatment. No significant deterioration in renal function normally occurs. Treatment may be continued provided renal function is normal, oedema is absent and the 24-hour protein excretion does not exceed 2 g (5). Heavy proteinuria and nephrotic syndrome due to membranous GN should respond to cessation of drug, but may take months or years to resolve (18). Immunofluorescence reveals granular subepithelial deposits of predominantly IgG and on electronmicroscopy, electron dense deposits are seen. IgM nephropathy (19) and minimal change nephropathy (20) have also been reported. If haematuria occurs, therapy should be withdrawn immediately as this may indicate rapidly progressive (crescentic) glomerulonephritis due to drug induced Goodpastures syndrome or lupus erythematosus or other causes. Goodpastures syndrome (with dyspnoea, haemoptysis, pleural effusions, gross haematuria and oliguria) may be associated with the presence of anti-glomerular basement membrane antibodies and haemoptysis and usually requires treatment with high dose corticosteroids. Occasionally circulating antimyeloperoxidase antibodies have been detected in such cases (21). This rare complication may be fatal in 50% of cases (22) and return of renal function to normal in the survivors is unlikely. DPN has been associated with anti-DNA (or anti-histone) antibodies leading to a syndrome of drug-induced lupus erythematosus. Occasionally, anti-double stranded DNA antibodies are produced which can induce significant lupus renal disease and proteinuria. DPN has also been implicated in drug-induced acute interstitial nephritis (23).

Renal biopsy is indicated in patients who develop toxicity on top of pre-existing renal disease or who have declining renal function. Monitoring of patients receiving penicillamine must continue long term, as the renal complications tend to occur several months into treatment.

Immunosuppressant drugs

Methotrexate

Methotrexate (MTX) is used commonly as the anchor drug in the treatment of rheumatoid arthritis both alone and in combination with sulphasalazine (SSA) and/or hydroxychloroquine (HC). Triple therapy with MTX/SSA/HC has been shown to be efficacious in patients previously failing MTX alone (24, Table 28.3). It is also used in the treatment of spondyloarthropathies, connective tissue diseases such as systemic lupus erythematosus and vasculitidies including Wegener's granulomatosus. MTX reduces purine biosynthesis via inhibition of the enzyme dihydrofolate reductase (DHFR) and other folate-dependent enzymes. Via inhibition of the enzyme 5-aminoimidazole-carboxamide-ribinucleotide-transformylase, MTX increases adenosine release leading to inhibition of neutrophil chemotaxis and other anti-inflammatory effects. MTX is normally given orally once a week, but can also be given parenterally if there is concern regarding bioavailibility or in order to prevent gastric toxicity. MTX and its metabolites are mainly eliminated via the kidney hence the dose of MTX must

Table 28.3 Results of triple therapy for patients with suboptimal response to MTX

Variable	Initial	Follow-up	p
ESR (mm/h)	30.3	19	0.06
Morning stiffness (min)	104	28	0.03
Swollen joint score	29.7	11.7	0.001
Tender joint score	30.1	10.4	0.001
Patient global status	4.1	2.6	0.03
Physician global	5.1	3.1	0.009

be reduced in renal impairment (5) and its use is contra-indicated in the presence of significant renal disease. Calculation of creatinine clearance in patients with renal impairment and at risk groups such as the elderly can guide dosage reduction (25). It is probable that all NSAIDs, including aspirin, decrease MTX clearance. Using microdialysis techniques in rats, time-concentration area under the curves for MTX and its major metabolite, 7-hydroxymethotrexate (7-OH-MTX) have been shown to increase about twofold in the presence of naproxen (26). Although clinical effects are uncommon with low dose MTX (27), the effect may be significant in patients receiving higher weekly maintenance doses (28). In addition, combination therapy with MTX and aspirin has been shown to be associated with deterioration in renal function as measured by plasma clearance of radiolabelled EDTA and mercaptoacetyltiglyceride (29). Combination therapy with sulphasalazine is not associated with an increase in toxicity (7).

The most common major side effects of MTX therapy are marrow suppression, hepatotoxicity and pneumonitis. Renal toxicity is very rare but the risk is increased in patients with pre-existing renal impairment and reduced renal clearance.

Leflunomide

Leflunomide, licensed for use in RA in 1999, is likely to be increasingly used in patients with difficult disease, which has not responded to combination therapy with sulphasalazine and methotrexate. The mechanism of action is via an active metabolite that inhibits the enzyme dihyoorotate dehydrogenase, which is involved in *de novo* pyrimidine synthesis that is especially required by activated lymphocytes. This leads to an antiproliferative effect. The active metabolite is further metabolized and then renally excreted.

At present leflunomide is contra-indicated in patients with moderate to severe renal insufficiency because of lack of clinical experience in this patient group; however, leflunomide has no measurable effect on renal function (30). Studies have indicated a beneficial effect on a subset of RA patients with elevated baseline uric acid levels. This may be due to a uricosuric effect on the proximal tubule. Proteinuria is not a recognized side effect of leflunomide. Leflunomide can induce a global rise in blood pressure, especially in patients with pre-existing hypertension. The mechanism for this is unknown.

Azathioprine

Azathioprine (AZA) is used in the treatment of rheumatoid arthritis, systemic lupus and vasculitis. AZA interferes with adenine and guanine ribonucleotides via suppression of inosinic acid synthesis (31). AZA is cleaved to 6-mercaptopurine (6-MP) which is metabolized inside cells to thioinosinic and thioguanylic acid through the action of hypoxanthine phosphoribosyltransferase (HGPRT). These secondary intracellular metabolites are responsible for the effect of AZA, making measurement of blood or plasma levels of AZA unlikely to be very useful. Xanthine oxidase is also involved in AZA metabolism and is inhibited by allopurinol leading to accumulation and increased toxicity of AZA and its metabolites. Therefore the dose of AZA needs to be greatly reduced in cases of co-administration. There are two distinct populations of AZA metabolisers: fast and slow, leading to a fourfold variation in the rate of clearance. In addition, the enzyme which metabolizes 6-MP (thiopurine methyltransferase) exhibits genetic polymorphism with a small subset of the population producing low levels. This leads to increased toxicity (usually bone marrow suppression) on low doses of AZA in these patients. The principle toxicities of AZA include marrow suppression and gastrointestinal upset. The dose of AZA should be reduced in severe renal impairment (5). AZA can rarely induce a hypersensitivity reaction, which in severe case manifests as multiple organ failure (32). Patients present with fever, hypotension and oliguria a few days after commencing AZA or increasing the dose. The reaction may be due to cytokine or mediator release induced by AZA (33). A case has been reported of a patient who developed end-stage renal failure following AZA hypersensitivity mimicking Goodpasture's syndrome (34). In a separate case report, a patient developed fever, hepatitis and acute interstitial nephritis after three weeks of AZA therapy, which recurred on recommencing the drug (35).

Cyclophosphamide

Cyclophosphamide (CTX) pulse therapy (usually intravenous) is commonly used for the management of severe SLE, systemic sclerosis and vasculitis. In some diseases such as Wegener's granulomatosis, continuous oral CTX is used to maintain disease control although it is generally thought that this method of administration is associated with a greater incidence of toxicity (36). Active metabolites of CTX produced in the liver prevent lymphocyte replication via DNA cross-linking (37). The kidney excretes CTX and its metabolites, therefore the dose of CTX must be reduced if renal impairment is present (5). Allopurinol and cimetidine inhibit hepatic microsomal enzymes, resulting in increased CTX toxicity. The frequency of toxicity in rheumatic patients limits the use of CTX in this group of patients. The most common toxic effects include gastrointestinal upset, increased risk of malignancy, infertility, cumulative bone marrow toxicity and haemorrhagic cystitis. The urological toxicity of CTX is due to its metabolite acrolein, which is excreted in the urine. The risk of haemorrhagic cystitis can be reduced by co-administration of mesna with each pulse (38) and assuring adequate patient hydration, neither of which is possible with continuous oral administration. Observational studies have reported a tenfold increase in the risk of bladder cancer following oral therapy with CTX (39), and the increased risk continues up to 17 years after discontinuation of oral CTX (40). The development of nonglomerular haematuria during CTX therapy is associated with an increased risk of subsequent bladder malignancy (41) and these patients should be followed long-term. Rarely renal cell carcinoma may develop following CTX therapy (42).

Chlorambucil

Chlorambucil is used occasionally in patients with rheumatic disease and vasculitis which is resistant to other therapy. Chlorambucil is metabolized to phenylacetic acid mustard, which cross links DNA inhibiting replication. Chlorambucil and its metabolites are renally excreted and therefore caution is required when prescribing for patients with renal impairment (5). The most common side effects are cumulative marrow suppression and infertility. There is an increased risk of haematological malignancy with prolonged use but no reported risk of urological tumours.

Mycophenolate mofetil

Mycophenolate is commonly used in combination with other immunosuppressive agents to prevent renal graft rejection. Recently it has been used in patients with severe resistant RA, SLE and juvenile arthritis although it is not licensed and is not being pursued for these indications in the UK. Mycophenolate is metabolized to the active metabolite mycophenolic acid (MPA). The mechanism of action is via inhibition of the enzyme inosine monophosphate dehydrogenase (IMPDH) which leads to inhibition of cellular and humoral immunity. The major toxicity is marrow suppression and gastrointestinal upset. Mycophenolate has been shown to be effective in the treatment of renal complications of SLE (43). However, when used in the prevention of renal graft rejection, the presence of renal impairment is associated with a higher incidence of toxicity (44). Measurement of MPA concentrations may prevent toxicity in such cases.

Antibiotics

In line with the hypothesis that rheumatoid arthritis is caused by an infectious agent, some patients with RA resistant to other therapies have been treated with antibiotics. The antibiotics used have mechanisms of action in addition to their anti-microbial effects, and it is likely these may be responsible for the anti-rheumatic activity.

Dapsone

In vitro studies show that dapsone inhibits and production of prostaglandin E_2 and hence inhibits polymorphonuclear neutrophil (PMN) activity. Dapsone has shown efficacy in RA in some studies, but its use is limited by the incidence of haemolytic anaemia. Dapsone can induce an SLE like syndrome but has no direct renal toxicity. Administration is contra-indicated in the presence of glucose 6 phosphate dehydrogenase deficiency.

Rifampicin

Rifampicin affects lymphocyte function and suppresses T-cell function in animal studies. It has been shown to be of benefit when injected intra-articularly into effusions, but oral efficacy has not been demonstrated and therefore its use in RA is limited. Rifampicin can cause renal insufficiency and the dose must be reduced if renal impairment is present (5).

Tetracyclines

The tetracyclines have several effects including decreased phagocytosis by PMNs and monocytes, inhibition of lymphocyte proliferation and inhibition of interferon-gamma (IFNγ) production. In addition, tetracyclines inhibit matrix metalloproteinases, which are involved in cartilage destruction. The most promising results regarding efficacy were seen with minocycline; however its use has recently declined following reports of drug-induced lupus (45). The metabolites of tetracycline build up in renal failure and lead to vomiting and dehydration. Tetracycline metabolites also have an antianabolic effect which cause a rise in blood urea, further aggravating the uraemic state in renally impaired patients and can in some circumstances precipitate dialysis. Minocycline and doxycycline are safe in renal impairment. Tetracyclines (minocycline) have rarely been associated with interstial nephritis (46).

Biological therapy

New antirheumatic therapies are now becoming available that can directly target components of the immune response. These drugs consist of monoclonal antibodies or soluble receptors which target cytokines, mainly tumour necrosis factor α (TNFα) and interleukin-1 (IL-1).

Anti-TNFα therapy

There are currently three anti-TNFα therapies which are used in patients with rheumatoid arthritis. Etanercept (Immunex/Wyeth) and infliximab (Centocor/Schering-Plough) were licensed for RA in early 2000. Etanercept consists of a

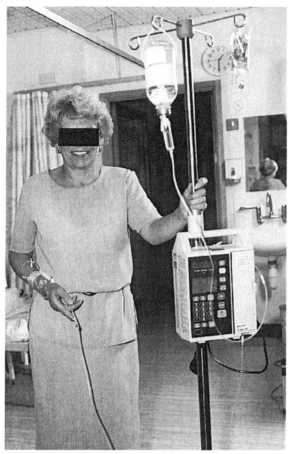

Fig. 28.1   Patient receiving intravenous infusion of infliximab during day case admission.

fusion protein of TNFα receptor and the Fc portion of a humanized immuno-globulin molecule. It is given subcutaneously twice a week. Infliximab is a chimeric human-mouse monoclonal antibody, which is given by intravenous infusion at 0, 2, 6 and then 8 weekly intervals (Fig. 28.1). Infliximab is given in combination with low dose methotrexate to reduce immune response by the patient to the non-humanized part of the molecule. The third anti-TNFα therapy, D2E7 (Knoll), a fully humanized monoclonal antibody, is currently undergoing phase three trials. The major side effects of these treatments are increased risk of infection, injection site/infusion reactions and potential increased risk of malignancy long-term. The most recent data suggest that over a two–three year follow-up, the risk of malignancy is not higher in the treated group when compared to untreated patients with RA (47, 48). There is no reported increased incidence of renal toxicity with these drugs during clinical trials; and they have not been used in patients with severe renal impairment during development.

Interleukin-1 inhibitor

An interleukin-1 receptor antagonist (IL–1ra, Amgen) has been submitted for approval. This is given by daily subcutaneous injections. No renal toxicity has been reported, but like the anti-TNFα therapies, it has not been tested in patients with renal impairment.

Drugs used for treatment of gout

Colchicine

Colchicine is used for the treatment of acute attacks of gout and for short-term prophylaxis during initiation of therapy with allopurinol in patients who are unable to tolerate NSAIDs or who are also receiving anticoagulants. It also has a prophylactic effect against recurrent attacks. Colchicine interrupts the inflammatory response to tissue deposition of urate crystals via various effects on neutrophils. It can cause renal damage and caution is recommended when prescribing in patients with renal impairment (5) The dose should be reduced in the presence of renal disease as it is renally excreted. Administration should be avoided if severe renal disease is present.

Allopurinol

Allopurinol, a xanthine-oxidase inhibitor, reduces the formation of uric acid from purines. It is used for the long-term prevention of attacks. Allopurinol can be used in the presence of renal impairment and urate stones (unlike uricosuric drugs). Allopurinol is renaly excreted so the dose needs to be reduced if renal impairment presents (5). Rarely acute interstitial nephritis leading to acute renal failure has been reported (49). In such cases, other features suggesting a hypersensitivity reaction may be present including arthralgia, fever, skin rash and evidence of abnormal liver function and eosinophillia on blood tests. Mild to moderate haematuria and proteinuria are usually present. Treatment includes drug withdrawal and corticosteroids. Allopurinol interacts with azathioprine and cyclophosphamide to increase the toxicity of these drugs.

Uricosuric drugs

Probenecid and sulphinpyrazone increase renal excretion of uric acid and are indicated for long-term prophylaxis in patients whose disease is resistant to allopurinol. These drugs are not effective in the presence of renal impairment and should not be used in the presence of urate stones. Cases of acute renal failure and nephrotic syndrome have been reported (5).

References

1. Samanta A., Webb C., Grindulis K.A., Fleming J. and Sheldon P.J. Sulphasalazine therapy in rheumatoid arthritis: qualitative changes in lymphocytes and correlation with clinical response. *Br J Rheum* 1992, 31(4): 259–63.

2. Kitas G.D., Farr M., Waterhouse I. and Bacon P.A. Influence of acetylator status on sulphasalazine efficacy and toxicity in patients with rheumatoid arthritis. *Scan J Rheum* 1992, 21(5): 220–5.

3. Amos R., Pullar T., Capell H. *et al.* Sulphasalazine for rheumatoid arthritis: toxicity in 774 patients monitored for one to 11 years. *Br Med J* 1986, 293: 420–3.

4. Dwarakanath A.D., Michael J. and Allan R.N. Sulphasalazine induced renal failure. *Gut* 1992, 33(7): 1006–7.

5. British National Formulary. 38. September 1999.

6. Helliwell P.S. Should testing for proteinuria be included in the monitoring schedule of sulphasalazine? *Br J Rheum* 1995, 34: 790–1.

7. Elkayam O., Yaron M., Zhukovsky G., Segal R. and Caspi D. Toxicity profile of dual methotrexate combinations with gold, hydroxychloroquine, sulphasalazine and minocycline in rheumatoid arthritis patients. *Rheum International* 1997, 17(2): 49–53.

8. Hall C.L., Fothergill N.J., Blackwell M.M., Harrison P.R., Mackenzie J.C. and MacIver A.G. The natural course of gold nephropathy: long term study of 21 patients. *Br Med J Clin Research* Ed. 1987, 296(6001): 745–8.

9. Saito T., Nishi S., Karasawa R., In H., Hayashi H., Ueno M., Ogino S., Sugiyama N., Suzuki S., Maruyama Y. *et al.* An ultrastructural study of glomerular basement membrane in rheumatoid arthritis patients with urinary abnormalities. *Clinical Nephrology* 1995, 43(6): 360–7.

10. Iesato K., Mori Y., Ueda S. *et al.* Renal tubular dysfunction as a complication of gold therapy in patients with rheumatoid arthritis. *Clin Nephrol* 1982, 17: 46.

11. Yarom R., Stein H., Peters P.D. *et al.* Nephrotic effect of parenteral and intra-articular gold. *Arch Pathol* 1975, 99: 36.

12. Madhok R., Capell H. and Waring R.H. Does sulphoxidation state predict gold toxicity in rheumatoid arthritis. *Br Med J* 1987, 294: 483.

13. Halla J.T., Cassidy J. and Hardin J.G. Sequential gold and penicillamine therapy in rheumatoid arthritis. *Am J Med* 1982, 72: 423.

14. Emery P., Panayi G.S., Huston G., Welsh K.I., Mitchell S.C., Shah R.R. *et al.* D-penicillamine induced toxicity in rheumatoid arthritis: the role of sulphoxidation status and HLA-DR3. *J Rheum* 1984, 11(5): 626–32.

15. Klouda P.T. *et al.* Strong association between idiopathic membranous nephropathy and HLA DR3. *Lancet* 1979, 2: 770–2.

16. Williams N.J., Ward J.R. and Reading J.C. Low dose D-penicillamine therapy in rheumatoid arthritis. *Arth Rheum* 1983, 26: 581–92.

17. Davison A.M., Dat A.T., Golding J.R. and Thompson D. Effects of penicillamine on the kidney. *Proc R Soc Med* 1977, 70(suppl 3): 109–12.

18. Hall C.L. The natural course of gold and penicillamine nephropathy: a long term study of 54 patients. *Advances in Experimental Medicine and Biology* 1989, 252: 247–56.

19. Rehan A. and Johnson K. IgM nephropathy associated with penicillamine. *Am J Nephrol* 1986, 6: 71.

20. Savill J.S., Chia Y. and Pusey C.D. Minimal change nephropathy and pemphigus vulgaris associated with penicillamine treatment of rheumatoid arthritis. *Clin Nephrol* 1988, 29: 267.
21. Gaskin G., Thompson E.M. and Pusey C.D. Goodpasture-like syndrome associated with anti-myeloperoxidase antibodies following penicillamine treatment. *Nephol Dial Transplant* 1995, 10: 1925.
22. Devogelaer J.P., Pirson Y., Vandenbroucke J.M., Cosyns J.P., Brichard S., and Nagant de Deuxchaisnes C. D-penicillamine induced crescentic glomerulonephritis: report and review of the literature. *J Rheum* 1987, 14(5): 1036–41.
23. Feehally J., Wheeler D.C., Mackay E.H. *et al.* Recurrent acute renal failure with interstitial nephritis due to D-penicillamine. *Renal Failure* 1987, 10: 55.
24. O'Dell J., Haire C., Erikson N., Drymalski W., Palmer W. and Maloley P. *et al.* Efficacy of triple DMARD therapy in patients with R.A. with suboptimal response to methotrexate. *J Rheum* 1996, 23 suppl 44: 72–4.
25. Bressolle F., Bologna C., Kinowski J., Arcos B., Sany J. and Combe B. Total and free methotrexate pharmacokinetics in elderly patients with rheumatoid arthritis. A comparison with young adults. *J Rheumatol* 1997, 24: 1903–9.
26. Ekstrom P.O., Giercksky K.E., Anderson A. and Slordal L. Alterations in methotrexate pharmacokinetics by naproxen in the rat as measured by microdialysis. *Life Sciences* 1997, 60(24): 359–64.
27. Combe B., Edno L., Lafforgue P. *et al.* Total and free methotrexate pharmacokinetics with and without piroxicam in rheumatoid arthritis patients. *Br J Rheum* 1995, 34: 421–8.
28. Kremer J.M. and Hamilton R.A. The effects of nonsteroidal anti-inflammatory drugs on maintenance doses but not at 7.5 mg. *J Rheum* 1995, 22(11): 2072–7.
29. Seideman P. and Muller-Suur R. Renal side effects of aspirin and low dose methotrexate in rheumatoid arthritis. *Annals of the rheumatic diseases* 1993, 52(8): 613–15.
30. Scott D.L., Whelton A., Smolen J.S., Weaver A., Emery P. and Strand V. Renal effects of leflunomide compared with other agents used to treat rheumatoid arthritis (R.A.). *Ann Rheum Dis* 1999, Abstract Supplement: S212.
31. Elion G.B. and Hitchings G.H. Azathioprine. *Handbook Exp Pharmacol* 1975, 38: 404–25.
32. Brown G., Boldt C., Webb J.G. and Halperin L. Azathioprine-induced multisystem organ failure and cardiogenic shock. *Pharmacotherapy* 1997, 17(4): 815–8.
33. Knowles S.R., Gupta A.K., Shear N.H. and Sauder D. Azathioprine hypersensitivity-like reactions — a case report and a review of the literature. *Clinical and Experimental Dermatology* 1995, 20(4): 353–6.
34. Stetter M., Schmidl M. and Krapf R. Azathioprine hypersensitivity mimicking Goodpasture's syndrome. *American Journal of Kidney Diseases* 1994, 23(6): 874–7.
35. Meys E., Devogelaer J.P., Geubel A., Rahier J., and Nagant de Deuxchaisnes C. Fever, hepatitis and acute interstitial nephritis in a patient with rheumatoid arthritis. Concurrent manifestations of azathioprine hypersensitivity. *J Rheum* 1992, 19(5): 807–9.
36. Guillevin L., Cordier J.F., Lhote F., Cohen P., Jarrousse B., Royer I. *et al.* A prospective multicenter, randomized trial comparing steroids and pulse cyclophosphamide versus steroids and oral cyclophosphamide in the treatment of generalized Wegner's granulomatosis. *Arth Rheum* 1997, 40(12): 2187–98.

37. Toskos G.C. Immunomodulatory treatments in patients with rheumatic diseases: mechanism of action. *Semin Arthritis Rheum* 1987, 17: 24–38.

38. Ehrlich R.M., Freedman A., Goldsobel A.B. and Stiehme E.R. The use of sodium-2-metcaptoethane sulfonate to prevent cyclophosphamide cystitis. *J Urol* 1984, 131: 960–2.

39. Kinlen J.H. Incidence of cancer in rheumatoid patients and other disorders with immunosuppressive treatment. *Am J Med* 1985, 78 (suppl 1A): 44–9.

40. Radis C.D., Kahl L.E., Baker G.L., Wasko M.C., Cash J.M., Gallatin A. *et al.* Effects of cyclophosphamide on the development of malignancy and on long-term survival of patients with rheumatoid arthritis. A 20-year follow-up study. *Arthritis Rheum* 1995, 38(8): 1120–7.

41. Talar-Williams C., Hijazi Y.M., Walther M.M., Linehan W.M., Hallahan C.W., Lubensky I. *et al.* Cyclophosphamide induced cystitis and bladder cancer in patients with Wegner's granulomatosis. *Ann Int Med* 1996, 124(5): 477–84.

42. Odeh M. Renal cell carcinoma associated with cyclophosphamide therapy for Wegner's granulomatosis. *Scan J. Rheum* 1996, 25(6): 391–3.

43. Dooley M.A., Cosio F.G., Nachman P.H., Falkenhain M.E., Hogan S.L., Falk R.J. *et al.* Mycophenolate mofetil therapy in lupus nephritis: clinical observations. *J Am Soc Nephr* 1999, 10(4): 833–9.

44. Butani L., Palmer J., Baluarte H.J. and Polinsky M.S. Adverse effects of mycophenylate mofetil in paediatric renal transplant recipients with presumed chronic rejection. *Transplantation* 1999, 68(1): 83–86.

45. Elkayam O., Yaron M. and Caspi D. Minocycline induced autoimmune syndromes: an overview. *Seminars in Arthritis and Rheumatism* 1999, 28(6): 392–7.

46. Wilkinson S.P., Stewart W.K., Spiers E.M. *et al.* Protacted systemic illness and interstitial nephritis due to minocycline. *Postgrad Med* 1989, 65: 53.

47. Kavanaugh A., Schaible T., DeWoody K., Marsters P., Dittrich K., Harriman G. and Malvern P.A. Long-term follow-up of patients treated with infliximab (anti-TNFα antibody) in clinical trials. *Arthritis Rheum* 1999, 42 (suppl): S401.

48. Moreland L., Cohen S., Baumgartner S., Schiff M., Tindall E. and Burge Birmingham. Long-term use of etanercept inpatients with DMARD-refractory rheumatoid arthritis. *Arthritis Rheum* 1999, 42 (suppl): S401.

49. Gelbart D.R., Weinstein A.B. and Fajardo L.F. Allopurinol induced interstitial nephritis. *Ann Intern Med* 1977, 86: 196.

PART IX

29

Rheumatologic diseases associated with interstitial nephritis

Alan D. Salama and Charles D. Pusey

Introduction

Tubulointerstitial nephritis (TIN) is an inflammatory renal condition in which the damage is focused on the tubules and interstitium. It is of considerable importance since tubulointerstitial damage more closely correlates with impairment of renal fuction than does the degree of glomerular damage (1). Interstitial inflammation may be secondary to glomerular injury, renovascular or metabolic disease, or may be initiated primarily within the interstitial compartment. The commoner causes of TIN are drug reactions, infections and an 'idiopathic' group. Many drugs used in rheumatology practice, particularly non-steroidal anti-inflammatory drugs, can lead to TIN; these are considered separately in Chapter 26. A number of systemic diseases are also associated with TIN, many as a result of autoimmune processes, in which tolerance to self-antigens is lost (2). Those disorders which may be encountered by rheumatologists will form the focus of this chapter (Table 29.1). Most descriptions of these patients are in case reports or small clinical series. As a result, no good trial data are available regarding treatment options.

Table 29.1   Associations of tubulointerstitial nephritis with systemic disease

Rheumatologic conditions associated with TIN
Systemic lupus erythematosus
Overlap syndrome/mixed connective tissue disease
Rheumatoid arthritis
Essential mixed cryoglobulinaemia
Sjogren's syndrome
Sarcoidosis
Tubulointerstitial nephritis and uveitis (TINU)
Primary systemic vasculitis

Clinical features

TIN may result in acute renal failure, accounting for up to 27% of cases presenting with renal failure and normal sized kidneys. More commonly, however, it may be chronic in nature (3). Many clinical features are common to TIN irrespective of its aetiology (Table 29.2). However, in the context of systemic disease, these features may be difficult to differentiate from those of the underlying condition. Furthermore, since suggestive clinical features can be absent or the diagnosis may not be suspected, renal biopsy is required to confirm the diagnosis (4).

Tubular damage occurs consequent to the interstitial inflammation and a number of functional tubular defects may develop, the pattern of which is dependent on the predominant region of the tubule affected (Table 29.3). If

Table 29.2 Presenting features and laboratory findings in TIN

Features	Findings
Fever	Renal impairment
Arthralgia	Eosinophilia
Rash*	Sterile pyuria
Flank tenderness	Haematuria
Gastrointestinal complaints	Proteinuria§
Hypertension	Casts (red cell and
Oedema	granular)
Oligoanuria	

* More common in drug-related cases.
§ Generally < 1 g/24 hours.
(Adapted from (4)).

Table 29.3 Sites of injury and patterns of tubular dysfunction in acute TIN

Site of injury	Tubular dysfunction	Clinical features
Proximal tubule	Decreased reabsorption of: Na^+, glucose, HCO_3^-, urate, PO_4^-, amino acids	Glycosuria, hypouricaemia, hypophosphataemia, aminoaciduria, alkaline urine, acidaemia*
Distal tubule	Decreased secretion of: Na^+, H^+ Decreased reabsorption of: Na^+.	Alkaline urine, acidaemia, hyperkalaemia, inability to preserve Na^{+**}
Medulla and papilla	Decreased reabsorption of: Na^+ Decreased concentrating ability	Polyuria, nocturia, inability to preserve Na^{+***}

* Proximal renal tubular acidosis. **Distal tubular acidosis. ***Nephrogenic diabetes insipidus.
(Adapted from (5)).

widespread interstitial inflammation is present, a mixture of defects may occur. These may result in presenting symptoms, such as renal tubular acidosis leading to hypokalaemic paralysis, or may be subclinical and only evident following specific investigations.

Investigations

Ultimately a renal biopsy is required to confirm a diagnosis of TIN, with samples sent for immunohistochemistry, electron microscopy and light microscopy. However, a number of findings suggest the diagnosis in the correct clinical setting.

Serum creatinine may be raised and is often the presenting feature. There may be evidence of systemic acidaemia, hypo- or hyper-kalaemia, hypophosphatemia or hypouricaemia. Fractional excretion of sodium may be raised, but is of use only in patients who have not received diuretics. Peripheral blood eosinophilia may be present, more commonly in cases of allergic aetiology (4). Immunological tests should be performed in all cases and may be helpful in the diagnosis of systemic disorders associated with TIN. Urine dipstick testing is generally positive for blood and protein, and can also reveal glucose, a low specific gravity and an alkaline pH. Analysis of the urinary sediment reveals both white and red blood cells, with casts of white cells and less commonly red cells. Eosinophiluria (>1% of total leucocytes) suggests an allergic aetiology, requires special staining methods, but is neither specific nor sensitive (6). A 24 hour urine collection usually shows non-nephrotic range proteinuria. This predominantly consists of low molecular weight proteins, such as β2-microglobulin and retinol-binding protein, which are freely filtered at the glomerulus and reabsorbed in health by the proximal tubules. Albumin makes up little of the measured proteinuria, in contrast to glomerular diseases (7). Imaging of the kidneys may reveal them to be enlarged with increased echogenicity on ultrasound scanning. Gallium-67 isotope scan may reveal strong renal uptake but is by no means specific, and should not be relied upon to exclude a diagnosis of TIN (6).

Suggested investigations in cases of TIN are shown in Table 29.4. Further tests may be required in specific cases.

Pathology

Regardless of the aetiology of TIN, there are a number of common pathological features. Acutely, there is oedema, tubular injury, and a cellular infiltrate (Fig. 29.1). This generally consists of lymphocytes (T and B cells), plasma cells, macrophages, and occasional granulocytes and NK cells. Granulomas may be present, as are eosinophils in certain forms of TIN. Chronically, there is persistent cellular infiltration, tubular atrophy, and interstitial fibrosis (8). Progression to chronicity with accompanying fibrosis may be rapid, occurring within weeks. Alternatively the inflammation may resolve spontaneously, without consequence. Most series have found a correlation between the degree of interstitial infiltrate

Table 29.4   Investigations in TIN

Suggested investigations in TIN

Blood
Urea, Creatinine, Electrolytes, Calcium, Phosphate, Uric acid, Chloride, Bicarbonate
Full blood count including eosinophil count
Immunology
ANCA, ANA, dsDNA, ENA
RhF, Cryoglobulins, Immunoglobulins, Complement
Serum ACE
Urine
Dipstick
Microscopy
Hansel's stain for eosinophils
Spot electrolytes, osmolality
24 hour collection for protein, including low molecular weight proteins
Creatinine clearance
Imaging
Ultrasound scanning
Renal Biopsy

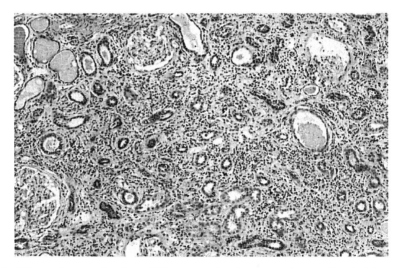

Fig. 29.1   Photomicrograph of renal biopsy section from a patient with tubulointerstitial nephritis and uveitis syndrome (TINU), showing a typical pattern of inflammation in the interstitum, with a heavy mononuclear cell infiltrate. There is loss of normal tubular architecture, with tubular atrophy and dilatation, large casts within the tubular lumens and interstitial expansion and oedema. The glomeruli are uninvolved. (H and E ×75).

and the severity of renal impairment, and between the degree of infiltration and the long-term outcome, although others have not (4, 9–11). Factors determining the outcome of interstitial inflammation, with repair and resolution or atrophy and fibrosis, remain poorly defined.

From human studies and animal models, tubular damage is known to occur through activity of the different effector arms of the immune response (8). It may be due to antibody or immune complex deposition, but is more commonly due to cellular immunity in the form of delayed type hypersensitivity reactions and cytotoxic effector cells. Antibodies may directly bind the tubular basement membrane (TBM), as in the rare anti-TBM disease, or may be directed against other unknown antigens in the tubulointerstitium. Such antigens may be a structural part of the tubule, may be secreted by it, or may be part of the urinary filtrate. In antibody mediated TIN there is usually linear deposition of immunoglobulin on the TBM, and in immune complex mediated TIN there are granular deposits.

Delayed type hypersensitivity (DTH) reactions and granulomas are found in TIN (Fig. 29.2), but in few of them is the T cell antigen known. Both CD4+ and CD8+ T cells are found, in varying proportions. Some are in an activated state, as evidenced by expression of CD25 (IL-2-receptor α chain) and MHC class II antigens on their cell surface (12, 13). Only in allograft rejection is it known that T cells can directly mediate tubular damage. In other circumstances where T cell infiltration is predominant the evidence that they act as orchestrators of disease is circumstantial. However, T cell numbers do correlate with serum creatinine at presentation and the degree of chronic tubulointerstitial damage (11).

Recently it has been suggested that infection with Epstein-Barr virus (EBV) may be a common cause of chronic 'idiopathic' interstitial nephritis (14) (and see Sjogren's syndrome below). EBV viral DNA was found in the tubulointerstitium in renal biopsy specimens from patients with chronic 'idiopathic' TIN. Furthermore the EBV receptor (CD21) was identified on proximal tubular cells. Viral particles were not identified in drug-related TIN. These data suggest, but do not prove, a causal role for EBV in inducing or perpetuating chronic interstitial inflammation. The role of EBV in acute TIN, and in TIN associated with different diseases, requires further clarification.

Systemic lupus erythematosus (SLE)

In patients with SLE, tubulointerstitial nephritis generally occurs in association with glomerular lesions. TIN may be seen in any of the WHO classes of lupus nephritis, although it occurs more commonly in grades III and IV (15), and in patients with more active disease (16). There are occasional reports of patients with SLE in whom TIN occurs in isolation, and in whom it is responsible for either acute or chronic renal failure (17–21). These patients generally have active disease, with positive ANA and DNA binding, but a 'benign' urine sediment. One reported patient was asymptomatic from his lupus, and had renal tubular

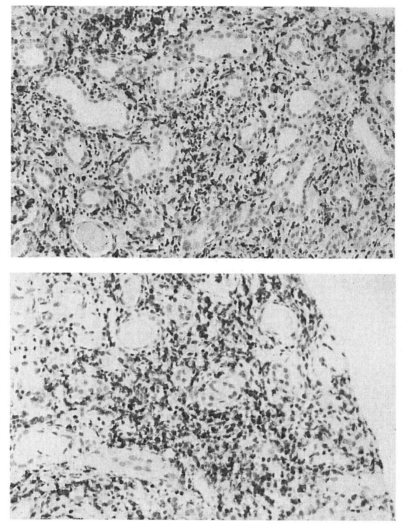

Fig. 29.2 (a) Photomicrograph of renal biopsy section from a patient with tubulointerstitial nephritis, stained for macrophages with anti-CD68. There is a marked increase in macrophage numbers, with widespread infiltration throughout the interstitium. (H and E ×190.) (b) Photomicrograph of renal biopsy section from a patient with tubulointerstitial nephritis stained for the presence of CD3, a pan T cell marker. There is a heavy, patchy infiltration of T cells surrounding the tubules, with evidence of tubular cell damage (tubulitis). (H and E ×190.)

acidosis as the only manifestation of disease (19). Functional disturbances in tubular function are common in patients with SLE, with up to 80% having some abnormality of tubular concentrating ability, urinary acidification or proximal tubular cell reabsorptive capacity (22). There is no clear correlation between the functional tubular abnormalities and renal histology. It is apparent that tubulointerstitial damage in treated patients with SLE is a better predictor of outcome than glomerular lesions (10).

Immune complex deposits along the TBM on renal biopsy are found in approximately half the cases of lupus nephritis (23). Deposits are similar to those found elsewhere in SLE, that is to say they consist of IgG, IgM, C1q, C3, C5-9 and rarely IgA. However, there may be greater variability in the composition of deposits in the interstitium than elsewhere (16). Interstitial capillary immune deposits are almost exclusive to SLE (24). There is a report of linear deposition of IgG, suggesting anti–TBM antibodies, in association with TIN in a child with SLE (25).

In one series, the severity of glomerular damage was found to correlate with the tubulointerstitial deposits, with more deposits occurring in association with increasing glomerular proliferation (16). Paradoxically, the severity of interstitial inflammation does not generally correlate with the extent of tubulointerstitial deposits (22). Thus, mechanisms other than antibody deposition are probably operating to induce tubular damage. There is strong evidence for cellular immunity in SLE-related TIN. There is a predominant T cell infiltrate, with mainly CD8+ cells in areas of tubulitis (11), and upregulation of MHC class I and II antigens and the co-stimulatory molecule CD40 on renal tubular cells. In one case of SLE-related TIN, significant numbers of interstitial mast cells were also found (17). Interestingly, an important role has recently been ascribed to interstitial mast cells in tubulointerstitial disease, fibrosis and renal dysfunction (26). Mast cell numbers in the interstitium correlate with the degree of renal dysfunction, intensity of tubulointerstitial injury and fibrosis in patients with various types of chronic glomerulonephritis, including SLE. Mast cells are known to secrete pro-fibrotic mediators including TNF-α and TGF-β, suggesting that they may play a role in chronic tubulointerstitial damage. Their role in primary tubulointerstitial disease remains to be defined.

Treatment and outcome

In those cases of isolated SLE-related TIN, treatment has been variable, and the number of reports are too few to allow specific recommendations to be made. In six of the eight patients reported, medium to high doses of corticosteroids were used with improvement of renal function in four. One of the responders received cyclophosphamide in addition to the steroids, but subsequently died from sepsis. In two others no immunosuppressive treatment was given and there was an improvement in renal function, although not back to normal. One patient was monitored for 3 years and followed a relatively benign course, with no sign of renal deterioration (21). It may therefore be advisable to observe such patients and treat only if the renal function deteriorates. In cases of TIN secondary to glomerular disease, treatment options are dictated by the severity of glomerulonephritis and have been reviewed elsewhere (27).

Overlap syndromes/mixed connective tissue disease

A rheumatological overlap syndrome with features of SLE, systemic sclerosis and polymyositis, and characterized by the presence of extractable nuclear antigens (ENA) was first described by Sharp in 1972 (28). Its definition has undergone some revision, and it may more truly represent a transitional syndrome which polarizes to one or other condition with time. Thus MCTD is now more properly identified, in association with antibodies to U1-RNP, in patients with synovitis, myositis, Raynaud's phenomenon, hand oedema and acrocyanosis (29). Renal involvement in this condition is commoner than originally thought, occurring in up to 25% of cases (28, 30, 31). Glomerular and vascular pathology predominate (mimicking that in SLE and scleroderma respectively), with membranous glomerulonephritis being the commonest glomerular lesion. Up to 20% of patients had evidence of interstitial disease (32, 33), although this was often secondary to glomerular lesions (32). Tubular immune deposits of IgG and C3 have also been reported (34). Serologic studies do not predict those with renal disease. Treatment has generally been with steroids, in regimens as used for SLE.

Rheumatoid arthritis

Rheumatoid arthritis is a chronic inflammatory autoimmune disease which, despite its multisystem involvement, rarely affects the kidney. The commoner pathologies are mesangioproliferative glomerulonephritis, amyloidosis and membranous glomerulonephritis (often secondary to drug therapy). In a few cases tubulointerstitial nephritis is found, and this is generally ascribed to therapy with non-steroidal anti-inflammatory drugs, gold or penicillamine (35). However, not all the patients with RA and TIN are reported to be on drug treatment. Detailed drug histories are not always available, and it is therefore difficult to exclude covert drug ingestion. In some reports, careful exclusion of secondary Sjögren's disease has not been carried out. The association of interstitial changes with mesangial expansion in a number of series, suggests that both lesions may be secondary to a single aetiological agent; whether this is a drug or RA itself remains unclear (36). Treatment has generally involved removal of the offending agents.

Essential mixed cryoglobulinaemia

Essential mixed cryoglobulinaemia (EMC) is characterized by circulating immunoglobulins capable of precipitating in the cold. In type II ECM the immunoglobulins are a mixture of a monoclonal IgM rheumatoid factor (RF) and polyclonal IgG bound to the RF. Many cases are associated with chronic hepatitis C infection. In EMC, the most common renal lesion is a mesangiocapillary glomerulonephritis, and this is often accompanied by interstitial inflammation. In some cases, immune complex deposits containing IgG, IgM and C3 are extensive and are associated with progressive chronic damage. Rheumatoid factor activity can be demonstrated within the deposits (24). Interstitial infiltration by predominantly CD8+ T cells is also found, associated with tubular injury. However, in many cases these changes more likely reflect the glomerular and vascular damage (37). In cases of severe renal involvement, treatment has been with plasmapheresis, steroids and cytotoxic agents. In hepatitis C associated cases there may be an additional role for alpha interferon or other anti-viral agents. This is covered in more detail in Chapter 23.

Sjögren's syndrome

Sjögren's syndrome (SS) is an autoimmune condition in which there is cellular infiltration of the exocrine glands, notably the salivary and lacrimal glands, giving rise to the characteristic clinical features. The condition may occur in isolation (primary SS) or in association with other autoimmune diseases, such as rheumatoid arthritis or SLE (secondary SS).

Renal involvement is well recognized but infrequent, and is often subclinical, with between 2 and 26% of patients developing overt disease (29). Renal impairment is generally mild but may be severe and result in acute or chronic renal failure (38). Urinary abnormalities are minor, with occasional leukocytes and modest proteinuria. The most common histological abnormality is tubulointerstitial nephritis with a predominant lymphocytic infiltrate, consisting mostly of T cells (15, 39). Tubular atrophy, nephrocalcinosis, interstitial oedema and fibrosis occur to variable extents. By contrast, glomerular changes are rare. Latent tubular abnormalities are reported to occur in 20–85% of patients (40–42). Tubulointerstitial immune deposits have been reported (40, 43), although they are generally absent. Areas of tubular atrophy and fibrosis appear to coincide with those in which immunoglobulin deposits are found, suggesting a possible aetiological role for antibodies in tubulointerstitial inflammation (43). Rarely, immune complex-mediated glomerulonephritis may also occur, with membranous or membranoproliferative types predominating.

Functional renal tubular defects, such as renal tubular acidosis, nephrogenic diabetes insipidus and Fanconi's syndrome may occur in up to 50% of cases (40, 41). Their presence does not appear to correlate with the histological findings, and may be subclinical. They tend to be more common in younger patients with chronic disease and impaired renal function (44). The most common tubular abnormality, and a sensitive indicator of renal involvement in SS, is a defect in concentrating ability, which occurs in up to 80% of patients (44). Renal tubular acidosis may be distal or proximal, with the former being commoner (42, 44). The patients are generally asymptomatic, and the diagnosis is established by finding hyperchloraemic acidosis with hypokalaemia. In about 30% of cases the defect is latent and only apparent after an acid-load test (45). Less often, the biochemical abnormalities may lead to symptoms which are the presenting features of undiagnosed SS (46). Hypergammaglobulinaemia itself does not appear to be sufficient to induce renal tubular acidosis (47, 48); however, specific anti-tubular antibodies may be able to induce such tubular defects (40, 49), localizing to particular tubular segments. Alternatively, the interstitial cellular infiltrate may be responsible, as is thought to be the case in the salivary and lacrimal glands (46).

An aetiological role for Epstein-Barr virus has been suggested in this condition. Viral DNA has been found in the salivary glands, peripheral blood mononuclear cells and renal tubules, in patients with SS, along with the viral cell receptor CD21 (14, 50, 51). EBV DNA has also been found in other cases of chronic tubulointerstitial nephritis, suggesting that there may be a more generalized role for this virus in initiating or perpetuating interstitial inflammation (14).

Treatment and outcome

Tubulointerstitial nephritis resulting in mild stable renal impairment may be left untreated without further deterioration. Treatment of isolated distal renal tubular acidosis is with sodium bicarbonate and potassium supplements. Renal tubular acidosis as well as interstitial inflammation may respond to long-term low-dose steroid therapy (52). Higher doses of steroids, such as pulsed methylprednisolone, may be required in cases showing a rapid evolution to uraemia (53). In some cases an additional immunosuppressive agent such as cyclophosphamide has been used, with marked improvement in renal function. Despite resolution of interstitial inflammation following treatment, tubular fibrosis appeared to develop in areas associated with TBM immune deposits (43). Secondary SS in association with SLE is generally treated with drug regimens appropriate for SLE.

Tubulointerstitial nephritis and uveitis (TINU) syndrome

In 1975, Dobrin *et al.* described two children who presented with acute renal failure secondary to eosinophilic interstitial nephritis. They also had bilateral uveitis, bone marrow granulomas, hypergammaglobulinaemia and an acute phase response. No evidence for any aetiological agent was found so it was proposed that this was a new syndrome (54), appropriately termed tubulointerstitial nephritis and uveitis (TINU). Since then there have been several reports of the association of interstitial nephritis and uveitis (55–59), though not always with granulomas. TINU remains a diagnosis of exclusion, since other systemic conditions may be associated with interstitial nephritis and uveitis, for example sarcoidosis, Sjögren's syndrome and Wegener's granulomatosis. Whether this syndrome represents a form fruste of sarcoidosis or Sjögren's, or is truly a separate entity, remains to be clarified (60, 61). In some cases of TINU, criteria for primary Sjögren's may also be fulfilled, with evidence of exocrine gland infiltration (59). The uveitis may occur at any time in relation to the nephritis, and has a tendency to relapse, unlike the tubulointerstitial lesions (56). Females are more commonly affected. Early reports tended to be mostly of children, although it is now apparent that all ages are susceptible (57, 58).

Non-specific symptoms of lethargy, myalgia, anorexia, weight loss and fever are common. Urinary abnormalities consist of proteinuria, leucocyturia, and tubular defects leading to glycosuria, aminoaciduria and impaired concentrating ability (56). Hypergammaglobulinaemia and an acute phase response seem to be universal. In some cases autoantibodies are found, including rheumatoid factors, ANA and more recently anti-neutrophil cytoplasm antibodies (ANCA) (62,63). Histological changes consist of interstitial cellular infiltration, with tubular atrophy and fibrosis (Fig. 29.1). Immune deposits along the TBM are generally absent. The cells are mostly T lymphocytes, in an activated state (64), but eosinophils occasionally predominate, as originally described (54). A genetic predisposition is possible, since TINU has been reported to occur in twins (65), and a suggestion of HLA-disease linkage has been made, with HLA-A24 being found in all four patients in one series (66).

Associations with infectious agents including chlamydia (67) have been reported. There is also an animal model in which both uveitis and granulomatous TIN are produced following inoculation with mycoplasma like organisms (MLO) obtained from patients with chronic uveitis (68).

Treatment and outcome

Renal recovery is the general rule, often without treatment (56). In a number of case reports, corticosteroids were given and recovery was ascribed to the treatment (57,62). The uveitis generally requires therapy with topical or systemic corticosteroids, and has a tendency to follow a relapsing-remitting course.

Sarcoidosis

Sarcoidosis is a chronic multisystem granulomatous disorder, commoner in young black women, with a variable presentation and unknown aetiology. Impaired renal function in sarcoidosis is rare, occurring in only 1–2% of patients (69). A much higher incidence of renal involvement, of up to 25%, is found in autopsy series (70,71). Renal involvement is generally due to nephrocalcinosis, nephrolithiasis and dehydration consequent to hypercalcaemia (72). Hypercalcaemia and hypercalcuria occur in 10% of patients, and are associated with reversible impairment in renal function (73). Nephrocalcinosis occurs in up to a third of those with hypercalcaemia.

However, interstitial nephritis in the absence of hypercalcaemia was first described by Berger and Relman in 1955 and has been reported in a number of patients subsequently (74–78). In a large series from Australia, only 1.3% of patients with sarcoidosis had interstitial nephritis; however, in smaller series in which renal disease was specifically looked for, the incidence was 5.5–40% (75, 79, 80). Glomerular disease and vasculitis may occur in sarcoidosis although they are rarer than interstitial nephritis (70,71). Renal granulomas, containing epithelioid and giant cells, are common and often surrounded by an inflammatory infiltrate consisting mostly of lymphocytes and plasma cells (Fig. 29.3). The granulomas are typically in the cortex, but can occur throughout the renal parenchyma. No association between the number of renal granulomas and the serum calcium has been found (80). The lymphocytes are mostly CD4+ T cells

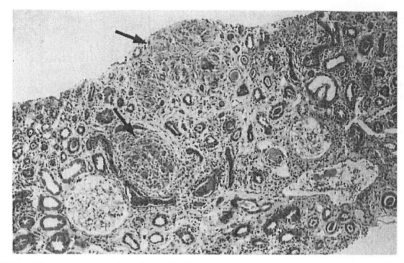

Fig. 29.3 Photomicrograph of renal biopsy section from a patient with sarcoidosis showing a granulomatous interstitial nephritis. There is a mononuclear cell infiltrate and two large non-caseating granulomas (arrows). Red cells can be seen within the tubular lumens. There is marked separation of the tubules, with tubular atrophy and interstitial oedema. The glomeruli are normal. (H and E ×75.)

(12), mirroring those found in other sarcoid granulomas. No immune deposits are seen. In one series of patients with such granulomatous interstitial nephritis, only 7% had normal renal function and 45% had severe renal failure (GFR < 20 ml/min) (77).

Presentation may be following routine renal function testing, or with polyuria or haematuria (81, 82). More commonly it follows other systemic symptoms of sarcoidosis (60, 78) (see Table 29.5). Patients may have mildly active urinary sediment, proteinuria, tubular defects such as reduced concentrating ability, and renal impairment. Levels of serum angiotensin converting enzyme may be normal, as can gallium scintigraphy, although it has been found to be positive in some cases of active granulomatous nephritis (60). Patients with sarcoidosis and granulomatous interstitial nephritis tend to be older male patients, with no racial bias (76).

Treatment and outcome

In patients with severe renal failure, corticosteroid therapy results in significantly improved renal function in 85% of cases (77). In some instances dialysis dependent patients may recover independent renal function (78). Up to 28% relapsed in Simonsen's series, and progressed towards end-stage renal disease. Relapse has also been noted in a renal transplant patient despite immunosuppression (83), and in other patients upon cessation or rapid reduction of steroids (77, 78, 82). Treatment generally consisted of 60 mg of prednisolone, lasting for between six

Table 29.5 Clinical features and investigations in patients with sarcoid granulomatous interstitial nephritis

Clinical features (in descending order of frequency)	Investigations
Hilar lymphadenopathy	Anaemia
Pulmonary infiltrates	Haematuria
Fever	Granular casts
Hepatomegaly	Renal glycosuria
Lymphadenopathy	Proteinuria (<2g/24 hours)
Ocular involvement	Sterile pyuria
Hypertension	Concentration defects
Splenomegaly	(urine specific
Arthropathy	gravity <1.007)
Rash	Renal tubular acidosis
Sinus involvement	

Adapted from (78) and (76).

weeks and four years. In a few reports steroid sparing agents were tried, with apparent success (77, 84). In some relapses re-institution of treatment resulted in improved renal function. In those with moderately impaired function (GFR 20–80 mls/min), steroids had a less dramatic effect with 65% improving and about a third left with unchanged renal function. It appears that those treated with lower doses of steroids fared worse. Steroid therapy is also beneficial in reversing tubular dysfunction, manifested by diabetes insipidus and renal glycosuria (76). In patients undergoing repeat biopsies following steroid therapy, granulomas and mononuclear infiltrates had regressed but there was evidence of fibrosis and scarring (72, 74). This could explain why many patients who respond to steroid therapy may have residual renal impairment up to 30 months later (78). Thus it would seem advisable to treat patients with a prolonged course of moderate to high doses of steroids in the first instance, and gradually taper the dose, whilst remaining vigilant for signs of relapse. In cases where steroids are contraindicated chlorambucil or methotrexate have been used (85).

Systemic vasculitis and tubulointerstitial nephritis

Anti-neutrophil cytoplasmic antibodies (ANCA) are serologic markers of pauci-immune glomerulonephritis (GN), whether it is limited to the kidney or associated with other systemic manifestations as in Wegener's granulomatosis (WG), microscopic polyangiitis (MP) or Churg Strauss syndrome (CSS). Interstitial inflammation in cases of pauci-immune GN is common, and this may develop into granulomatous TIN, as seen in WG (86) and CSS (along with eosinophilic infiltration) (87). Isolated interstitial nephritis associated with ANCA is recognized but uncommon (88, 89). In one series, 11% of patients with WG and MP had evidence of interstitial nephritis without glomerular involvement. Four of these six cases had ANCA (88) and in none of them was the clinical diagnosis considered to be TIN. Cases of severe eosinophilic TIN in association with ANCA, but lacking sufficient criteria for a diagnosis of Churg Strauss syndrome, have been reported (90–92). ANCA have also been reported in some patients thought to have TINU (90–92). In our series of patients presenting with acute TIN, two have ANCA (representing 10%) one of which was associated with anti-MPO antibody. Neither had features of systemic vasculitis, nor have they gone on to develop them. Thus ANCA may also be associated with TIN, possibly as a nonspecific autoimmune phenomenon, without evidence of vasculitis.

Treatment and outcome

Treatment of ANCA associated systemic vasculitidies has been extensively covered elsewhere (93). Isolated TIN associated with systemic vasculitis has generally been treated with similar, although less intensive, regimens. In Cameron's series (88), half the patients were treated with steroids alone, and the other half had additional cyclophosphamide or azathioprine. Overall half of the patients had residual renal impairment and the rest remained on dialysis, with two subsequently dying. In cases of CSS with TIN, steroids were used alone in milder forms of the disease, but combined with additional immunosuppressive treatment in more severe cases.

Conclusions

Tubulointerstitial nephritis may occur in a number of systemic diseases, albeit infrequently, and lead to acute or chronic renal impairment. It is a diagnosis which requires a high index of suspicion and a confirmatory renal biopsy. It may be associated with a range of functional tubular abnormalities which are often sub-clinical in nature. The inflammatory reaction generally responds to immunosuppressive treatment with corticosteroids, although this may not prevent subsequent tubular atrophy and interstitial fibrosis. Little is known regarding the immunological stimulus which triggers this condition, or the factors involved in progression or resolution.

Acknowledgements

ADS is an MRC Training Fellow. We are grateful to Dr T. Cook for providing the histopathology specimens.

References

1. Ong A.C.M. and Fine L.G. Loss of glomerular function and tubulointerstitial fibrosis: cause or effect? *Kidney International* 1994, 45: 345–51.
2. Neilson E.G. Interstitial nephritis: another kissing disease? *Journal of Clinical Investigation* 1999, 104: 1671–2.
3. Farrington K., Levison D., Greenwood R., Cattell W. and Baker L. Renal biopsy in patients with unexplained renal impairment and normal kidney size. *Quarterly Journal of Medicine* 1989, 70: 221–3.
4. Buysen J.G.M., Houthoff H.J., Krediet R.T. and Arisz L. Acute interstitial nephritis: A clinical and morphological study in 27 patients. *Nephrology Dialysis Transplantation* 1990, 5: 94–7.
5. Eknoyan G. Acute tubulointerstitial nephritis. In: Schrier R.W. and Gottschalk C.W., eds. *Diseases of the Kidney*. Sixth edn. Boston: Little, Brown and Company, 1997, 1249–65.
6. Ten R.M., Torres V.E., Milliner D.S., Schwab T.R., Holley K.E. and Gleich G.J. Acute interstitial nephritis: Immunologic and clinical aspects. *Mayo Clinic Proceedings* 1988, 63: 921–30.
7. Fogazzi G.B. and Fenili D. Urinanalysis and microscopy. In: Davidson A.M., Cameron J.S., Grunfeld J.-P., Kerr D.N.S., Ritz E., Winearls C.G., eds. *Oxford Textbook of Clinical Nephrology*. Oxford: Oxford Medical Publications, 1998, 21–38.
8. Kelly C.J., Tomaszewski J.E. and Neilson E.G. Immunopathogenic mechanisms of tubulointerstitial injury. In: Tisher C.C., Brenner B.M., eds. *Renal Pathology: with clinical and functional correlations*. Second edn. Philadelphia: J.B. Lippincott Company, 1994, 699–722.
9. Laberke H.G. and Bohle A. Acute interstitial nephritis. Correlation between clinical and morphological findings. *Clinical Nephrology* 1980, 14: 263.
10. Esdaile J.M., Levington C., Federgreen W., Hayslett J.P. and Kashgarian M. The clinical and renal biopsy predictors of long-term outcome in lupus nephritis: A study of 87 patients and a review of the literature. *Quarterly Journal of Medicine* 1989, 269: 779–833.
11. Alexopoulos E., Camerson J.S. and Hartley B.H. Lupus nephritis: correlation of interstitial cells with glomerular function. *Kidney International* 1990, 37: 100–109.
12. Boucher A., Droz D., Adafer E. and Noel L.H. Characterisation of mononuclear cell subsets in renal cellular interstitial infiltrates. *Kidney International* 1986, 29: 1043–49.
13. Kobayashi Y., Honda M., Yoshikawa N. and Ito H. Immunological study in sixteen children with acute tubulointerstitial nephritis. *Clinical Nephrology* 1998, 50: 14–20.
14. Becker J.L., Miller F., Nuovo G.J., Josepovitz C., Schubach W.H. and Nord E.P. Epstein-Barr virus infection in proximal tubule cells: possible role in chronic interstitial nephritis. *Journal of Clinical Investigation* 1999, 104: 1673–81.
15. D'Agati V.D. Renal disease in systemic lupus erythematosus, mixed connective tissue disease, sjogren's syndrome and rheumatoid arthritis. In: Jennette J.C., Olson J.L., Schwartz M.M. and Silva F.G., eds. *Heptinstall's Pathology of the Kidney* Fifth edn. Philadelphia: Lippincott-Raven, 1998, 541–624.
16. Park M.H., D'Agati V.D., Appel G.B. and Pirani C.L. Tubulointerstitial disease in lupus nephritis: relationship to immune deposits, interstitial inflammation, glomerular changes, renal function, and prognosis. *Nephron* 1986, 44: 309–19.
17. Case records of the MGH. Case-2. *New England Journal of Medicine* 1976, 294: 100–105.

18. Cunningham E., Provost T., Brentjens J., Reichlin M. and Venuto R.C. Acute renal failure secondary to interstitial lupus nephritis. *Archives of Internal Medicine* 1978, 138: 1560–61.

19. Disler P.B., Lewin J.R., Laidley L. and Meyers A.M. Systemic lupus erythematosus with pure interstitial disease: a case report. *Kidney International* 1978, 13: 428.

20. Tron F., Ganeval D. and Droz D. Immunologically mediated acute renal failure of non-glomerular origin in the course of systemic lupus erythematosus: report of two cases. *American Journal of Medicine* 1979, 67: 529–32.

21. Gur H., Koplvic Y. and Gross D.J. Chronic predominant interstitial nephritis in a patient with systemic lupus erythematosus: a follow up of three years and review of the literature. *Annals of Rheumatic Disease* 1987, 46: 617–23.

22. Yeung C.K., Wong K.L., Ng R.P. and Ng W.L. Tubular dysfunction in systemic lupus erythematosus. *Nephron* 1984, 36: 84–8.

23. Colvin R.B. and Fang L.S.T. Interstitial Nephritis. In: Tisher C.C. and Brenner B.M., eds. *Renal Pathology: with clinical and functional correlations.* Second edn. Philadelphia: J.B. Lippincott Company, 1994: 723–68.

24. Lehman D.H., Wilson C.B. and Dixon F.J. Extraglomerular immunoglobulin deposits in human nephritis. *American Journal of Medicine* 1975, 58: 765–86.

25. Makker S.P. Tubular basement membrane antibody-induced interstitial nephritis in systemic lupus erythematosus. *American Journal of Medicine* 1980, 69: 949–52.

26. Hiromura K., Kurosawa M., Yano S. and Naruse T. Tubulointerstitial mast cell infiltration in glomerulonephritis. *American Journal of Kidney Disease* 1998, 32: 593–99.

27. Cameron J.S. Systemic Lupus Erythematosus. In: Neilson E.G., Couser W.G., eds. *Immunologic renal diseases.* Philadelphia: Lippincott-Raven, 1997, 1055–98.

28. Sharp G.C., Irvin W.S., Tam E.M., Gould R.G. and Holman H.R. Mixed connective tissue disease: an apparently distinct rheumatic disease syndrome associated with a specific antibody to an extractable nuclear antigen (ENA). *American Journal of Medicine* 1972, 52: 148.

29. Morrow J., Nelson J.L., Watts R. and Isenberg D. *Autoimmune rheumatic disease.* Second edn. Oxford: Oxford University Press, 1999.

30. Sullivan W.D., Hurst D.J., Harmon C.E. *et al.* A prospective evaluation emphasising pulmonary involvement in patients with mixed connective tissue disease. *Medicine* 1984, 63: 92–107.

31. Bennett R.M. Mixed connective tissue disease and other overlap syndromes. In: Kelley W.N., Harris E.D., Ruddy S. and Sledge C.B. eds. *Textbook of Rheumatology.* Fifth edn. Philadelphia: W.B. Saunders, 1997: 1065–78.

32. Kitridou R.C., Akmal M., Turkel S.B., Ehresmann G.R., Quismorio F.P. and Massry S.G. Renal involvement in mixed connective tissue disease: A longitudinal clinicopathologic study. *Seminars in Arthritis and Rheumatism* 1986, 16: 135–45.

33. Bennet R.M. Mixed connective tissue disease. In: Grishman E., Churg J., Needle M.A., Venkataseshan V.S., eds. *The kidney in collagen vascular disease.* New York: Raven Press, 1993: 167–77.

34. Silverstein R. and Vergne-Marini P. The kidney in mixed connective tissue disease and Sjogren's syndrome. In: Suki W.N., Eknoyan G, eds. *The kidney in systemic disease.* Second edn. New York: A Wiley Medical Publication, 1981: 77–97.

35. Helkin H.J., Korpela M.M., Mustonen J.T. and Pasternack A.I. Renal biopsy findings and clinicopathologic correlations in rheumatoid arthritis. *Arthritis and Rheumatism* 1995, 38: 242–47.

36. Sellers L., Siamopoulos K., Wilkinson R., Leohapand T. and Morley A.R. Renal biopsy appearances in rheumatoid disease. *Clinical Nephrology* 1983, 20: 114–20.
37. Schwartz M.M. The dysproteinaemias and amyloidosis. In: Jennette J.C., Olson J.L., Schwartz M.M., Silva F.G., eds. *Heptinstall's Pathology of the Kidney.* Philadelphia: Lippincott-Raven, 1998, 1321–69.
38. Rayadurg J. and Koch A.E. Renal insufficiency from interstitial nephritis in primary Sjogren's syndrome. *Journal of Rheumatology* 1990, 17: 1714–18.
39. Tu W.H., Shearn M.A., Lee J.C. and Hopper J. Interstitial nephritis in Sjogren's syndrome. *Annals of Internal Medicine* 1968, 69: 1163–70.
40. Talal N., Zisman E. and Schur P.H. Renal tubular acidosis, glomerulonephritis and immunologic factors in Sjogren's syndrome. *Arthritis and Rheumatism* 1968, 11: 774–86.
41. Siamopoulos K.C., Mavridis A.K., Elisaf M., Drosos A.A. and Moutsopoulos H.M. Kidney involvement in primary Sjogren's syndrome. *Scandinavian Journal of Rheumatology* 1986, 61: 156–60.
42. Pokorny G., Sonkodi S., Ivanyi B. *et al.* Renal involvement in patients with primary Sjogren's syndrome. *Scandinavian Journal of Rheumatology* 1989, 18: 231–34.
43. Winer R.L., Cohen A.H., Sawhney A.S. and Gorman J.T. Sjogren's syndrome with immune-complex tubulointerstitial disease. *Clinical Immunology and Immunopathology* 1977, 8: 494–503.
44. Shiozawa S., Shiozawa K., Shimizu S., Nakada M., Isobe T. and Fujita T. Clinical studies of renal disease in Sjogren's syndrome. *Annals of Rheumatic Diseases* 1987, 46: 768–72.
45. Shearn M.A. and Tu W.H. Latent renal tubular acidosis in Sjogrens syndrome. *Annals of Rheumatic Diseases* 1968, 27: 27–32.
46. Christensen K.S. Hypokalaemic paralysis in Sjogren's syndrome secondary to renal tubular acidosis. *Scandinavian Journal of Rheumatology* 1985, 14: 58–60.
47. Mason A.M.S. and Golding P.L. Hyperglobulinaemic renal tubular acidosis: a report of nine cases. *British Medical Journal* 1970, 3: 143–146.
48. Shioji R., Furuyama T., Ondodera S., Saito H., Ito H. and Sasaki Y. Sjogren's syndrome and renal tubular acidosis. *American Journal of Medicine* 1970, 48: 456–463.
49. Pasternack A. and Linder E. Renal tubular acidosis: An immunopathological study on four patients. *Clinical and Experimental Immunology* 1970, 7: 115–123.
50. Saito I., Servenius B., Compton T. and Fox R.I. Detection of Epstein-Barr virus DNA by polymerase chain reaction in blood and tissue biopsies from patients with Sjogren's syndrome. *Journal of Experimental Medicine* 1989, 169: 2191–2198.
51. Mariette X., Gozlan J., Clerc D., Bisson M. and Marinet F. Detection of Epstein-Barr virus DNA by in situ hybridization and polymerase chain reaction in salivary gland biopsy specimens from patients with Sjogren's syndrome. *American Journal of Medicine* 1991, 90: 286–94.
52. El-Mallakh R.S., Bryan R.K., Masi A.T., Kelly C.E. and Rakowski K.J. Long-term low-dose glucocorticoid therapy associated with remission of overt renal tubular acidosis in Sjogren's syndrome. *American Journal of Medicine* 1985, 79: 509–14.
53. Rosenberg A.M., Dyck R.F. and George D.H. Intravenous pulse methylprednisolone for the treatment of a child with Sjogren's nephropathy. *Journal of Rheumatology* 1990, 17: 391–4.
54. Dobrin R.S., Vernier R.L. and Fish A.J. Acute eosinophilic interstitial nephritis and renal failure with bone marrow-lymph node granulomas and anterior uveitis. *American Journal of Medicine* 1975, 59: 325–33.

55. Steinman T.I. and Silva P. Acute interstitial nephritis and iritis. *American Journal of Medicine* 1984, 77: 189–91.
56. Vanhaesebrouck P., Carton D., De Bel C., Praet M. and Proesmans W. Acute tubulointerstitial nephritis and uveitis syndrome (TINU syndrome). *Nephron* 1985, 40: 418–22.
57. Cacoub P., Deray G., Le Hoang P. *et al.* Idiopathic acute interstitial nephritis associated with anterior uveitis in adults. *Clinical Nephrology* 1989, 31: 307–10.
58. Salu P., Stempels N., Vanden Houte K. and Verbeelen D. Acute tubulointerstitial nephritis and uveitis syndrome in the elderly. *British Journal of Ophthalmology* 1990, 74: 53–5.
59. Vidal E., Rogues A.M. and Aldigier J.C. The TINU syndrome or the Sjogren's syndrome. *Annals of Internal Medicine* 1992, 116: 93.
60. van Dorp W.T., Lobatto K.J., Weening J.J. and Valentijn R.M. Renal failure due to granulomatous interstitial nephritis after pulmonary sarcoidosis. *Nephrology Dialysis Transplantation* 1987, 2: 573–5.
61. Segev A., Ben-Chitrit S., Orion Y. *et al.* Acute eosinophilic interstitial nephritis and uveitis (TINU syndrome) associated with granulomatous hepatitis. *Clinical Nephrology* 1999, 51: 310–13.
62. Okada K., Okamoto Y., Kagami S. *et al.* Acute interstitial nephritis and uveitis with bone marrow granulomas and anti-neutrophil cytoplasmic antibodies. *American Journal of Nephrology* 1995, 15: 337–42.
63. Chen H.-C., Sheu M.-M., Tsai J.-H. and Lai Y.-H. Acute tubulo-interstitial nephritis and uveitis with anti-neutrophil cytoplasmic antibodies in an adult: an autoimmune disorder? *Nephron* 1998, 78: 372.
64. Yoshioka K., Takemura T., Kanasaki M., Akano N. and Maki S. Acute tubulointerstitial nephritis and uveitis syndrome: activated immune cell infiltration in the kidney. *Paediatric Nephrology* 1991, 5: 232–4.
65. Gianviti A., Greco M., Barsotti P. and Rizzoni G. Acute tubulointerstitial nephritis occurring with a one year lapse in identical twins. *Paediatric Nephrology* 1994, 8: 427–30.
66. Iitsuka T., Yamaguchi N., Kobayashi M., Nakamura H., Usuki Y. and Koyama A. HLA tissue types in patients with acute tubulointerstitial nephritis accompanying uveitis. *Japanese Journal of Nephrology* 1993, 35: 723–31.
67. Stapp R., Mihatsch M.S., Matter L. and Streali R.A. Acute tubulointerstitial nephritis with uveitis in a patient with serologic evidence for chlamydia infection. *Klinische Wochenschrift* 1990, 68: 971–5.
68. Johnson L., Wirostko E. and Wirostko B. Murine chronic tubulointerstitial nephritis: induction by human uveitis mycoplasma-like organisms. *Pathology* 1994, 26: 464–70.
69. Cavallo T. Tubulointerstitial nephritis. In: Jennette J.C., Olson J.L., Schwartz M.M., Silva F.G., eds. *Heptinstall's Pathology of the Kidney*. Philadelphia: Lippincott-Raven, 1998, 667–723.
70. Ricker W. and Clark M. Sarcoidosis: A clinicopathologic review of three hundred cases including twenty-two autopsies. *American Journal of Clinical Pathology* 1949, 19: 725–49.
71. Longscope W.T. and Freiman D.G. A study of sarcoidosis based on a combined investigation of 160 cases including 30 autopsies from the Johns Hopkins Hospital and Massachusetts General Hospital. *Medicine* 1952, 31: 132–140.

72. Muther R.S., McCarron D.A. and Bennett W.M. Renal manifestations of sarcoidosis. *Archives of Internal Medicine* 1981, 141: 643–5.

73. Singer F.R. and Adams J.S. Abnormal calcium homeostasis in sarcoidosis. *New England Journal of Medicine* 1986, 315: 755–7.

74. Berger K.W. and Relamn A.S. Renal impairment due to sarcoid infiltration of the kidney. Report of a case proved by renal biopsies before and after treatment with cortisone. *New England Journal of Medicine* 1955, 252: 44–49.

75. Lebacq E., Verhaegen H. and Desmet V. Renal involvement in sarcoidosis. *Postgraduate Medical Journal* 1970, 46: 526–9.

76. Muther R.S., McCarron D.A. and Bennett W.M. Granulomatous sarcoid nephritis: A cause of multiple renal tubular abnormalitis. *Clinical Nephrology* 1980, 14: 190–7.

77. Simonsen O. and Thysell H. Sarcoidosis with normocalcaemic granulomatous nephritis: five case reports and a review of 24 cases in the literature. *Nephron* 1985, 40: 411–17.

78. Singer D.R. and Evans D.J. Renal impairment in sarcoidosis: granulomatous nephritis as an isolated cause (two case reports and review of the literature). *Clinical Nephrology* 1986, 26: 250–6.

79. Richmond J.M., Chambers B., D'Apice A.J.F., Whitworth J.A. and Kincaid-Smith P. Renal disease in sarcoidosis. *Medical Journal of Australia* 1981, 2: 36–37.

80. MacSerraigh E.T., Doyle C.T., Twomey M. and O'Sullivan D.J. Sarcoidosis with renal involvement. *Postgraduate Medical Journal* 1978, 54: 528–32.

81. Williams P.F., Thomson D. and Anderton J.L. Reversible renal failure due to isolated renal sarcoidosis. *Nephron* 1984, 37: 246–9.

82. Mills P.R., Burns A.P., Dorman A.M., Sweny P.J. and Moorhead J.F. Granulomatous sarcoid nephritis presenting as frank haematuria. *Nephrology Dialysis Transplantation*. 1994, 9: 1649–51.

83. Shen S.Y., Hall-Craggs M., Posner J.N. and Shabazz B. Recurrent sarcoid granulomatous nephritis and reactive tuberculin skin test in a renal transplant patient. *American Journal of Medicine* 1986, 80: 699–702.

84. Kelly C.J. and Neilson E.G. Tubulointerstitial diseases. In: Brenner B.M., ed. *Brenner and Rector's: The Kidney*. Philadelphia: W.B. Saunders company, 1996, 1655–79.

85. Israel H.L. The treatment of sarcoidosis. *Postgraduate Medical Journal* 1970, 46: 537–40.

86. Ronco P., Mougenot B., Bindi P., Vanhille P. and Mignon F. Clinicohistological features and long-term outcome of Wegener's granulomatosis. In: Sessa A., Meroni M., Battini G., eds. *Renal involvement in systemic vasculitis*. Contributions to Nephrology. Basal: Karger, 1991, 94: 47–57.

87. Clutterbuck E.J., Evans D.J. and Pusey C.D. Renal involvement in Churg-Strauss syndrome. *Nephrology Dialysis Transplantation*. 1990, 5: 161–67.

88. Cameron J.S. Renal vasculitis: Microscopic polyarteritis and Wegener's granulomatosis. In: Sessa A., Meroni M. and Battini G., eds. *Renal involvement in systemic vasculitis*. Contributions to Nephrology. Basel: Karger, 1991, 94: 38–46.

89. Lockwood C.M. Antineutrophil cytoplasmic antibodies: The nephrologist's perspective. *American Journal of Kidney Disease* 1991, 18: 171–4.

90. Okada K., Okamoto Y., Kagami S. *et al.* Acute tubulo-interstitial nephritis and uveitis with bone marrow granulomas and anti-neutrophil cytoplasmic antibodies. *American Journal of Nephrology* 1995, 15: 337–42.

91. Yamamoto T., Yoshihara S., Suzuki H., Nagase M., Oka M. and Hishida A. MPO-ANCA-positive cresentic necrotising glomerulonephritis and tubulointerstitial nephritis with renal eosinophilic infiltration and peripheral blood eosinophilia. *American Journal of Kidney Diseases* 1998, 31: 1032–37.

92. Chen H.C., Sheu M.M., Tsai J.H. and Lai Y.H. Acute tubulo–interstitial nephritis and uveitis with anti-neutrophil cytoplasmic antibodies in an adult: an autoimmune disorder? *Nephron* 1998, 78(3): 372.

93. Gaskin G. and Pusey C.D. Systemic vasculitis. In: Davidson A.M., Cameron J.S., Grunfeld J.-P., Kerr D.N.S., Ritz E., Winearls C.G., eds. *Oxford Textbook of Clinical Nephrology*. Oxford: Oxford Medical Publications, 1998: 877–910.

30

Gout, uric acid, and the kidney

J. Stewart Cameron

Introduction

The renal complications of the classical gout of middle-aged males have diminished in frequency and severity during the past half century, but this decline has high-lighted the minority of inherited forms of gout arising from disorders of purine metabolism or apparently monogenic urate transport abnormalities in the renal tubule, which carry a high prevalence of renal involvement. In addition, both rheumatologists and nephrologists now find themselves dealing with 'new' syndromes of gout in patients on dialysis, and after otherwise successful renal and cardiac transplantation. Finally a role for urate in the progression of both vascular disease and renal damage has re-emerged during the 1990s.

Uric acid

The human and primate end-product of purine metabolism (1, 2) is uric acid (trihydroxypurine), because we lack the promoter region of the gene coding for the hepatic enzyme uricase (3), which degrades insoluble uric acid to soluble allantoin. The biological value (if any) of failing to break down urate has been much debated: uric acid is a major anti-oxidant, providing more than half this activity in primate plasma (4). Approximately two-thirds of uric acid is eliminated by the kidney (5) and one-third by bacterial uricolysis in the gut, a ratio reversed in renal failure. Renal uric acid excretion varies from 3.5 to 7 mmol/24h/70 kg bodyweight (6,7) of which all but about 2 mmol/24h is derived from dietary purines. The ingestion of foods and drinks rich in purines is well-known to be high in subjects with 'classical' gout, a disorder of affluent societies, rare in women and children and in hard times (1,2,8). Normal plasma concentration ranges vary with the local diet and the method used, but using specific methods the mean UK plasma uric acid concentrations are 222 ± 42 (SD) µmol/l for females and 281 ± 41 µmol/l for males) (9). Non-specific methods (e.g. on an AutoAnalyser™) will give values higher than this, and unfortunately are commonly used in clinical practice.

Uric acid is toxic through insolubility and the inflammation engendered by resulting crystals within tissues (8,10–12), identifiable by the characteristic angle of rotation at which a change from yellow to blue occurs on examination under polarized light. Urate crystals activate the complement system, and inflammatory cells phagocytose the negatively-charged crystals, with release of chemotactic and inflammatory mediators (13, 14).

Handling of urate by the human kidney

Urate is an organic anion freely filterable at the glomerulus (1,15) but the details of its handling by the human proximal tubule remain only partially understood (16–18). Handling of urate is complete by the end of the proximal tubule, during which urate transport is bidirectional, with (in humans) a net reabsorption of around 90% of filtered urate, the fractional excretion (FE_{ur}) thus being about 10% (16,17). Net reabsorption is slightly higher in males (92%, (FE_{ur} 8%) than in fertile females (88%, FE_{ur} 12%) and is lower in children (70–85%, FE_{ur} 15–30%). Net secretion of urate (FE urate > GFR) can be observed on occasion in humans, and secretion is part of normal tubular handling of urate (1,2,16–19). Since tubular handling differs greatly between species, animal studies can tell us little (18,19), and models proposed for humans have relied heavily on inferences from pharmacological manipulation of urate excretion (20–23). The resultant four-component model (24) (Figure 30.1) however now appears insecure in the light of studies of uric acid transport in brush border membrane (BBM) vesicles

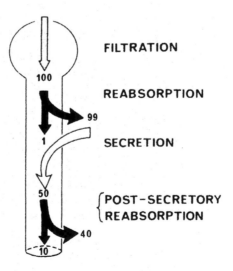

Fig. 30.1 The 'classical' four-component model of the handing of urate in the mammalian renal tubule (for details see text). This model was evolved from a combination of micropuncture studies in species such as rat and dog which show, like humans, net reabsorption of urate; and pharmacological studies in intact humans using pyrazinoic acid and/or probenecid. The significance of these pharmacological interpretations, however, has been thrown into doubt by recent findings from mammalian and human brush border vesicles (see text).

from the proximal tubule (25–27), which have shown that pyrazinamide does not inhibit secretion of urate, but enchances tubular reabsorption (26). An anion channel in the BBM which subserves reabsorption of urate has been described (23,25,26) and now cloned (28). There is little information on urate transport in basolateral membranes from human kidneys, but evidence suggests at least a voltage-sensitive pathway (29,30). The level of FE_{ur} is set by genetic factors (30,31) but how this is expressed in terms of reabsorption or secretion is unknown.

Endogenous and exogenous factors affecting uric acid handling by the human kidney

Many factors can alter renal tubular handling of urate/uric acid, and hence the plasma urate concentration (Table 30.1). This may be mediated through direct effects upon one of the urate transporters, or though contraction or expansion of plasma volume (1,2,32) via effects on renal haemodynamics and sodium reabsorption, which is indirectly coupled to urate reabsorption. Treatment with diuretics currently accounts for over 50% of new attacks of gout (33,34). The proportion of elderly females in this group is unusually high, and the mode of clinical pre-

Table 30.1 Substances that alter renal tubular handling of urate

Endogenous	Exogenous
Substances that decrease urate excretion	
Lactate	salicylate (low doses)
β-hydroxybutyrate	pyrazinamide
α-ketoglutarate	nicotinate
acetoacetate	ethambutol
	Lead
	Beryllium
	diuretics*
	cyclosporine
Substances that increase urate excretion	
Pregnancy*	saline infusion*
	probenecid
	sulphinpyrazone
	benzbromarone
	Some AT receptor antagonists 1 (Figure 1)
	phenylbutazone
	radiocontrast agents
	mega dose vitamin C
	high dose salicylate (>3G)
	fenofibrate

* Through effects on circulating volume and renal perfusion; thiazide and loop diuretics are uricosuric initially, but lead to urate retention during chronic use from volume depletion.

sentation often atypical, which can lead to misdiagnosis (35). Overproduction of lactate and ketone bodies may explain in part the hyperuricaemia associated with status epilepticus or with excessive alcohol consumption (36,37).

Most 'uricosuric' and some other drugs have a biphasic effect on urate excretion: at low doses they promote urate retention and at high doses induce uricosuria (38); benzbromarone and sulphinpyrazone are exceptions however (39,40). This does not usually matter, because the commonly employed dosages are always uricosuric, but *(acetyl)salicylate* is important in that low doses may be given long term, causing urate retention rather than uricosuria. Some angiotensin II receptor (AT1) anatagonists are uricosuric, which probably results not from intra-renal vasodilatation (in which case all ACE inhibitors would be uricosuric), but from interaction with the renal tubular brush border anion transporter (41).

A rise in FE_{ur} is less important, although crystalluria, stones and occasionally even acute renal failure are risks (42). *Circulatory volume expansion* tends to increase urate clearance as in early pregnancy SIADH (syndrome of inappropriate ADH secretion), and some malignant diseases (43–45).

Classical gout as a disorder of low renal urate excretion and purine overload

The risk of an attack of gout is directly related to the plasma urate concentration, from negligible at 300 μmol/l to almost certain, given time, at 600 μmol/l or greater. There is strong evidence that in almost all middle-aged, predominantly male patients with gout, hyperuricaemia results from an inherited polygenic decrease in FE_{ur} (mean 5.4%) (1,2,6,16,24), amplified by a large intake of dietary purine; endogenous production of urate is normal (5,7). This results in a higher plasma urate concentration for the same excretion of uric acid in the urine compared to controls (Fig. 30.2). Some races (such as Polynesians of either sexes) show much lower FE_{ur} and higher plasma urate concentrations than Caucasians (46–48) and have a high prevalence of clinical gout. The male:female difference in FE_{ur}, hyperuricaemia and gout up to the menopause may be the result of an influence of oestrogens on tubular handling of urate (49). After the menopause, uric acid concentrations are similar in men and women (50) and hormone replacement therapy lowers post-menopausal hyperuricaemia (51).

'Gouty nephropathy': chronic renal disease in classical gout

Until 40–50 years ago, renal disease and renal failure appear to have been common in typical male gout of middle age, almost all patients showing some renal involvement; and in 20–80% it was the attributed cause of death (52–55). Today renal failure is rare in this type of gout, and renal function is almost always normal when corrected for age, (as in symptomless hyperuricaemia) although differing views of the effects of age and concomitant vascular disease have led to different interpretations of these data (36,45,56–59). In the absence of

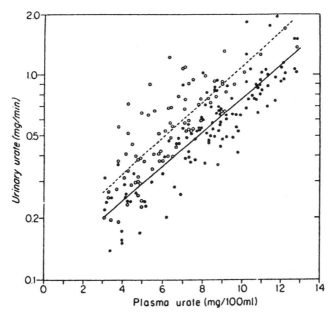

Fig. 30.2 Excretion of urate in normal subjects and in patients with 'classical' gout. As an expression of the reduced FE_{ur}, at any level of urinary excretion of urate (vertical axis, mg/min) the plasma urate concentration (mg/dl, horizontal axis; 10 mg/dl = 520 µmol/l) is set higher in the gouty subjects. The concentration of plasma urate and the amount of urate in the urine along the line of relationship are set by variations in purine intake above 0.25 mg/min (~2 mmol/24h). Note that the vertical axis has been logarithmically transformed to straighten the line of relationship (data from Simkin P.A. Urate excretion in normal and gouty men. *Adv Exp Med Biol* 1977;76B:41–45; reproduced with permission).

hypertension, renal function remains stable (60,61) but abnormalities of urinary sediment and mild proteinuria may be found in many patients.

The reasons for this change in the prevalence of renal failure and gross tophaceous articular gout remain uncertain. Renal damage can follow vascular disease (57) or deposition of crystalline urate within the kidney (10,62). There has been a decline in purine intake on the one hand, and more effective treatment first with uricosuric agents and then with allopurinol. This last hypothesis is strengthened by the fact that even today, when occasional patients with long-neglected gout are seen, their joint tophi can be just as severe as in the historical period. Another factor may have been a decline in the incidence of occult chronic lead intoxication (see below).

Thus the nature of 'gouty nephropathy' – or even its existence as such (63–66) – has been the subject of recent debate. Confusion has arisen because today we can recognize at least four varieties of 'gout':

(1) Middle-aged males with so-called 'classical' gout: the great majority. Production and excretion of urate are normal but FE_{ur} is low. Renal function

is normal for age and remains so. Renal tophi are rare today.

(2) Lead intoxication, with secondary gout and renal failure from chronic interstitial nephritis (64,67,68). Production and excretion of urate are normal but
FE_{ur} is low, and renal urate tophi are sometimes present. Was common, now
rarer but may be more common than supposed.

(3) Familial gout of precocious onset in either sex associated with a very low
FE_{ur} (5% or less), in which there is a high incidence of early progressive
renal disease. Production and excretion of uric acid are normal or low
(1,2,16,69,70) and renal tophi rare.

(4) Inherited disorders of purine metabolism (1,2,16,69,70) with acutely or chronically raised urate production and excretion. Also arises from disorders of
myelopoiesis. FE_{ur} is normal, but extensive intra-renal crystal deposits or
stones are often present.

In the past many cases of supposed 'primary' gout with severe renal involvement fell into one of the last three categories, which accounts for statements that
5–15% of supposed 'classical' primary gout were over-producers of urate.
Whenever the conjunction of gout and renal damage is seen today, these secondary types of gout should be looked for. This is especially important when the
patient is a young adult or a child, above all if female.

Intrarenal urate/uric acid deposits

The only specific feature of *chronic* gouty nephropathy is the interstitial tophus
of sodium urate crystals (Fig. 30.3) (52–55); these could originate from ambient

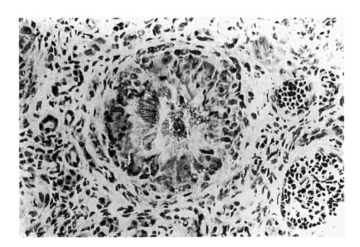

Fig. 30.3 Crystals of monosodium urate within a largely-destroyed renal tubule, surrounded by a cellular reaction, which may contain giant cells. This appearance is now
rarely seen except in gouty patients with urate overproduction (such as from HRPT
deficiency), or in acute hyperuricaemic renal failure. Exactly how these renal tophi form
has been the subject of controversy (see text).

plasma urate, with deposition into the interstitium of the kidney of needle-shaped sodium urate (62,71) or from erosion of precipitated amorphous uric acid crystals out of the tubules into the interstitium, with subsequent transformation to sodium urate (16,52); both can induce inflammation and could interact (71). Appropriate treatment if the former is true is to lower the plasma urate concentration by any means. If however the initial event is the intratubular deposition of uric acid crystals, then uricosuric agents are contraindicated.

Acute hyperuricaemic nephropathy (72–75) arises when a large load of urate transits through the kidney; volume contraction, a low urine flow rate and an acid urine will all decrease the solubility of the uric acid. Precipitation of uric acid crystals occurs within the tubular lumen with tubular blockage and ingestion of crystals leading to tubular necrosis, inflammation, and acute renal failure. Sludged uric acid may also fill the ureters. The kidneys are enlarged, very 'bright' on ultrasonography, the urine volume is low and contains massive amounts of uric acid crystals. This syndrome is most commonly seen when myeloid tumours undergo sudden lysis under treatment, although it has been recorded occasionally following treatment of solid tumours and spontaneously in myeloblastic disease. Large amounts of nucleic acid are released and rapidly and degraded into urate, so that the plasma urate exceeds even 1000 μmol/l. Gross overproduction of urate with hyperuricaemia and acute renal failure is seen also in HPRT deficiency (see below) and in all the various causes of rhabdomyolysis together with high plasma phosphate concentrations and myoglobinuria, so the role of hyperuricaemia in the acute renal failure is not clear. Finally, acute urate nephropathy can be precipiated by the uricosuric agents in Table 30.1, but in the absence of underlying urate overproduction this is rare.

Other histological features

Usually, only sclerosing changes in intra-renal vessels and interstitial fibrosis together with tubular atrophy and secondary glomerulosclerosis are present, *without* urate crystals (78,79). This could represent a consequence of primary renovascular pathology (57), but could result from previous crystal deposition with subsequent lysis of the crystals, for which there is experimental evidence. Needle renal biopsies rarely sample the medulla, where deposits of urate are more prominent. Also, aqueous formalin dissolves urate crystals out, and unlike the acinar uric acid crystals, amorphous deposits leave no 'spaces' behind by which they can be identified, so that histological specimens from gouty patients should be snap-frozen in liquid nitrogen, or immersed in 100% alcohol.

Gout as an association of renal failure

During progressive renal failure from any cause, the glomerular filtration rate falls and the plasma urate concentration rises, but clinical gout secondary to chronic renal failure is rare (80–82). It has been suggested that this arises from depressed phagocytosis, and patients who have had gouty attacks before they entered end-stage renal disease often stop having attacks when they start dialysis (82). However, this explanation sits uneasily with the acute inflammation seen in pseudo-gout from precipitation of calcium pyrophophate crystals, which is common in untreated or poorly treated uraemia.

The rise in plasma urate concentration flattens off above 400–500 μmol/l, despite further decline in the glomerular filtration rate. This apparent anomaly arises from first a fall in total uric acid excretion (62), although a decline in urate production is controversial (7,83); second, a rise in extra-renal excretion through uricolysis in the gut from a normal one-third to two-thirds (5,83); and lastly a progressive increase in FE_{ur} from 10% up to as high as 85% in advanced renal failure (22,84,85). The mechanisms underlying this rise are not clear (22,85,86), but one important clinical consequence is that uricosuric agents such as probenecid and benzbromarone become ineffective as the plasma creatinine rises above 250–300 μmol/l (see below). It has been suggested that urate handing in patients with polycystic kidneys differs from other uraemics, but further studies fail to confirm this (87).

Thus, if a patient with chronic renal impairment or on dialysis develops gout, some variety of 'secondary' gout is likely to be present.

Lead intoxication

Hyperuricaemia and 'saturnine' gout have long been recognized as complications of chronic lead intoxication (67,68,88), principally from industrial exposure but also from leaching of lead into wine from lead glass decanters or ceramic glazes, in drinkers of 'moonshine' whiskey contaminated with lead in the Eastern USA (68), and in children exposed to the lead oxide from peeling paint on timber houses in Australia (89). The FE_{ur} is reduced through an unknown mechanism, perhaps related to extra-cellular volume contraction from associated hyporeninaemic hypoaldosteronism.

Patients with non-gouty chronic renal failure who then develop gout but have no recorded exposure to lead have, however, an increased body burden of lead (90,91), as do patients with evident gout who then develop renal failure (92). It may be that chronic lead poisoning plays a larger role in the genesis of otherwise obscure chronic renal failure than has been realized (64,93,94), although this has been contested (95). Lead urate crystals may serve as nucleation sites for monosodium urate, and the enzyme guanase is inhibited by lead (96). The increased tubular reabsorption of urate is probably a secondary phenomenon, and the interstitial nephritis the result of direct toxicity.

Familial hyperuricaemia, gout and renal failure

This constellation has been known for 30 years (97) but only recently has received much attention (69,70,98–106) and is usually termed *Familial juvenile hyperuricaemic nephropathy (FJHN)*, since gout itself is an inconsistent feature (69,70,99,100). Onset is in childhood, adolescence, or early adult life and renal failure is often recognized between 20 and 40 years of age. The sex incidence is equal and there is no association with obesity. It is inherited as an autosomal dominant but the nature and location of the responsible gene is unknown (101,102) except in a single Japanese family, in which the gene appeared to lie near 16p12 (103), a region known not to be involved in British Caucasian patients (104)[1]. The majority of patients are normotensive, and hypertension is usually of late onset in those with renal dysfunction (69,70).

Cardinal features are hyperuricaemia and extreme renal hypoexcretion of urate (mean FE_{ur} 5.1%), disproportionate to the age, sex or degree of renal dysfunction. However, as renal failure begins this low FE_{ur} increases, so that in early uraemia the FE_{ur} becomes normal for a while which can confuse diagnosis (98). Symptomless members of families should be screened also, and some – even children – will be found already not only with low FE_{ur}, but also reduced renal function (105).

The kidney may be almost normal on histology, but usually shows non-specific patchy areas of tubular atrophy and fibrosis, with focal interstitial infiltration of lymphocytes and histiocytes and globally sclerosed glomeruli (100,106,107). Uric acid crystals are rarely present (100,108,109) but the absence of crystals does not exclude their presence in the past.

Thus the manner in which the renal failure, the low FE_{ur} and hyperuricemia may relate to one another in FJHN is not yet clear (101). A reduced FE_{ur} for age and sex precedes the fall in GFR in otherwise apparently healthy family members (69,70,105). Urate production is normal, and the molecular defect for FJHN perhaps lies in the gene coding for one of the anion transporters in the proximal tubular, or an increased transtubular flux of urate (or some other anion) may be the toxic event (8). It has been suggested also that renal vasoconstriction and decreased renal blood flow, perhaps from purinergic vasocontrictors in the afferent glomerular arterioles may underly the problem (99,110,111).

Three families with associated autosomal dominant nephronophthisis-medullary cystic disease have been reported (109,112,113), but we found no evidence of linkage between FJHN and the locus for recessive familial juvenile nephronophthisis on chromosome 2p13 (102) in other families.

Inherited disorders of purine production and salvage

HPRT deficiency and the kidney

HPRT catalyses the salvage transfer of the phosphoribosyl moiety of PP–ribose-P to hypoxanthine and guanine to form IMP and GMP respectively, and in subjects genetically deficient in HPRT there is a lack of feed-back control of synthesis accompanied by rapid catabolism of purine bases to uric acid (1,2,114–117). The gene is located at Xq26–q27.2 (117) and the condition inherited in a sex-linked dominant fashion. Male hemizygotes show a broad spectrum of presentation from complete deficits with the *Lesch-Nyhan syndrome*: an infant with spasticity and pyramidal tract signs, compulsive self-mutilation, choreo-athetosis and developmental retardation (114–120), to the much commoner partial defects with normal neurological findings, associated only with uric acid overproduction and its consequences, who present later in adolescence or early adulthood (1,114,115,117–120). A variety of mutations have been described (121) a third of which are *de novo* mutations. All but two female carrier heterozygotes studied have been clinically and biochemically normal (122,123).

Severe forms present in infancy with crystalluria, acute renal failure and gout (1,117,124–126). Plasma uric acid is grossly elevated, often in excess of 1000 μmol/l. The kidneys show intra-renal urate deposition and are 'bright' on ultrasound examination and excretion of urate (114,115,125) and hypoxanthine (125,126) is elevated. In other patients the symptoms are at first exclusively neurological, and only the later appearance of gout or renal complications may draw attention to the underlying metabolic defect (114,115,117). The true diagnosis may remain unsuspected also in patients with partial deficiencies, who present as severe juvenile gout without any neurological abnormalities (125,126). The HPRT deficiency can be confirmed by studies in lysed or (preferably) intact red cells (118,126) and antenatal diagnosis is possible. The long-term prognosis is good in children and adolescents with the partial defect who are treated, but patients with the full Lesch-Nyhan syndrome rarely survive beyond adolescence; death is usually due to aspiration pneumonia or renal failure (118,119).

Phosphoribosyl pyrophosphate synthetase (PRPS) superactivity

This rare X-linked condition has been reported in only a few dozen families. The enzyme PRPS catalyses the transfer of the pyrophosphate group of ATP to ribose-5-phosphate to form PP-ribose-P. Two-thirds of patients presented with severe gout or kidney stones in adolescence or early adulthood (127,129). As in HPRT deficiency, the severity of the phenotypic expression varies from a neonatal presentation with severe neurodevelopmental retardation, dysmorphic features and inherited nerve deafness, to milder forms presenting later in childhood or early adult life with uric acid crystalluria or gout (125,128,130). Gout in the mother is common since female heterozygotes have urate overproduction; also sometimes deafness. Thus, it should be suspected particularly in male children whose mothers have gout.

Glycogen storage disease type I

This results from a deficiency of the enzyme glucose-6-phosphatase, and leads to secondary hyperuricaemia and hyperuricosuria which may present as acute renal failure in infancy, childhood or early adult life, or later as gout (1,2,114). This must be considered also when there is evidence of uric acid overproduction in the face of normal purine enzymes. The purine overproduction arises from a combination of accelerated ATP breakdown and increased synthesis, and the associated lactic acidosis reduces the FE_{ur} (1).

How should we treat patients with the various forms of chronic gouty nephropathy?

Classical gouty nephropathy of middle age

NSAIDs should be avoided for *acute* attacks of gout in those with reduced renal function, and colchicine used instead. However, this drug is far from ideal, slow to act and intra-articular cortidosteroids will give much-needed and immediate relief. It is obvious that management of the *chronic* disease should first address issues such as diet, obesity, smoking and alcohol intake. Beer is a potent source of purine through RNA in yeast. Control of hypertension again scarcely needs emphasis, but as in almost all areas of medicine is rarely controlled effectively in practice. The hypouricaemia induced by AT1 antagonists could be exploited at this point (131), but there are insufficient data as yet to judge whether this carries real advantages.

Because of doubt as to the origin of the intra-renal urate, it is best to reduce urate production using allopurinol, which, however, must be used with care in patients with renal impairment. Its active metabolite oxypurinol is handled by the human kidney in a fashion akin to uric acid (132,133) and thus, unlike its parent drug which is freely filtered and excreted, oxypurinol is actively reabsorbed in the tubule. Even in patients with normal kidney function, oxypurinol has a long half-life and its clearance will be affected by all the events outlined in Table 30.1, especially plasma volume contraction from any cause, including diuretics (134,135) which delay excretion. Thus, in advanced renal failure the dose of allopurinol must be reduced to as little as 100 mg daily or even 100 mg three times weekly (136) the objective being to keep the plasma oxypurinol concentration around 100 μmol/l (134,136,137). One study described poor response to allopurinol in heavy drinkers (138) and related this to the combined effect of ethanol in impairing urate excretion as well as increasing its production (37,139).

Administration of chronic low-dose colchicine seems to be effective in preventing attacks of gout (139) even athough it does not alter plasma urate concentrations and no formal trial data are available. Uricosuric agents become ineffective at a plasma creatinine concentration of 250–300 μmol/l, but probenecid remains an effective agent for lowering plasma urate at lesser degrees of renal impairment. Benzbromarone seems to be more effective in moderate to severe uraemia (140), but is not licensed in the USA or the UK and has to be obtained from the Sanofi corporation in France. Azapropazone is another possibility, whose retention in renal failure does not seem to be enhanced by frusemide (141). To complicate things further, uricosuric drugs such as probenecid may also interfere with the tubular transport of diuretics such as frusemide (142).

Lead-associated nephropathy

All the above applies, but if lead intoxication is identified the question of avoiding further exposure, and removing the lead using edetate arises. Details of this

fusion may be reponsible for the low FE_{ur} (111), but the association is probably not specific and in most studies the association of urate with vascular events disappears when other risk factors such as hypertension, smoking or hyperlipidemia are taken into account. Post-menopausal women are protected from vascular disease by treatment with oestrogens, and as well as lowering lipids, plasma urate concentrations are reduced (50). It has been suggested also that hyperuricaemia is important in the appearance and progression of renal impairment in hypertensive patients with symptomless hyperuricaemia (176). This suggestion was made more attractive by the finding of actual urate crystals in the medulla of patients dying with uraemia from various renal disorders (177,178). However, careful prospective studies (61,179) failed to show any effect of lowering plasma urate in patients with hypertension or polycystic kidneys. Thus, at the moment there is no indication to treat symptomless patients to reduce hyperuricaemia, whatever their level of renal function. Attention should be directed to other well-recognized risk factors for progression of vascular and renal disease until more data are available.

Notes

[1] A further family with FJHN in which the gene appears to lie close to 16p12 has been reported also from the Czech Republic.

References

1. Stone T.W. and Simmonds H.A. *Purines: basic and clinical aspects.* Kluwer, London, 1991.
2. Becker M.A. and Roessler B.J. Hyperuricemia and gout. In: C.R. Scriver, A.L. Beaudet, W.S. Sly and D. Valle (eds). *The metabolic and molecular bases of inherited disease, 7th* edn. pp. 1655–77. McGraw-Hill, New York, 1995.
3. Wu X.W., Muzny D.M., Lee G.C. and Caskey C.T. Two independent mutational events in the loss of urate oxidase during hominid evolution. *J Molec Evolution,* 1992, 34: 78–84.
4. Becker B.F. Towards the physiological function of uric acid. *Free Radical Biol Med,* 1993, 14: 615–31.
5. Sørensen L.B. and Levinson D.J. Origin and extrarenal elimination of uric acid in man. *Nephron,* 1975, 14: 7–20.
6. Löffler W., Simmonds H.A. and Grobner W. Gout and uric acid nephropathy: some new aspects in diagnosis and treatment. *Klin Wschr,* 1983, 61: 1233–9.
7. Löffler W. *et al.* Uric acid production and turnover in patients with gout and renal insufficiency of rare origin. *Klin Wschr,* 1987, 65: 6–7.
8. Gresser U. and Zöllner N. (eds) *Urate deposition in man and its clinical consequences.* Springer-Verlag, Berlin, 1991.
9. Simmonds H.A., Duley J.A. and Davies P.M. Analysis of purines and pyrimidines in blood, urine and other physiological fluid. In F. Hommes (ed.): *Techniques in diagnostic human biochemical genetics. A laboratory manual.* pp. 397–425. Wiley Liss, New York, 1991.
10. Cameron J.S. and Simmonds H.A. Uric acid, gout and the kidney. *J Clin Pathol,* 1981, 34: 1245–54.

11. Roberge C.J., Gaudry M., de Medicis R., Lussier A., Poubelle P.E. and Naccache P.H. Crystal-induced neutrophil activation. IV specific inhibition of tyrosine phosphorylation by colchicine. *J Clin Invest*, 1993, 92: 1722–9.

12. Terkeltaub R.A. Gout and mechanisms of crystal-induced inflammation. *Curr Op Rheumatol*, 1993, 5: 510–6.

13. Terkeltaub R., Zacharie C., Santoro D., Martin J., Peveri P. and Matsuchima K. Monocyte-derived neutrophil chemotactic factor/interleukin 8 is a potential mediator of crystal-induced inflammation. *Arthritis Rheum*, 1991, 34: 894–903.

14. Di Giovine F.S., Malawista S.E., Thornton E. and Dutt G.W. Urate crystals stimulate production of tumor necrosis factor from human blood monocytes and synovial cells. Cytokine mRNA and protein kinetics and cellular distribution. *J clin Invest*, 1991, 87: 1375–81.

15. Kovarsky J., Holmes E., and Kelley W.N. Absence of significant urate binding to plasma proteins. *J Lab Clin Med*, 1979, 93: 85–91.

16. Cameron J.S., Moro F., and Simmonds H.A. Uric acid and the kidney. In: *Oxford Textbook of Clinical Nephrology*, Davison A.M., Camerson J.S., Grünfeld J-P., Kerr D.N.S., Ritz E., Winearls C. (eds). Pp. 1157–73. London, Oxford University Press, 1998.

17. Wortman R.L. Uric acid and gout. In: D.W., Seldin, G. Giebisch (eds) *The kidney: physiology and pathophysiology*, pp. 2971–91. Raven Press, New York, 1992.

18. Roch-Ramel F. Renal excretion of uric acid in mammals. *Clin Nephrol*, 1979, 12: 1–6.

19. Danzler W.H. Comparative aspects of renal urate transport. *Kidney Int*, 1996, 49: 1549–51.

20. Diamond H.S. Interpretation of pharmacologic manipulation of urate transport in man. *Nephron*, 1989, 51: 1–5.

21. Roch-Ramel F., and Weiner I.M. Renal excretion of urate: factors determining the action of drugs. *Kidney Int*, 1980, 18: 665–76.

22. Colussi G., Rombola G., De Ferrari M.E., Rolando P., Surian M., Malberti F., and Minetti L. Pharmacological evaluation of urate handling in humans: pyrazinamide test vs. combined pyrazinamide and probenecid administration. *Nephrol Dial Transplant*, 1987, 2: 10–16.

23. Roch-Ramel F. Renal transport of organic ions. *Curr Opin Nephrol Hypertens*, 1998, 7: 517–24.

24. Levinson D.J. and Sørensen L.B. Renal handling of uric acid in normal and gouty subjects: evidence for a 4-component system. *Ann Rheum Dis*, 1980, 39: 173–9.

25. Aronson P.S. The renal tubule: a model for diversity of anion exchangers and stilbene-sensitive anion transporters. *Annu Rev Physiol*, 1989, 51: 419–41.

26. Roch-Ramel F., Werner D. and Guisan B. Urate transport in brush-border membrane of human kidney. *Am J Physiol*, 1994, 266: F797–F805.

27. Maesaka J.K. and Fishbane S. Regulation of renal urate excretion: a critical review. *Am J Kidney Dis*, 1998, 32: 917–33.

28. Spitzenberger F., Grabeler J. and Schröder H.-E. Molecular characteristics of renal ion transport systems – cloning of a putative urate transporter/channel from cultured LLC-PK1 kidney epithelial cells and human kidney. *Cell Mol Biol Letters*, 1999, 4: 475–6.

29. Polkowski C.A. and Grassl S.M. Uric acid transport in rat renal basolateral membrane vesicles. *Biochim Biophys Acta*, 1993, 1146: 145–52.

30. Emmerson B.T., Nagel S.L., Duffy D.L. and Martin N.G. Genetic control of the renal clearance of urate: a study of twins. *Ann Rheum Dis*, 1992, 51: 375–7.

31. Short E.M. Hyperuricemia and gout. In: King R.A., Rutter J.I., Mitulsky A.E. (eds) *The genetic basis of common diseases*, pp. 482–506, Oxford University Press, London, 1992.

32. Nuki G., Watson M.L., Williams B.C., Simmonds H.A. and Wallace R.C. Congenital chloride losing enteropathy associated with tophaceous gouty arthritis. *Adv Exp Med Biol*, 1992, 309A: 203–9.

33. Lowe J., Gray J., Henry D.A. and Lawson D.H. Adverse reactions to frusemide in hospital patients. *Br Med J*, 1979, 2: 360–2.

34. Meyers O.L. and Monteagudo F.S.E. Gout in females: analysis of 92 patients. *Clin Exp Rheumatol*, 1985, 3: 105–9.

35. Platt P.N. and Dick W.C. Diuretic-induced gout: the beginnings of an epidemic. *The Practitioner*, 1985, 229: 281–4.

36. Gibson T., Highton J., Simmonds H.A. and Potter C.F. Hypertension, renal function, and gout. *Postgrad Med J*, 1979, 55(suppl 3): 21–5.

37. Faller J. and Fox I.H. Ethanol-induced hyperuricaemia. Evidence for increased urate production by activation of adenine nucleotide turnover. *N Engl J Med*, 1982, 307: 1598–1602.

38. Yü, T.-F. and Gutman A.B. Paradoxical retention of uric acid by uricosuric drugs in low dosage. *Proc Soc Exp Biol Med*, 1955, 90: 542–7.

39. Walter-Sack I. Benzbromarone disposition and uricosuric action: evidence for hydroxylation instead of debromination to benzarone. *Klin Wschr*, 1988, 66: 160–6.

40. Sommers D.K. and Schoenman H.S. Drug interactions with urate excretion in man. *Europ J Pharmacol*, 1987, 32: 499–502.

41. Edwards R.M., Trizna W., Stack E.J. and Weinstock J. Interaction of nonpetide antgiotensin II receptor antagonists with the urate trasporter in rat renal brushborder membranes. *J Pharmacol Exp Ther*, 1996, 276: 125–9.

42. Keidar S., Kohan R., Levy J., Grenadier E., Palant A. and Ben-Ari. Non-oliguric acute renal failure after treatment with sulfinpyrazone. *Clin Nephrol*, 1982, 17: 266–7.

43. Prospert F., Soupart A., Brimioulle S. and Decaux G. Evidence of defective tubular reabsorption and normal secretion of uric acid in the syndrome of inappropriate secretion of antidiuretic hormone. *Nephron*, 1993, 64: 189–92.

44. Maesaka J.K., Venkatesan J., Piccione J.M., Decker R., Driesbach A.W. and Wetherington J.D. Abnormal urate transport in patients with intracranial disease. *Am J Kidney Dis*, 1992, 19: 10–15.

45. Beck L.H. Hypouricemia in the syndrome of inappropriate secretion of antidiuretic hormone. *N Engl J Med*, 1979, 301: 526–30.

46. Gibson T., Waterworth P., Hatfield P., Robinson G. and Bremner K. Hyperuricaemia, gout and kidney function in young New Zealand Maori men. *Br J Rheumatol*, 1984, 23: 276–82.

47. Simmonds H.A., McBride M.B., Hatfield P.J., Grahame R., McCaskey J. and Jackson M. Polynesian women are also at risk for hyperuricaemia and gout because of a defect in renal urate handling. *Br J Rheumatol*, 1994, 33: 932–7.

48. McBride M.B., Simmonds H.A., Hatfield P.J., Grahame R., McCaskey J. and Jackson M. Renal urate hypoexcretion in Polynesian women is not as severe as in United Kingdom (UK) women with familial juvenile hyperuricaemic nephropathy. *Adv Exp Med Biol*, 1995, 310: 35–8.

49. Nicholls A., Snaith M.L. and Scott T.J. Effect of oestrogen therapy on plasma and urinary levels of uric acid. *Br Med J*, 1972, 1: 449–53.

50. Mikkelsen W.N., Dodge H.J. and Valkenburg H. The distribution of serum uric acid values in a population unselected as to gout and hypertension. *Am J Med*, 1965, 39: 242–51.

51. Sumino H., Ichikawa S., Kanda T., Nakamura T. and Skamaki T. Reduction of serum uric acid by hormone replacement therapy in postmenopausal women with hyperuricaemia. *Lancet*, 1999, 354: 650 (letter).

52. Brown J. and Mallory G.K. Renal changes in gout. *N Engl J Med*, 1950, 243: 325–9.

53. Talbott J.H. and Terplan K.L. The kidney in gout. *Medicine (Baltimore)*, 1960, 39: 405–67.

54. Gonick H.C., Rubini M.E., Gleason I.O. and Sommers S.C. The renal lesions in gout. *Ann Intern Med*, 1965, 62: 667–74.

55. Barlow K.A. and Beilin L.S. Renal disease in primary gout. *Q J Med*, 1968, 37: 79–96.

56. Klinenberg J.R., Gonick H.C. and Dornfeld L. Renal function abnormalities in patients with symptomless hyperuricemia. *Arthritis Rheum*, 1975, 18: 725–30.

57. Yü T.-F. and Berger, L. Impaired renal function in gout. Its association with hypertensive vascular disease and intrinsic renal disease. *Am J Med*, 1982, 72: 95–9.

58. Tarng D.C., Lin H.Y., Shyong M.L., Wang J.S., Yang W.C. and Hyang T.P. Renal function in gout patients. *Am J Nephrol*, 1995, 15: 31–7.

59. Gibson T., Highton J., Potter C. and Simmonds H.A. Renal impairment and gout. *Ann Rheum Dis*, 1980, 39: 417–23.

60. Berger L. and Yü T.-F. Renal function in gout. An analysis of 524 gouty subjects including long term follow-up studies. *Am J Med*, 1975, 59: 605–13.

61. Fessel W.J. Renal outcomes of gout and hyperuricemia. *Am J Med*, 1979, 67: 74–82.

62. Emmerson B.T. and Row G. An evaluation of the pathogenesis of the gouty kidney. *Kidney Int*, 1975, 8: 65–71.

63. Reif M.C., Constatinier A. and Levitt M.F. Chronic gouty nephropathy: a vanishing syndrome. *N Engl J Med*, 1981, 304: 535–6.

64. Porter G. Gouty nephropathy. Fact or fiction? *Am J Kidney Dis*, 1983, 2: 553–4.

65. Beck L.H. Requiem for gouty nephropathy. *Kidney Int*, 1986, 30: 280–7.

66. Nickeleit V. and Mihatsch M.J. Uric acid nephropathy and end-stage renal disease –review of a non-disease. *Nephrol Dial Transplant*, 1997, 12: 1832–8.

67. Bennett W.M. Lead nephropathy. *Kidney Int*, 1985, 28: 212–20.

68. Wedeen R. and de Broe M.E. Heavy metals and the kidney. In: *Oxford Textbook of Clinical Nephrology*, 2nd edn. Eds Davison A.M., Cameron J.S., Grünfeld J.P., Kerr D.N.S., Ritz E., Winearls C. Oxford University Press, Oxford, 1998, pp. 1175–89.

69. Cameron J.S., Moro F. and Simmonds H.A. Gout, uric acid and purine metabolism in pediatric nephrology. *Pediatr Nephrol*, 1993, 7: 105–18.

70. Cameron J.S., Moro F., McBride M. and Simmonds H.A. Inherited disorders of purine metabolism and transport. In: *Oxford Textbook of Clinical Nephrology* 2nd edn. Eds Davison A.M., Cameron J.S., Grünfeld J.P., Kerr D.N.S., Ritz E. and Winearls C. Oxford University Press, Oxford, 1998, pp. 2469–82.

71. Stavric B., Johnson W.J. and Grice H.C. Uric acid nephropathy: an experimental model. *Proc Soc Exp Biol Med*, 1969, 130: 512–16.

72. Anonymous (editorial). Tumour lysis syndrome. *Lancet*, 1981, ii: 849.

73. Dykman D., Simon E.E. and Avioli LV. Hyperuricemia and uric acid nephropathy. *Arch Intern Med*, 1987, 147: 1341–5.

74. Conger J.D. Acute uric acid nephropathy. *Med Clin N Amer*, 1990, 74: 859–71.

75. Kanwar Y.S. and Manaligod J.R. Leukemic urate nephropathy. *Arch Pathol*, 1975, 99: 467–72.

76. Jones D.P., Mahmoud H. and Chesney R.W. Tumor lysis syndrome: pathogenesis and management. *Pediatr Nephrol*, 1985, 9: 206–12.

77. Andreoli S.P., Clark J.H., McGuire W.A. and Bernstein J.M. Purine excretion during tumor lysis syndrome children with acute lymphocytic leukemia receiving allopurinol: relationship to renal failure. *J Pediatr*, 1986, 109: 292–8.

78. Oliva H. and Barat A. Histopathology of the kidney in in percutaneous biopsy in gout. In: *The kidney in gout and hyperuricemia*, eds Yü T, Berger L. Futura Publishing Co., New York, 1982, pp. 175–94.

79. Pardo V., Perez-Stable E. and Fisher E.R. Ultrastructural studies in hypertension. III. Gouty nephropathy. *Lab Invest*, 1968, 18: 143–50.

80. Vecchio P.C. and Emmerson B.T. Gout due to renal disease. *Br J Rheumatol*, 1992, 31: 63–5.

81. Richet G., Mignon F. and Ardaillou R. Goutte secondaire des néphropathies chroniques. *Presse Méd*, 1965, 73: 633–8.

82. Ifudu O., Tan C.C., Dulin A.L., Delano B.G. and Friedman E.A. Gouty arthritis in end-stage renal disease: clinical course and rarity of new cases. *Am J Kidney Dis*, 1994, 23: 347–51.

83. Sørensen L.B. Gout secondary to chronic renal disease: studies on urate metabolism. *Ann Rheum Dis*, 1980, 39: 424–30.

84. Danovich G.M., Weinberger J. and Berlyne G.M. Uric acid in advanced renal failure. *Clin Sci*, 1972, 43: 331–41.

85. Steele T.H. and Rieselbach R.E. The contribution of residual nephrons within the chronically diseased kidney to urate homeostasis in man. *Am J Med*, 1967, 43: 876–86.

86. Boumendil-Podevin E.F., Podevin R.A. and Richet G. Uricosuric agents in uremic sera. Identification of indoxyl sulfate and hippuric acid. *J Clin Invest*, 1975, 55: 1142–52.

87. Kaehny W.D., Tangel D.J., Johnson A.M., Kimberling W.J., Schrier R.W. and Gabow P.A. Uric acid handling in autosomal dominant polycystic kidney disease with normal filtration rates. *Am J Med*, 1990, 89: 49–52.

88. Richet G., Albahary C., Ardaillou R., Sultan C. and Morel-Maroger L. Le rein du saturnisme chronique. *Revue Française d'Études Cliniques et Biologiques*, 1964, 9: 188–96.

89. Emmerson B.T. Identification of the causes of persistent hyperuricaemia. *Lancet*, 1991, 337: 1461–63.

90. Colleoni N. and D'Amico G. Chronic lead accumulation as a possible cause of renal failure in gouty patients. *Nephron*, 1986, 44: 32–5.

91. Koster J., Erhardt A., Stoeppler M. and Ritz E. Mobilizable lead in patients with chronic renal failure. *Europ J Clin Invest*, 1989, 19: 228–33.

92. Miranda-Carús E., Mateos F.A., Sanz A.G., Herero E., Ramos T. and Puig J.G. Purine metabolism in patients with gout: the role of lead. *Nephron*, 1997, 75: 327–35.

93. Batuman V., Maesaka J.K., Haddad B. and Wedeen R.P. The role of lead in gout nephropathy. *N Engl J Med*, 1981, 304: 520–23.

94. Lin J.C. and Huang P.T. Body lead and stores and urate excretion in men with chronic renal failure. *J Rheumatol*, 1994, 21: 705–09.

95. Nuyts G.D., Daelemans R.A., Jorens Ph G., Elserviers M.M., Van de Vyver F.L. and De Broe M.E. Does lead play a role in the development of chronic renal disease? *Nephrol Dial Transplant*, 1991, 6: 307–15.

96. Farkas W.R., Stanawitz T. and Schneider M. Saturnine gout: lead-induced formation of guanine crystals. *Science*, 1978, 199: 786–88.
97. Duncan H. and Dixon A.StJ. Gout, familial hyperuricaemia, and renal disease. *Q J Med*, 1960, 29: 127–36.
98. Calabrese G., Simmonds H.A., Cameron J.S. and Davies P.M. Precocious familial gout with reduced fractional excretion of urate and normal purine enzymes. *Q J Med*, 1990, 75: 441–50.
99. Puig J.G., Michán A.D., Jiménez M.L., Pérez de Ayala C., Mateos F.A., Capitàn C.F., de Miguel E. and Gijón J.B. Familial gout. Clinical spectrum and uric acid metabolism. *Arch Intern Med*, 1991, 151: 726–32.
100. Reiter L., Brown M.A. and Edmonds J. Familial hyperuricemic nephropathy. *Am J Kidney Dis*, 1995, 25: 235–41.
101. Cameron J.S., Moro F. and Simmonds H.A. What is the pathogenesis of familial juvenile gouty nephropathy? *Adv Exp Med Biol*, 1991, 309A: 185–91.
102. Moro F., Noam I., Cameron J.S., Simmonds H.A., McBride M.B., Mathew C.P., Ogg C.S., Puig J.G., Miranda M.E. and Matoes F.A. Mapping the gene for familial juvenile hyperuricaemic nephropathy. *Pharmacy World Sci*, 1993, 15: F23.
103. Kamatani N., Moritani M., Yamanaka H., Takeuchi F., Hosoya T. and Itakura M. Localization of a gene for familial juvenile hyperuricemic nephropathy (FJHN) causing underexcretion-type gout to 16p12 by genome-wide linkage analysis of a large family. *Arthr Rheum* 2000 43: 925–9.
104. Marinaki A. and Simmonds H.A. (unpublished observations), 1999.
105. McBride M.B., Rigden S., Haycock G.B., Dalton N., van t'Hoff W., Rees L., Raman G.V., Moro F., Ogg C.S., Cameron J.S. and Simmonds H.A. Presymptomatic detection of familial juvenile hyperuricaemic nephropathy in children. *Pediatr Nephrol*, 1998, 12: 357–64.
106. Simmonds H.A., Cameron J.S., Potter C.F., Warren D., Gibson T. and Farebrother, D. Renal Failure in young subjects with familial gout. *Adv Exp Med Biol*, 1980, 122A: 15–20.
107. Richmond J.M., Kincaid-Smith P., Whitworth J.A. and Becker G.J. Familial urate nephropathy, *Clini Nephrol*, 1981, 16: 163–68.
108. Farebrother D.A., Pincott J.R., Simmonds H.A., Warren D.J., Dillon M.J. and Cameron J.S. Uric acid crystal-induced nephropathy: evidence for a specific renal lesion in a gouty family. *J Pathol*, 1981, 135: 159–68.
109. Murakami T., Kawakami H., Nakatsuda K., Jojima K., Nohno H. and Matsuzaki H. Underexcretory-type hyperuricemia, disproportionate to the reduced glomerular filtration rate, in two boys with mild proteinuria. *Nephron*, 1990, 56: 439–42.
110. Puig J.G., Miranda M.E., Mateos F.A., Picazo M.L., Jiménez M.L., Calvin T.S. and Gil A.A. Hereditary nephropathy associated with hyperuricaemia and gout *Arch Intern Med*, 1993, 153: 357–65.
111. Messerli F.H., Fröhlich E.D., Dreslinski G.R., Suarez D.H. and Aristumo G.G. Serum uric acid in essential hypertension: an indicator of renal vascular involvement. *Am J Med*, 1990, 93: 817–21.
112. Burke J.R., Inglis J.S., Craswell P.W., Mitchell K.R. and Emmerson B.T. Juvenile nephronophthisis and medullary cystic disease–the same disease (report of a large family with medullary cystic disease associated with gout and epilepsy). *Clin Nephrol*, 1982, 18: 1–8.
113. Thompson G.R., Weiss J.J., Goldman R.T. and Rigg G.A. Familial occurrence of hyperuricemia, gout and medullary cystic disease. *Arch Intern Med*, 1978, 138: 1614–17.

114. Wyngaarden J.M. and Kelley W.N. *Gout and hyperuricemia*. New York, Grune and Stratton, 1976.

115. Simmonds H.A. Purine and pyrimidine disorders. Chapter 6. In: J.B. Holton (ed.), *The Inherited Metabolic Diseases*, PP. 297–350. Edinburgh, Churchill Livingstone, 1994.

116. Watts R.W.E. Defects of tetrahydrobiopterin synthesis and their possible relationship to a disorder of purine metabolism, the Lesch-Nyhan syndrome. *Adv Enzyme Reg*, 1985, 23: 25–58.

117. Rossiter B.J.F. and Kaskey T. Hypoxanthine guanine phsophoribosyl transferase deficiency. In: C.R., Scriver A.L., Beaudet W.S., Sly and D. Valle (eds). *Metabolic and molecular bases of inherited disease*, 7th Ed. Pp. 1679–1705. McGraw-Hill, New York, 1995.

118. Page T. and Nyhan W.L. The spectrum of HPRT deficiency: an update. *Adv Exp Med Biol*, 1989, 253A: 129–33.

119. McCarthy G. Practical aspects of the management of the Lesch–Nyhan syndrome. *British Inherited Disease Group Newsletter*, 1992, 6: 14–16.

120. Nyhan W.L. and Wong D.F. New approaches to understanding Lesch–Nyhan disease. *N Engl J Med*, 1996, 334: 1602–04.

121. Davidson B.L., Tarle S.A., Van Antwerp M., Gibbs D.A., Watts R.W., Kelley W.N. and Palella T.D. Identification of 17 independent mutations responsible for human hypoxanthine-guanine phosphoribosyltransferase (HPRT) deficiency. *Am J Hum Genet*, 1991, 48: 951–55.

122. Van Bogaert P., Ceballos I., Desguerre I., Telvi L., Kamoun P. and Ponsot G. Lesch-Nyhan syndrome in a girl. *J Inher Metab Dis*, 1992, 15: 790–91.

123. Ogasawara N., Stout J.T., Goto H. Sonta A.-I., Matsumoto A. and Caskey C.T. Molecular analysis of a female Lesch–Nyhan patient. *J Clin Invest*, 1989, 84: 1024–27.

124. Stapleton F.B. Uric acid nephropathy. In: C.M. Edelmann Jr (ed.) *Pediatric Renal Disease*, 2nd edn., pp. 1647–59. Little, Brown, Boston, 1992.

125. Simmonds H.A. When and how does one search for inborn errors of purine and pyrimidine metabolism? *Pharmacy World Sci*, 1994, 16: 139–48.

126. Simmonds H.A., Cameron J.S., Barratt T.M., Dillon M.J., Meadow S.R. and Trompeter R.S. Purine enzyme defects as a cause of acute renal failure in childhood. *Pediatr Nephrol*, 1989, 3: 433–7.

127. Zoref E., de Vries A. and Sperling O. Mutant feedback resistant phosphoribosylpyrophosphate synthetase associated with purine overproduction and gout. *J Clin Invest*, 1975, 56: 1093–99.

128. Roessler B.J., Golovoy N., Palella T.D., Heidler S. and Becker M.A. Identification of distinct PRPS1 (figure 1) mutations in two patients with X-linked phosphoribosyl pyrophosphate synthetase superactivity. *Adv Exp Med Biol*, 1991, 309B: 125–28.

129. Ishizuka T., Iizasa T., Taira M., Ishijima S., Sonoda T., Shimada H., Nagatake N. and Tatibana M. Promoter regions of the human X-linked housekeeping genes PRPS1 and PRPS2 encoding phosphoribosylpyrophosphate synthetase subunit I and II. *Biochim Biophys Acta*, 1992, 1130: 139–48.

130. Christen H.-J., Hanefeld F., Duley J.A. and Simmonds H.A. Distinct neurological syndrome in two brothers with hyperuricaemia. *Lancet*, 1992, 340: 1167–8.

131. Shahainfar S., Simpson R.L., Carides A.D., Thyagarajan B., Nakagawa Y., Parks J.H. and Coe F.L. for the Losartan uric acid study group. Safety of losartan in

hypertensive patients with diuretic–induced hyperuricemia. *Kidney Int*, 1999, 56: 1879–85.

132. Elion G.B., Yü T.-F., Gutman A.B. and Hitchings G.H. Renal clearance of oxipurinol, the chief metabolite of allopurinol. *Am J Med*, 1968, 45: 69–77.

133. Graham S., Day R.O., Wong H., McLachlan A.J., Bergendal L., Miners J.O. and Birkett D.J. Pharmacodynamics of oxypurinol after administration of allopurinol to healthy subjects. *Br J Clin Pharmacol*, 1996, 41: 299–304.

134. Hande K.R., Noone R.M. and Stone W.E. Severe allopurinol toxicity. Description and guidelines for prevention in patients with renal insufficiency. *Am J Med*, 1984, 76: 47–56.

135. Hande K.R. Evaluation of thiazide–allopurinol interaction. *Am J Med Sci*, 1986, 292: 213–16.

136. Cameron J.S. and Simmonds H.A. Use and abuse of allopurinol. *Br Med J*, 1987, 294: 1504–05.

137. Simmonds H.A., Cameron J.S., Morris G.S. and Davies P.M. Allopurinol in renal failure and the tumour lysis syndrome. *Clin Chim Acta*, 1986, 160: 189–95.

138. Ralston S.H., Capell H.A. and Sturrock R.D. Alcohol and response to treatment of gout. *Br Med J*, 1988, 296: 1641–2.

139. Yü T.F. The efficacy of colchicine prophylaxis in articular gout – a reappraisal after 20 years. *Sem Arthritis Rheum*, 1982, 12: 256–63.

140. Grahame R, Simmonds H.A., McBride M.B. and Marsh F.P. How should we treat tophacous gout in patients with allopurinol sensitivity? *Adv Exp Med Biol*, 1998, 431: 19–23.

141. Williamson P.J., Ene M.D. and Roberts C.J.C. A study of potential interactions between azapropazone and frusemide in man. *Br J Clin Pharmacol*, 1984, 18: 619–23.

142. Bidiville J. and Roch-Ramel F. Competition of organic ions for furosemide and *p*-aminohippurate secretion in the rabbit. *J Pharmacol Exp Ther*, 1986, 237: 636–43.

143. Moro F., Simmonds H.A., McBride M.B., Cameron J.S., Williams D.G. and Ogg C.S. Does allopurinol ameliorate progression in familial juvenile gouty nephropathy (FJGN)? *Adv Exp Med Biol*, 1991, 309A: 199–202.

144. Gibson T., Rodgers V., Potter C. and Simmonds H.A. Allopurinol treatment and its effect on renal function in gout: a controlled study. *Ann Rheum Dis*, 1982, 41: 59–65.

145. Yakota N., Yamanaka H., Yamamoto Y., Fujimoto S. and Tanaka K. Autosomal dominantly transmission of gouty arthritis with renal disease in a large Japanese family. *Ann Rheum Dis*, 1991, 50: 108–11.

146. Miranda M.E. on behalf of the Spanish group for the study of FNAH. The influence of allopurinol on renal deterioration in familial nepropathy (*sic*) associated with hyperuricemia (FNAH). *Purine and Pyrimidine metabolism in man VIII*. A. Sahota, M. Taylor (eds). Plenum Press, New York, 1994, pp. 61–4.

147. Gomez G.A., Stutzman L. and Ming Chu T. Xanthine nephropathy during chemotherapy in deficiency of hypoxanthine-guanine phosphoribosyl transferase. *Arch Intern Med*, 1978, 138: 1017–19.

148. Brock W.A., Golden J. and Kaplan G.W. Xanthine calculi in the Lesch Nyhan syndrome. *J Urol*, 1983, 130: 157–9.

149. Kenney I.J. Renal sonography in long standing Lesch-Nyhan syndrome. *Clin Radiol*, 1991, 43: 39–41.

150. Ablin A., Stephens B.G., Hirata T., Wilson K. and Williams H.E. Nephropathy, xanthinuria, and orotic aciduria complicating Burkitt's lymphoma treated with chemotherapy and allopurinol. *Metabolism*, 1972, 21: 771–5.

151. Hande K.R., Hixon C.V. and Chabner B.A. Postchemotherapy purine excretion in lymphoma patients receiving allopurinol. *Cancer Res*, 1981, 41: 2273–9.
152. Flury W., Ruch H.R. and Montandon A. Zur Behandlung der Hyperurikämie nach Nierentransplantation. *Schweiz Med Wschr*, 1977, 107, 1339–41.
153. Kahl L.E., Thompson M.E., and Griffith B.P. Gout in the heart transplant recipient: physiologic puzzle and therapeutic challenge. *Am J Med*, 1989, 87: 286–94.
154. Burack D.A., Griffith B.P. and Thompson M.E. Hyperuricemia and gout amongst heart transplant recipients receiving cyclosporine. *Am J Med*, 1992, 92: 141–6.
155. Lin H-Y., Rocher L.L., McQuillan M.M., Schmaltz S., Palella T.D. and Fox I.H. Cyclosporine-induced hyperuricemia and gout. *N Engl J Med*, 1989, 321: 287–92.
156. Baethge B.A., Work J., Landreneau M.D. and McDonald J.C. Tophaceous gout in patients with renal transplants treated with cyclosporine A. *J Rheumatol*, 1993, 20: 718–20.
157. Steidel K., Brandis M., Kramer M. Leititis J.U. and Zimmerhackl L.B. Cyclosporine inhibits renal uric acid transport in renal transplants not in children treated for nephrotic syndrome. *Renal Failure*, 1990, 12: 193–98.
158. Cohen M.R., Proximal gout following renal transplantation. *Arthritis Rheum*, 1994, 37: 1709–10.
159. Noordzij T.C., Leunissen K.M. and van Hooff J.P. Renal handlign of plasma urate and incidence of gouty arthritis during cyclosproine and diuretic use. *Transplantation*, 1991, 52: 64–7.
160. Marcén R., Gallego N, Orofino L., Gamez C, Estepa M.R., Sabater J., Teruel J.L. and Ortuño J. Impairment of tubular secretion of urate in renal transplant patients on cyclosporine. *Nephron*, 1995, 70: 307–13.
161. Zürcher R.M., Bock H.A. and Thiel G. Hyperuricaemia in cyclosporin-treated patients: a GFR-related effect. *Nephrol Dial Transplant*, 1996, 11: 153–8.
162. Chocair P., Duley J., Simmonds H.A., Cameron J.S., Ianhez L., Arap S. and Sabbaga E. Low-dose allopurinol plus azathioprine/cyclosporin/prednisolone, a novel immunosuppressive regimen. *Lancet*, 1993, 342: 83–4.
163. Raman V., Sharman V.L. and Lee H.A., Azathioprine and allopurinol: a potentially dangerous combination. *J Int Med*, 1990, 228: 69–71.
164. Jacobs F., Mamzer-Bruneel M.F., Skhiri H., Rherevet E., Legendre C. and Kries H. Safety of the mycophenolate-allopurinol combination in kidney transplant recipeints with gout. *Transplantation*, 1997, 64: 1087–8.
165. Gaudiano V., Baganato C, Santarsai G. and Lopez T. Efficacia del micofenolato mofetile in associazione con allopurinolo in pazienti con trapianto di rene e iperuricemia. *Giorn Ital Nefrol*, 1999, 16: 479 (letter).
166. Zürcher R.M., Bock H.A. and Thiel G. Excellent uricosuric efficacy of benzbromarone in cyclosporin-A-Treated renal transplant patients: a prospective study. *Nephrol Dialysis Transplant*, 1994, 9: 548–51.
167. Rozenberg S., Roche B., Dorent R., Koeger A.C., Borget C., Wrona N and Bourgeois P. Urate oxidase for the treatment of tophacous gout in heart transplant recipients. A report of three cases. *Revue du Rheumatisme*, 195, 62: 392–94.
168. Simmonds H.A., Nephrolithiasis in the context of purine metabolism. In: G Wolfram (ed) *Genetic and therapeutic aspects of purine metabolism*, pp. 79–93. Springer Verlag, Berlin, 1989.
169. Riese R.J., Sakhaee K., Uric acid nephrolithiasis: pathogenesis and treatment. *J Urol*, 1992, 148: 765–71.

170. Pak Poy RK. Urinary pH in gout. *Aust Ann Med*, 1965, 14: 35–9.

171. Sperling O. Renal hypouricemia: classification tubular defect and clinical consequences. *Contr Nephrol*, 1992, 100: 1–14.

172. Yim J-J., Oh K.H., Chin H., Ahn C., Kim S.H., Han J.S., Kim S. and Lee J.S. Exercise-induced acute renal failure in a patient with congenital renal hypouricaemia. *Nephrol Dial Transplant*, 1998, 13: 994–7.

173. Campion, E.W., Glynn R.J. and DeLabry L.O. Asymptomatic hyperuricemia. Risks and consequences in the normative aging study. *Am J Med*, 1987, 82: 421–26.

174. Rigby A.S. and Wood P.H.N. Serum uric acid and gout–what does this herald for the population? *Clin Exp Rheumatol*, 1994, 12: 395–400.

175. Freedman D.S., Wiliamson D.F., Gunter E.W. and Byers T. Relation of serum uric acid to mortality and ischemic heart disease. *Am J Epdemiol*, 1995, 141: 637–44.

176. Johnson R.J., Kivilghn S.D. Kim Y-G., Suga S. and Fogo A.B. Reappraisal of the pathogenesis and consequences of hyperuricemia in hypertension, cardiovascular disease, and renal disease. *Am J Kidney Dis*, 1999, 33: 225–34.

177. Verger D., Leroux-Robert C., Ganter P. and Richet G. Les tophus goutteux de la médullaire rénale des urémiques chroniques. *Nephron*, 1967, 4: 356–70.

178. Östberg Y. Renal urate deposits in chronic renal failure. *Acta Med Scand*, 1968, 183: 197–201.

179. Rosenfeld J.B., Effect of long term allopurinol administration on serial glomerular filtration rate in normotensive and hypertensive hyperuricemic subjects. *Adv Exp Med Biol*, 1974, 41B: 581–86.

180. Stibůrková, B., Majewski, J., Šebesta, I., Zhang, W., Ott, J., and Kmoch, S. Familial Juvenile Hyperuricemic Nephropathy: localization of the gene on chromosome 16.p112- and evidence of genetic heterogeneity. *Am J Hum Genet* 2000, 66: 1989–1994.

31

Dialysis arthropathy

Megan Griffith and Edwina Brown

Introduction

Transplantation is the treatment of choice in renal replacement therapy, but for an increasing number of patients this is no longer an option due to age, comorbidity, sensitization from previous transplants, etc. In combination with the lack of donor organs this is resulting in a large population of patients on long-term dialysis. The incidence of joint problems is high in these patients, with joint symptoms occurring in up to 69% of patients on maintenance haemodialysis for more than three months (Brown and Gower 1982). Dialysis related arthropathy is common, affecting 97% of patients who have been on haemodialysis with cuprophane membranes for more than 10 years (Sethi *et al.* 1990); this population is also prone to other arthropathies seen in the general population such as gout, pseudo-gout, infection, haemarthroses, connective tissue disease, avascular necrosis, and osteoporosis. This chapter will focus on dialysis arthropathy as many of these other arthropathies are described in detail elsewhere in this volume.

Dialysis related amyloidosis is a severe arthropathy which increases in frequency with age and time spent on dialysis (van Ypersele *et al.* 1991). In 1980 amyloid was identified in tissue from carpel tunnel biopsies of haemodialysis patients (Assenat *et al.* 1980), and in 1985 the main constituent of 'dialysis amyloid' was found to be β2-microglobulin (Gejyo *et al.* 1985). Since that time there have been a number of advances in understanding the biochemistry and ultrastructure of dialysis amyloid (Argiles *et al.* 1989; Miyata *et al.* 1996a-c; Inoue *et al.* 1997); however, controversy still remains over the pathogenesis. The presentation, diagnosis, pathogenesis and treatment will be discussed.

Presentation

Amyloid arthropathy and fractures

Dialysis amyloidosis has a predilection for bones and soft tissue around joints. β2-microglobulin deposits in cartilage, and then subsequently extends to capsule and to synovium and finally to bone. The lesions are initially paucicellular, but later macrophage infiltration occurs (Argiles *et al.* 1994; Garber *et al.* 1999). Patients present with pain and stiffness in the joints: symptoms usually start in the shoulder joints and are often bilateral. Symptoms then spread to other peripheral joints such as knees, ankles and wrists and the disease runs a chronic progressive course culminating in restricted movement of joints and disability (Brown *et al.* 1986; Bardin 1996). The pain may be worse at night, and exacerbated by haemodialysis (van Ypersele 1988). Effusions may develop, and usually, but not invariably, synovial fluid contains low numbers of inflammatory cells (Bardin 1996; Ferrari *et al.* 1997). Destructive spondyloarthropathy occurs, particularly of the cervical spine (Allain *et al.* 1988; Kroner *et al.* 1991; Fututake *et al.* 1997), and lumbar region (Marcelli *et al.* 1996). Patients usually present with arthalgias, and there is often severe narrowing of the spinal canal secondary to β2-microglobulin deposition in the intervertebral discs, facet joints and associated ligaments. This can result in compressive polyneuropathies, cord compression and even death (Kroner *et al.* 1991; Danesh *et al.* 1999). Bone invasion occurs late, resulting in bone cysts and pathological fractures (van Ypersele *et al.* 1988; Campistol 1990; and Koch 1992).

Carpel tunnel syndrome

Soft tissue involvement results in carpel tunnel syndrome which is often the first presenting complaint of β2-microglobulin amyloidosis. This has been observed after only a few years on dialysis and is almost invariable after 20 years of dialysis (Charra *et al.* 1988; van Ypersele *et al.* 1988; and Bardin 1996). It is characterized by burning pain, numbness and tingling in the thumb, index, middle, and lateral half of the ring finger and palm. As the median nerve is further compressed, atrophy of the muscles of the thenar eminence develops with loss of apposition of the thumb. The pain is worse at night and during haemodialysis, and can be elicited by tapping over the wrist (Tinel's sign) or compression of the wrist (Phaleus sign). The treatment, as for other non-reversible forms of carpel tunnel syndrome, is surgical. Although most of the material found at operation is fibrous, deposits of β2-microglobulin are found in up to 70% of cases (van Ypersele *et al.* 1988, Chary-Valckenaere *et al.* 1998). Rarely amyloid deposits are found in the ulnar nerve giving rise to a corresponding syndrome (Guyon's syndrome), of pain and tingling over the palmer surface and the medial half of the ring finger and the little finger (Borgatti *et al.* 1991).

Visceral involvement

Visceral involvement of many organs has been found at post-mortem; deposits in the vasculature are the most common, and result in focal thickening of vessel walls and thrombosis. Larger visceral deposition is also found, although it is often asymptomatic. Dialysis amyloid preferentially deposits in certain organs, particularly heart (80%) and gastrointestinal tract (78%), but has also been found in lung (59%), liver (41%), kidneys (33%) and spleen (5%) (Jadoul *et al.* 1999). Heart failure can be a severe and occasionally fatal complication (Kawano *et al.* 1998). Gastrointestinal involvement presents with bleeding, bowel perforation, chronic diarrhoea, or pseudo-obstruction, the degree of β2-amyloid deposition increasing according to time spent on dialysis (Jimenez *et al.* 1998).

Diagnosis

The precise diagnosis of β2-amyloidosis depends on histological confirmation of amyloid deposits. Material from joints is rarely available, although patients may often have had a preceding carpel tunnel syndrome and undergone surgical re-section with positive histology. Biopsies of asymptomatic structures such as rectum are largely unhelpful (Koch 1992). There are particular radiological fea-tures of β2-amyloid deposition, which help to differentiate it from other causes of arthropathy in dialysis patients. The joints most commonly involved are wrists, shoulders and hips. Swelling of soft tissue occurs with the development of bone cysts, which increase in number and size over time. There is preserva-tion or widening of the joint space, which differentiates cysts secondary to dialy-sis amyloidosis from osteoarthritis associated cysts (Maldague *et al.* 1996). Jadoul and van Ypersele have drawn up criteria for the specific diagnosis of amyloid arthropathy, Table 31.1, (Jadoul *et al.* 1999); however, it is rare to have all the required features, hence this can be insensitive. Ultrasound is a potentially more sensitive method of detection, as soft tissue changes precede bony involvement. A number of studies have found a correlation between thickening of shoulder tendons and hip capsules with the length of time on haemodialysis, and a corre-lation with symptoms of dialysis related amyloid (Kay *et al.* 1992; Jadoul *et al.* 1993; Cardinal *et al.* 1995). Ultrasound can also be used to follow the develop-ment of dialysis amyloid in affected patients.

A potentially more specific investigation for amyloid is the SAP (serum amyloid P component) scan. Amyloid fibrils bind the plasma serum amyloid protein P component; thus, by using a radiolabelled form of this, amyloid de-posits can be detected (Figure 31.1). This has proved extremely useful in the di-agnosis and follow-up of other types of amyloid in which the amyloid deposits have been found to be a lot more dynamic than previously thought (Gillmore *et al.* 1997). SAP scans have confirmed deposits in all sits of histologically confirmed disease in both haemodialysis and CAPD patients (Nelson *et al.* 1991;

Table 31.1 Radiological features specific for B2 amyloid arthropathy

Cysts	Must be >10 mm in hip and shoulder, or >5 mm in wrists. Must be situated outside areas prone to synovial inclusions, i.e. femoral neck and weight-bearing areas of the acetabulum, or be increasing in diameter by 30% per annum.
Joints	At least 2 joints must be affected. At least 2 defects must be present in one of these if both affected joints are wrists.
Joint space	Next to the lesion must be normal.

(Adapted from Jadoul and van Ypersele 1999).

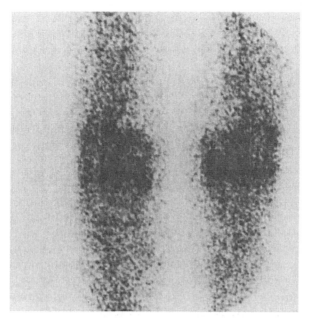

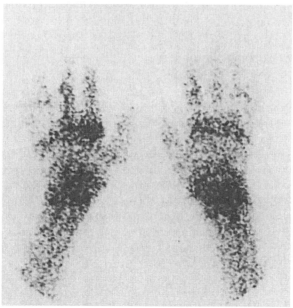

Fig. 31.1 I123-labelled serum amyloid P component scans in a patient who has under-gone haemodialysis for 16 years and who had developed carpel tunnel syndrome and large joint arthralgia typical of β2-microglobulin amyloidosis. There is uptake of tracer into amyloid deposits in the wrists and small joints of the hands (below) and in both knees (above). *Courtesy of Professor Philip Hawkins, National Amyloidosis Centre, Royal Free Hospital, London.*

Tan *et al.* 1999). Hip and shoulder deposits were less than expected from the clinical syndromes of the patients; this may reflect a lack of sensitivity for detecting β2-microglobulin in these specific areas. Many of the amyloid deposits were asymptomatic, an observation also made in post-mortem studies (Jadoul *et al.* 1997).

β2-microglobulin scintigraphy, with I^{131} labelled β2-microglobulin, is a potentially sensitive and specific screening method for detecting larger deposits of amyloid; however, the high levels of radiation limit its use (Floege *et al.* 1990). A possible alternative is ^{111}Indium DTPA labelled β2-microglobulin, but this remains to be validated (Schaeffer *et al.* 1996).

Pathogenesis

The main component of dialysis amyloid was identified as β2-microglobulin in 1985 (Geyjo *et al.* 1985); however the precise mechanisms by which it precipitates into amyloid fibrils are still not clear. The quantity of β2-microglobulin is likely to be important; β2-microglobulin is excreted mainly via the kidneys, and levels of β2-microglobulin rise as the glomerular filtration rate falls. When approaching end-stage renal disease a small decrease in glomerular filtration rate can substantially increase serum levels of β2-microglobulin (Kabanda 1994; McCarthy 1994). Acidosis is likely to be another contributory factor. In patients with chronic renal failure, the level of bicarbonate is inversely correlated with level of β2-microglobulin, and cells *in vitro* have been shown to produce and release more β2-microglobulin in acidotic conditions (Sonikian *et al.* 1996). Age is an independent factor which is negatively correlated with β2-microglobulin levels (Kabanda *et al.* 1994).

Whether or not β2-microglobulin is modified before it is able to form fibrils is another area of controversy. Linke *et al.* (1989) initially reported isolation of a truncated form of β2-microglobulin in amyloid deposits; this proteolysis of the N terminal of the molecule renders it more hydrophobic and could potentially initiate its deposition as amyloid fibrils. However, most of the β2-microglobulin in amyloid deposits has not been modified in this way (Argiles *et al.* 1995). Other forms of β2-microglobulin have been characterized, although they are not specific for amyloid deposits. Carboxymethyllysine, pentosidine, deoxyglucosone and imidazolone have all been identified in advanced glycation end products formed from β2-microglobulin (Miyata *et al.* 1996a and b; Niwa 1997; Motomiya *et al.* 1998). These modifications may result in cross-linking of the protein and amyloid formation, or the modification may occur to β2-microglobulin already present in amyloid deposits; this has been found to render the β2-microglobulin chemotactic and the resultant influx of monocytes are then stimulated to produce proinflammatory cytokines (Miyata *et al.* 1994; 1996c). Monocyte infiltration only occurs in the late symptomatic stage of dialysis amyloidosis, and the pro-inflammatory effect of the modified β2-microglobulin on these cells may contribute to the tissue damage that occurs. The β2-microglobulin molecules are associated with the surface of the amyloid fibrils (Inoue *et al.* 1997). A recent study has also shown that macrophages internalize the β2-microglobulin but that the lysosomes into which the β2-microglobulin is taken up are not effective in processing and clearing the β2-microglobulin, suggesting that a failure of clearance of the β2-microglobulin may also contribute to pathogenesis (Garcia–Garcia *et al.* 1999). β2-microglobulin has an affinity for collagen which may explain its deposition in joints and bones (Homma *et al.* 1989). Modification of β2-microglobulin by advanced glycation end products also increases its affinity for collagen (Hou *et al.* 1997). Other molecules, such as keratan sulphate, have also been found in close association with β2-microglobulin and may also account for its non-uniform deposition in the body (Athanasou *et al.* 1995).

Prevention/treatment

Transplantation is the most effective treatment for dialysis amyloid. Not only do the symptoms resolve but the radiological changes fail to progress. (Jadoul *et al.* 1989; Bardin *et al.* 1995; Mourad and Argiles 1996; Tan *et al.* 1996). This was initially attributed to the anti-inflammatory effects of high dose steroids used, but it soon became clear that the remission continued after steroids had been decreased or withdrawn. Bone cysts tend to persist (Jadoul *et al.* 1989; Mourad and Argiles 1996), although Tan *et al.* found that in 4/5 patients the cysts had decreased in size and there was ossification in the cyst walls (Tan *et al.* 1996). Tan *et al.* also found a decrease in measured articular amyloid in SAP scans in 8/9 transplanted patients, suggesting regression of the amyloid. However, any such regression must be extremely slow, as deposits persist for many years post-transplantation (Sethi *et al.* 1989; Jadoul *et al.* 1996). Presumably this is also the reason that dialysis amyloid recurs very quickly after transplant failure and return to dialysis (Mourad and Argiles 1996).

It was speculated that chronic ambulatory peritoneal dialysis (CAPD) may be protective, as better clearance of β2-microglobulin occurs with CAPD compared to haemodialysis (Sethi *et al.* 1988), and bioincompatible haemodialysis membranes have been implicated in raised levels of β2-microglobulin (DeBroe *et al.* 1987). However, clinical and post-mortem studies suggest that the incidence is similar in both groups (Benz *et al.* 1988; Jadoul *et al.* 1997). β2-microglobulin amyloidosis has also been reported in patients with chronic renal failure pre-dialysis (Zingraff *et al.* 1990). High flux haemodialysis membranes such as AN69 or polysulphone produce significantly greater clearance of β2-microglobulin and lower serum levels in patients (Marowka and Schiffl 1993; van Ypersele and Jadoul 1996). There are reports of improvements in symptoms after changing to high flux membranes (Hardouin *et al.* 1988), and it is currently our practice to use these membranes in patients with symptomatic dialysis arthropathy, although controlled long-term data is still needed to confirm these improvements.

Symptomatic treatment with analgesics is important. Non-steroidal anti-inflammatory drugs can be effective in reducing symptoms although they must be used cautiously in dialysis patients who have an increased risk of developing gastrointestinal complications; and a proton pump inhibitor should be prescribed concurrently. Low dose prednisolone is also helpful for those with more severe symptoms (Bardin 1994). However once steroids have been started it is extremely difficult to withdraw them, hence the long-term risks of steroid treatment, especially osteoporosis, must be taken into account before beginning treatment.

Surgical options should always be considered. Carpel tunnel syndromes should be operated on early to prevent permanent neuropathies. Joint replacements can be carried out for pathological fractures (Campistol *et al.* 1990). Others have also claimed successful results for various surgical procedures in severe shoulder pain, including synovectomy, resection of the coracoacromial ligament, curettage of cysts and ceramic implantation (Okutsu *et al.* 1991; Tekenaka *et al.* 1992). These procedures should be carried out by specialists in the field, and, in view of the progressive nature of the disease, longer-term follow-up is required before these can be generally recommended.

Conclusion

In summary, dialysis arthropathy is an unremitting, disabling disease whose incidence will increase with the increasing survival of patients on long-term dialysis. Advances made in understanding its pathogenesis are important as they may lead to therapeutic interventions to prevent the development of amyloidosis, and to treat those patients who are already affected. Treatment should include consideration of the available dialysis options such as the use of high flux membranes, in conjunction with symptomatic medical treatment and assessment by surgeons specializing in this field.

References

Allain T.J., Stevens P.E., Bridges L.R. *et al.* (1988). Dialysis myelopathy: quadriparesis due to extradural amyloid of β2-microglobulin origin. *British Medical Journal*, 296, 752–3.

Argiles A., Mourad G., Alexrud-Cavadore C. *et al.* (1989). High molecular weight proteins in haemodialysis associated amyloidosis. *Clinical Science*, 76: 547–52.

Argiles A., Mourad G. Kerr P.G. *et al.* (1994). Cells surrounding haemodialysis-associated amyloid deposits are mainly macrophages. *Nephrology, Dialysis Transplantation*, 9, 662–7.

Argiles A., Garcia-Garcia M., Derancourt J. *et al.* (1995). β2-microglobulin isoforms in healthy individuals and in amyloid deposits. *Kidney International*, 48: 1397–405.

Assenat H., Calemard E., Charra B. *et al.* (1980). Hemodialyse. Syndrome du canal carpien et substance amyloid. *La Nouvelle Presse Medicale*, 24: 1715.

Athanasou N.A. Puddle B. and Sallie B. (1995). Highly sulphated glycosaminoglycans in articular cartilage and other tissues containing β2-microglobulin dialysis amyloid deposits. *Nephrology, Dialysis, Transplantation*, 10: 1672–8.

Bardin T. (1994). Low dose prednisolone in dialysis-related arthropathy. *Revue du Rheumatism* (English Edition), 61: 97S–100S.

Bardin T. (1996). Arthropathy and carpel tunnel syndrome of β2-microglobulin amyloidosis. In *Dialysis amyloid* (ed. C. van Ypersele and T.P. Drueke), pp. 71–97. Oxford University Press.

Bardin T., Lebail-Darne J.L., Zingraff J. *et al.* (1995). Dialysis arthropathy: outcome after renal transplantation. *American Journal of Medicine*, 99: 243–8.

Benz R.L., Siegfried J.W. and Teehan B.P. (1988). Carpel tunnel syndrome in dialysis patients: comparison between continuous ambulatory peritoneal dialysis and haemodialysis populations. *American Journal of Kidney Disease*, 9: 473–6.

Borgatti P.P., Lusenti T., Franco V., Anelli A. and Brancaccio D. (1991). Guyon's syndrome in a long term haemodialysis patient. *Nephrology, Dialysis and Transplantation*, 6: 734–5.

Brown E.A. and Gower P.E. (1982). Joint problems in patients on maintenance haemodialysis. *Clinical Nephrology*, 18: 247–50.

Brown E.A., Arnold I. and Gower P.E. (1986). Dialysis arthropathy: complication of long term treatment with haemodialysis. *British Medical Journal*, 292: 163–6.

Campistol J.M., Sole M., Munoz-Gomez J. *et al.* (1990). Pathological fractures in patients who have amyloidosis associated with dialysis. *Journal of Bone and Joint Surgery*, 72-A: 568–74.

Cardinal E., Buckwalter K.A., Braunstein E.M. *et al.* (1995). Amyloidosis in the shoulder of patients on chronic haemodialysis: sonographic findings. *American Journal of Roentgenology*, 166: 153–6.

Charra B., Calemard E. and Laurent G. (1988). Chronic renal failure treatment duration and mode: their relevance to the late dialysis periarticular syndrome. *Blood Purification*, 6: 117–24.

Chary-Valckenaere I., Kessler M., Mainard D. *et al.* (1998). Amyloid and non-amyloid carpel tunnel syndrome in patients receiving chronic renal dialysis. *Journal of Rheumatology*, 25: 1164–70.

Danesh F.R., Klinlmann J., Yokoo H. *et al.* (1999). Fatal cervical spondyloarthropathy in a haemodialysis patient with severe systemic deposition of β2-microglobulin amyloid. *American Journal of Kidney Disease*, 33: 563–6.

DeBroe M.E., Nouwen J., Waeleghem J.P. (1987). On the mechanisms and site of production of β2-microglobulin during haemodialysis. *Nephrology, Dialysis, Transplantation*, 2: 124–5.

Ferrari A.J., Rothfuss S. and Schumacher H.R. Jr (1997). Dialysis arthropathy: identification and evaluation of a subset of patients with unexplained inflammatory effusions. *Journal of Rheumatology*, 24: 1780–6.

Floege J., Durchert W., Brandis A. *et al.* (1990). Imaging of dialysis related amyloid (AB-amyloid) deposits with 131–I–β2-microglobulin. *Kidney International*, 38: 1169–76.

Fututake T., Takagi K., Kuwabara S. *et al.* (1997). Destructive spondyloarthropathy of the cervical spine in haemodialysed patients. *No-To-Shinkei*, 49: 713–22.

Garber C., Jadoul M., Noel H. *et al.* (1999). Histological characteristics of sternoclavicular beta-2-microglobulin amyloidosis and clues for its histiogenesis. *Kidney International*, 55: 1983–90.

Garcia-Garcia M., Argiles A., Gouin-Charnet A. *et al.* (1999). Impaired lysosomal processing of B2-microglobulin by infiltrating macrophages in dialysis amyloidosis. *Kidney International*, 55: 899–906.

Geyjo F., Yamada T., Odani S. *et al.* (1985). A new form of amyloid protein associated with chronic haemodialysis was identified as β2-microglobulin. *Biochemistry Biophysics Research Communication*, 129: 701–6.

Gillmore J.D., Hawkins P.N. and Pepys M.B. (1997). Amyloidosis: a review of recent diagnostic and therapeutic developments. *British Journal of Haematology*, 99: 245–56.

Hardouin P., Flipo R.M., Foissac-Gegoux P. *et al.* (1988). Dialysis-related β2-microglobulin amyloid arthropathy. Improvements of clinical symptoms after a switch of dialysis membranes. *Clinical Rheumatology*, 7: 41–5.

Homma N., Geyjo F., Isemura P. *et al.* (1989). Collagen-binding affinity of Beta-2-microglobulin, a preprotein of haemodialysis-associated amyloidosis. *Nephron*, 53: 37–40.

Hou F.F., Chertow G.M., Kay J. *et al.* (1997). Interaction between β2-microglobulin and advanced glycation end products in the development of dialysis-related amyloidosis. *Kidney International*, 51: 1514–19.

Inoue S., Kuroiwa M., Ohashi K. *et al.* (1997). Ultrastructural organisation of haemodialysis-associated β2-microglobulin amyloid fibrils. *Kidney International*, 52: 1543–9.

Jadoul M., Malgem J., Pirson Y. *et al.* (1989). Effect of renal transplantation on the radiological signs of dialysis amyloid osteoarthropathy. *Clinical Nephrology*, 32: 194–7.

Jadoul M., Malgem J., Van de Berg B. *et al.* (1993). Ultrasonographic detection of thickened joint capsules and tendons as markers of dialysis-related amyloidosis: a cross-sectional and longitudinal study. *Nephrology Dialysis, Transplantation*, 8: 1104–9.

Jadoul M.C., Noel H., van-Ypersele-de Strihou C. (1996). Histological β-2-microglobulin-amyloidosis 10 years after a successful renal transplantation. *American Journal of Kidney Diseases*, 27: 888–90.

Jadoul M., Garbar C., Noel H. *et al.* (1997). Histological prevalence of B2-microglobulin amyloidosis in haemodialysis: a prospective post mortem study. *Kidney International*, 51: 1928–32.

Jadoul M., Garbar C., Vanholder R. *et al.* (1998). Prevalence of β2-microglobulin amyloidosis in CAPD patients compared with haemodialysis patients. *Kidney International*, 54: 956–9.

Jadoul M.C. and van-Ypersele-de Strihou C. (1999). β2-microglobulin amyloidosis. In *Complications of Long-term Dialysis* (eds E. Brown and P. Parfrey) p. 121–44. Oxford University Press, New York.

Jimenez R.E., Price D.A., Pinkus G.S., *et al.* (1998). Development of β2-microglobulin amyloidosis correlates with time on dialysis. *American Journal of Surgical Pathology*, 22: 729–35.

Kabanda A., Jadoul M., Pochet J.M. *et al.* (1994). Determinants of the serum concentrations of low molecular weight proteins in patients on maintenance haemodialysis. *Kidney International*, 45, 1689–96.

Kawano M., Muramoto H., Yamada M. *et al.* (1998). Fatal beta2-microglobulin amyloidosis in patients on haemodialysis. *American Journal of Kidney Disease*, 31, E4.

Kay J., Benson C.B., Lester S. *et al.* (1992). Utility of high-resolution ultrasound for the diagnosis of dialysis-related amyloidosis. *Arthritis and Rheumatism*, 35: 926–32.

Koch K.M. (1992). Dialysis related amyloidosis. *Kidney International*, 41: 1416–29.

Kroner G., Stabler A., Seiderer M. *et al.* (1991). β2-microglobulin related amyloidosis causing atlanto-axial spondyloarthropathy with spinal cord compression in haemodialysis patients: detection by MRI. *Nephrology, Dialysis, Transplantation*, S2: 91–5.

Linke R.P., Hampl H., Lobeck H. *et al.* (1989). Lysine-specific cleavage of β2-microglobulin in amyloid deposits associated with haemodialysis. *Kidney International*, 36: 675–81.

Maldague B., Malghem J. and Van de Berg B. (1996). Radiology of dialysis amyloidosis. In *Dialysis amyloid* (ed. C. van Ypersele and T.B. Drueke), Oxford University Press, 98–135.

Marcelli C., Perennou D., Cyteval C. *et al.* (1996). Amyloidosis-related cord compression in long-term haemodialysis patients. Three case reports. *Spine*, 21: 381–5.

Marowka C. and Schiffl H. (1993). Comparative evaluation of β2-microglobulin removal by haemodialysis membranes: a six year follow up. *Nephron*, 63: 368–9.

McCarthy J.T., Williams A.W. and Johnson W.J. (1994). Serum β2-microglobulin concentrations in dialysis patients: importance of intrinsic renal function. *Journal of Laboratory and Clinical Medicine*, 123: 495–505.

Miyata T., Inagi R., Iida Y. *et al.* (1994). Involvement of β2-microglobulin modified with advanced glycation end products in the pathogenesis of haemodialysis associated amyloidosis. *Journal of Clinical Investigation*, 93: 521–8.

Miyata T., Taneda S., Kawai R. *et al.* (1996a). Identification of pentosidine as a native structure for advanced glycation end products in β2-microglobulin containing amyloid fibrils in patients with dialysis-related amyloidosis. *Proceedings of the National Academy of Science USA*, 93: 2353–8.

Miyata T., Ueda Y., Shinzato T., Iida Y. *et al.* (1996b). Accumulation of albumin linked and free-form pentosidine in the circulation of uraemic patients with end-stage renal failure: Renal implications in the pathophysiology of pentosidine. *Journal of the American Society of Nephrology*, 7: 1198–1206.

Miyata T., Iida Y., Ueda Y. *et al.* (1996c). Monocyte/macrophage response to β2-microglobulin modified with advanced glycation end products. *Kidney International*, 49: 538–50.

Motomiya M., Oyama N., Iwamoto H. *et al.* (1998). N-(carboxymethyl 0 lysine in blood from maintenance haemodialysis patients may contribute to dialysis-related amyloidosis. *Kidney International*, 54: 1357–66.

Mourad G. and Argiles A. (1996). Renal transplantation relieves the symptoms but does not reverse β2-microglobulin amyloidosis. *Journal of the American Society of Nephrology*, 7, 798–804.

Nelson S.R., Hawkins P.N. and Richardson S. (1991). Imaging of haemodialysis-associated amyloidosis with ^{123}I-serum amyloid P component. *Lancet*, 338: 335–8.

Niwa T., Katsuzaki T., Miyazaki S. *et al.* (1997). Amyloid β2-microglobulin is modified with imidazolone, a novel advanced glycation end product, in dialysis-related amyloidosis. *Kidney International*, 51: 187–94.

Okutsu I., Ninomiya S., Takatori Y. *et al.* (1991). Endoscopic management of shoulder pain in long-term haemodialysis patients. *Nephrology, Dialysis, Transplantation*, 6: 117–19.

Schaeffer J., Floege J. and Koch K.M. (1996). Whole body scintigraphy. In: *Dialysis amyloid* (ed. C. van Ypersele and T.B. Drueke), Oxford University Press, 145–55.

Sethi D., Brown E. and Gower P.E. (1988). CAPD, protection against developing dialysis amyloid? *Nephron*, 50, 85–6.

Sethi D., Brown E., Cary N. *et al.* (1989). Persistence of dialysis amyloid after renal transplantation. *American Journal of Nephrology*, 9, 173–4.

Sethi D., Naunton Morgan T.C., Brown F.A. *et al.* (1990). Dialysis arthropathy: a clinical, biochemical, radiological and histological study of 36 patients. *Quarterly Journal of Medicine*, 282, 1061–82.

Sonikian M., Gogusev J., Zingraff J. *et al.* (1996). Potential effect of metabolic acidosis on β2-microglobulin generation: in vivo and in vitro studies. *Journal of the American Society of Nephrology*, 7: 350–60.

Takenaka R., Fukatsu A., Matsuo S. *et al.* (1992). Surgical treatment of haemodialysis-related shoulder arthropathy. *Clinical Nephrology*, 38: 224–30.

Tan S., Irish A., Winearls C. *et al.* (1996). Long term effect of renal transplantation on dialysis-related deposits and symptomatology. *Kidney International*, 50: 282–9.

Tan S.Y., Baillod R., Brown E. *et al.* (1999). Clinical, radiological and serum amyloid P component scintigraphic features of β2-microglobulin amyloidosis associated with continuous ambulatory peritoneal dialysis. *Nephrology, Dialysis Transplantation*, 14: 1467–71.

Van Ypersele de Strihou C., Honhon B., Vandenbroucke J.M. *et al.* (1988). Dialysis amyloidosis. In: *Advances in Nephrology*, Vol. 117 (ed. J.P. Grunfeld, J.F. Bach and J.L. Funck-Brentano), pp. 401–22. Year Book Medical Publishers.

Van Ypersele de Strihou C., Jadoul M., Malghem J. *et al.* (1991). Effect of dialysis membrane and patient's age on signs of dialysis related amyloidosis. *Kidney International*, 39, 1012–19.

Van Ypersele de Strihou C. and Jadoul M. (1996). Prevention and treatment β2-microglobulin amyloidosis. In *Dialysis amyloid* (ed. C. Van Ypersele and T.B. Drueke). Oxford University Press, p. 261–76.

Zingraff J.J., Noel L.H., Bardin T. *et al.* (1990). β2-microglobulin amyloidosis in chronic renal failure. *New England Journal of Medicine*, 323: 1070–1.

32

Rheumatological complications of renal disease and transplantation

Zunaid Karim, Cathy Lawson, and Paul Emery

Introduction

Renal manifestations of rheumatic disease occur commonly. These include renal osteodystrophy and dialysis associated arthropathy. Renal transplantation and its management can create a new series of rheumatic problems. Transplant can be complicated by continuing osteodystrophy, osteoporosis, and crystal arthropathy in addition to osteonecrosis, acute bone pain syndrome and reflex sympathetic dystrophy.

Renal osteodystrophy

Renal osteodystrophy encompasses a range of bone diseases including osteoporosis, osteomalacia, secondary hyperparathyroidism, aluminium toxicity, and β2-microglobulin amyloidosis.

Osteomalacia can produce generalized pain and may result in fractures. There may be an associated proximal myopathy. Reduced levels of 1,25 dihydroxyvitamin D3 occur as a result of reduced hydroxylation of its precursor, due to chronic renal failure but also by further inhibition through increased phosphate levels. As calcium levels fall, hyperparathyroidism develops, and calcium levels are then increased via bone resorption. Osteitis fibrosa develops as a result of secondary hyperparathyroidism, with osteopaenia and subperiosteal erosions.

β2-microglobulin amyloidosis is the consequence of β2-microglobulin protein deposition. It can produce carpal tunnel syndrome, shoulder arthropathy, bone cysts, femoral fractures and a destructive cervical spondyloarthropathy. It is more common in patients on long-term haemodialysis.[1]

Aluminium-induced bone disease may present as bone pain or a slow healing fracture. Both aluminium-containing phosphate binders and the dialysate can contribute to overload.

Markers of osteodystrophy

Serum alkaline phosphatase, immunoreactive parathyroid hormone (PTH) and aluminium levels are commonly used to evaluate osteodystrophy (Table 32.1).

Table 32.1 Biochemical features of aluminium-induced bone disease and secondary hyperparathyroidism. Levels of serum calcium and phosphate are not predictors of type or severity of bone disease

	Aluminium-induced bone disease	Secondary hyperparathyroidism
Alkaline phosphatase	Normal/Increased	Increased++
Parathyroid hormone	<2 times normal	>2 times normal
Serum aluminium (mcg/L)	Increased	Increased
Increase in aluminium level after desferrioxamine challenge	>150 mcg/L	<150 mcg/L

Secondary hyperparathyroidism is typically associated with very raised levels of alkaline phosphatase, high parathyroid hormone levels, a low basal aluminium level and desferrioxamine challenge producing less than 150 mcg/L increase in serum aluminium. Aluminium-induced bone disease, however, results in lower alkaline phosphatase levels, less than twice normal PTH levels, and an increase of more than 150 mcg/L in aluminium levels with desferrioxamine challenge.[1] Serum osteocalcin (bone gammacarboxylglutamic acid-protein) correlates with PTH and alkaline phosphatase before and after transplant and has been suggested as a confirmatory parameter of renal osteodystrophy.[2] It has been suggested that alkaline phosphatase may be an unreliable marker of bone resorption, as both cyclosporin A (CyA) and prednisolone can affect levels.[3,4]

Most radiological features appear late in disease (Fig. 32.1). Bone biopsy is often required to ascertain the type and severity of bone disease.

Prevention and treatment of renal osteodystrophy

Serum calcium levels should be kept higher than 2.5 mmol/L by oral calcium supplements and dialysate calcium. Dietary phosphate restriction should aim to keep phosphate levels below 1.4 mmol/L, along with phosphate binding agents and dialysis. Vitamin D supplementation is also employed. Aluminium toxicity is minimized by avoiding drugs containing aluminium, and restricting aluminium concentrations in the dialysate.

Refractory hyperparathyroidism in a patient on appropriate medication indicates the need for parathyroidectomy, and symptomatic aluminium toxicity necessitates desferrioxamine therapy. The shoulder arthropathy of β2-microglobulin amyloidosis is often resistant to conservative management and may require surgical intervention.[1]

Renal osteodystrophy after transplant

Most patients undergoing transplant already have evidence of renal osteodystrophy. Renal insufficiency post-transplant may cause ongoing hyperparathyroidism and osteomalacia, and in addition corticosteroids contribute to osteoporosis.

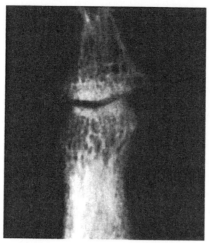

Fig. 32.1 Radiographs of a patient with renal osteodystrophy demonstrating (A) typical changes of subperiosteal erosion (inset), tuft resorption, vascular calcification, and a Brown Tumour in the proximal phalanx of the index finger; and (B) patchy osteosclerosis resulting in the classic 'rugger jersey' spine appearance.

Following renal transplant, metabolic changes occur with a reduction in PTH levels and an improvement in acidosis and vitamin D metabolism. There is then a slow resolution of parathyroid gland hyperplasia and hypersecretion. Osteomalacia and aluminium related bone disease usually improve, as is often the case with amyloid. Hypophosphataemia is considered a cause of persistent osteomalacia after successful transplant. This can be due to renal tubular phosphate handling dysfunction, treatment with corticosteroids, or phosphate-binding antacids.[5]

Assessment of renal osteodystrophy in transplant recipients is directed towards monitoring persistent hyperparathyroidism, and diagnosing osteonecrosis and osteopaenia.

Dialysis-related arthropathy

This may present with carpal tunnel syndrome, trigger finger, synovial hypertrophy and hand muscle wasting. Hand function in particular is found to decrease with time spent on dialysis.[6] Of historical note, the use of cuprophane membranes for dialysis was associated with a symmetrical polyarthritis, in nearly all patients on dialysis for more than ten years.[7] It resulted in lytic bone deposits of β2-microglobulin, and associated symptoms included shoulder impingement syndrome, carpal tunnel syndrome, and hip and knee pain.[8] Symptoms improved on changing to synthetic polyacrylonitrile membranes.[9]

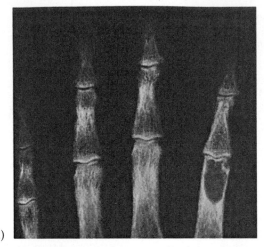

(A)

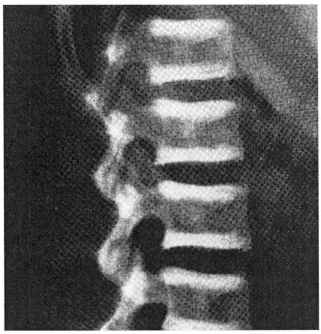

(B)

Fig. 32.1 Radiographs of a patient with renal osteodystrophy demonstrating (A) typical changes of subperiosteal erosion (inset), tuft resorption, vascular calcification, and a Brown Tumour in the proximal phalanx of the index finger; and (B) patchy osteosclerosis resulting in the classic 'rugger jersey' spine appearance.

Osteoporosis

Osteoporosis is common in renal transplant recipients and is predominantly related to corticosteroid use. High dose corticosteroids are commonly prescribed immediately post-transplant and during periods of rejection. The increased use of other immunosuppressive agents such as CyA and azathioprine has allowed for an overall reduction in corticosteroid use; however many transplant recipients develop osteoporotic fractures that reduce their quality of life.[10] Unfortunately the wide spectrum of bone disease in renal patients has often excluded them from studies of prevention and treatment of osteoporosis, leading to limited evidenced-based management guidelines.

Clinical features

There is a trend for bone mineral density (BMD) to be lower than normal at the time of transplant.[11] This may be due to previous corticosteroid use and long-standing metabolic acidosis.[1] In addition, BMD loss following transplant is more rapid than in other patient groups.[12]

The prevalence of lumbar osteopaenia and osteoporosis in renal transplant recipients has been calculated at 28.6% and 7.1% respectively, with a mean time post-transplant of 8.1 years.[13] Cross-sectional studies have revealed fracture prevalence to be 7–11% in non-diabetic transplant recipients, and up to 45% in diabetics.[14,15] These fractures commonly involve the vertebrae, long bones or metatarsals and occur relatively late in the transplant period.

Bone loss is greatest during the first six to twelve months[11,16,17] and predominantly affects cancellous (trabecular) bone.[10] This is consistent with a dominant corticosteroid effect. Bone loss continues in the first year with density declining by between 6 and 15%.[12,16] Losses in second and subsequent years of 1–2% have been demonstrated,[13,17] although one study has suggested no loss of bone after the second year in excess of the normal age and sex dependent decline.[11]

Pathogenesis

The pathogenesis of rapid bone loss post-transplant is multifactorial. It may relate to pre-existing hyperparathyroidism rendering cortical bone thin. Genetic factors may also be implicated, with patients who are homozygous recessive for the vitamin D receptor gene being shown to recover more bone in the 3–12 months after transplant than those who are heterozygous or homozygous dominant.[10] Other factors contributing to bone loss are uraemia, secondary hyperparathyroidism, aluminium accumulation, and osteomalacia.

Risk factors

Prednisolone dosage is the most important risk factor for bone loss,[13] with a significant correlation between daily prednisolone dose and the degree of vertebral bone loss. Initial PTH levels also correlate with bone loss; however, CyA, azathioprine dose and total daily Ca intake do not.[17] Vitamin D therapy and physical activity tend to counterbalance bone loss. It is suggested that when prednisolone dosage falls below 7.5 mg daily only normal BMD loss is apparent.[11] In contrast, most patients taking in excess of 10 mg daily will sustain bone loss.[10] Certain studies suggest a protective effect of CyA against corticosteroid-induced osteopaenia,[18-20] whereas others demonstrate a causal link between CyA and osteoporosis.[21-23] As acute graft rejection requiring high dose corticosteroid has the principal effect on bone loss post-transplant, cautious reduction of corticosteroid dosage to avoid rejection is likely overall to cause less reduction in BMD than rapid reduction leading to rejection.[17] The effect on BMD these drugs have by repression of active inflammatory disease is unclear.

Mechanism of action of drugs

All of the mechanisms by which corticosteroids increase bone resorption (Table 32.2) are exacerbated by chronic renal failure. They have a direct effect on the skeleton by inhibiting bone formation and accelerating resorption.[16] Corticosteroids inhibit calcium absorption from the GI tract, interfering with the action of 1,25-dihydroxy vitamin D. They induce urinary calcium loss possibly by a direct action on the tubules. These effects may lead to secondary hyperparathyroidism, with further resorption of skeletal calcium. Corticosteroids also suppress gonadotrophin secretion leading to diminished ovarian or testicular function. They reduce bioavailability of skeletal growth factors by inhibiting pituitary secretion of growth hormone. Corticosteroid myopathy has a negative effect on weight bearing activity, and may also increases the risk of falling, with subsequent fracture.

CyA and tacrolimus are thought to have their effect by increasing bone turnover and resorption, as well as decreasing gonadal steroid synthesis.[16] Tacrolimus may have an even greater effect on bone loss than CyA.[24]

Investigations and management

Patients awaiting transplant should be assessed at baseline with thoracic and lumbar spine radiographs, DEXA (Dual energy X-ray absorptiometry) scanning,

Table 32.2   Mechanism of action by which glucocorticoids contribute to osteoporosis

Site	Effect
Bone	Inhibit bone formation, accelerate resorption
GI tract	Inhibit calcium absorption
Kidney	Induce urinary calcium loss
Muscle	Myopathy; reduced weight-bearing activity, also increased risk of falls and subsequent fracture
Hypothalamic-Pituitary Axis	Inhibit secretion of growth hormone and gonadotrophin; reduced bioavailability of skeletal growth factors and reduced ovarian or testicular function

Table 32.3 Investigation and management of bone metabolism following transplant. Other markers currently under investigation include collagen products, D-pyridinoline and N-telopeptides

	Baseline	Post-transplant
Serum	Calcium, phosphate, alkaline phosphatase, parathyroid hormone, vitamin D, osteocalcin and testosterone	Every 6 months
Urine	Calcium	Every 6 months
Radiography	Lumbar spine and thorax	If suspicion of fracture
DEXA	Hip and lumbar spine	Every 6 months for 2 years, then annually

plus serum and urinary markers[10] (Table 32.3). Post-transplant, patients should be monitored with DEXA scanning and serum and urinary markers. Radiographs need only be repeated if a fracture is suspected.[16]

Therapy for reduced bone mass should be instituted during the waiting period, and for those with normal bone density, immediately post-transplant[10] (Table 32.4). As yet there are no data showing that pre-transplant therapy reduces the risk of fractures.

Calcitonin, bisphosphonates and hormone replacement therapy (HRT) have been shown to be beneficial in corticosteroid-induced osteoporosis. However, bisphosphonates are not recommended in moderate to severe renal insufficiency (creatinine clearance <30), as they are renally excreted. HRT improves BMD in corticosteroid-induced osteoporosis, and animal studies demonstrate prevention of CyA-induced bone loss by oestrogens.[10] Some authors suggest that HRT alone is not enough to prevent bone loss in the first year. Hypogonadal men should receive testosterone.

Table 32.4 Recommendations for preventing and managing osteoporosis

- Treat underlying disorders affecting bone and mineral metabolism
- Reduce immunosuppressive drugs to maintenance doses as rapidly as possible
- Use lowest maintenance doses of drugs possible
- Resume weight-bearing exercise as soon as possible
- Adequate dietary calcium (1000 mg daily for men, 1500 mg daily for post-menopausal women)
- Adequate vitamin D (400–800 IU daily)
- Minimize lifestyle risk factors for osteoporosis (smoking and alcohol)
- Avoid loop diuretics which increase urinary calcium excretion
- Monitor serum testosterone in men and supplement if hypogonadal
- Begin oestrogen replacement in post-menopausal and pre-menopausal amenorrhoeic women
- Consider bisphosphonates or calcitonin, if appropriate

Patients should receive the recommended daily allowance of calcium and vitamin D. Pharmacological doses of vitamin D have also been recommended to prevent corticosteroid and transplant-induced osteoporosis,[25–28] although hypercalcaemia can occur.

Osteonecrosis

Osteonecrosis is the result of impairment of blood supply, usually to the femoral head, which leads to cell death in components of cartilage and bone. This explains the frequently used terms of 'avascular necrosis' or 'aseptic osteonecrosis'. Prevalence in renal transplant recipients has been documented as up to 40%[1] in the past, with more recent data suggesting a prevalence of around 5%.[29] It most commonly affects the femoral head, but has also been described in the humeral head and distal femur.

High dose corticosteroids and pre-transplant hyperparathyroidism are risk factors for osteonecrosis. The prevalence of osteonecrosis in renal transplant recipients receiving high dose prednisolone (average 12.5 mg daily in the first year) has been calculated at 11.2%, compared with 5.1% in those receiving low (average 6.5 mg) dose.[30]

The introduction of CyA has led to lower doses of corticosteroid being used to treat episodes of rejection.[29] The incidence of osteonecrosis has subsequently reduced; however, a causal relationship between CyA therapy alone[31] and osteonecrosis of the femoral head has also been demonstrated. Other risk factors in transplant recipients are hyperlipidaemia and gout.

Patients are often asymptomatic, but can describe pain when weight-bearing and at rest. Later, they may notice a limp, or even later describe reduced range of movement.

Radiographs are often unhelpful in early stages, with bone scintigraphy and MRI used for diagnosis. MRI may detect lesions prior to symptoms (Fig. 32.2). The lack of a clear understanding of the natural history of asymptomatic lesions, in addition to cost and the complication rate of surgery, are against routine screening.[1,32]

Conservative therapy for symptomatic femoral head osteonecrosis usually fails[33] and surgical decompression is required.[1,34]

Fig. 32.2 This patient with established osteonecrosis of the right hip presented with recent onset left hip pain. Radiograph of the pelvis (A) demonstrated established osteonecrosis on the right with a normal appearance on the left. MRI in the same patient (B) revealed established osteonecrosis, with subchondral collapse and sclerosis, on the right and early changes on the left.

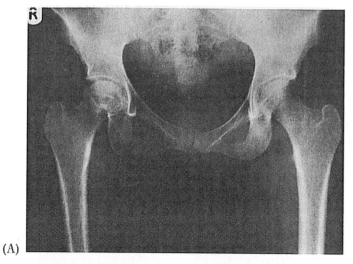

(A)

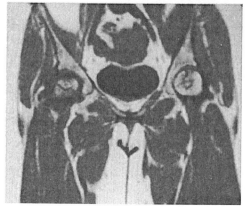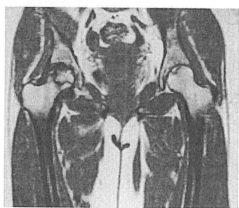

(B)

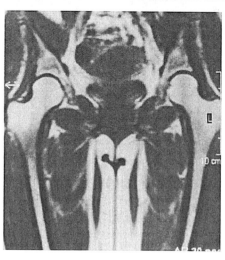

The frequency of arthroplasty for painful osteonecrosis of the hip, in renal transplant recipients, has been calculated at 2%. Although it is the treatment of choice with good symptom relief, there is often a poor functional outcome[29,35] as well as a high rate of early and late complications, compared with primary hip arthroplasty. Bilateral hip involvement, osteoporosis and high rates of skeletal re-modelling may contribute to higher failure rates in this group.[36]

Acute hot joint

An acute hot joint in transplant recipients presents difficult problems, both with regard to diagnosis and management. Painful joint effusions can occur during episodes of acute rejection, which resolve with treatment of the rejection. Radiography, and examination of synovial fluid may be helpful in the differential diagnosis (Table 32.5).

Gout

Sodium urate crystal deposition is more common in renal insufficiency than renal failure, and is rare in dialysis patients. Gout after transplant is due to persistent reduction in creatinine clearance and CyA use.[1]

Table 32.5   Acute hot joint. Radiographic and light microscopy (LM) features that may help diagnosis. Synovial fluid should always be cultured for bacteria and fungi

	Gout	Hydroxyapatite	Pseudogout	Sepsis
Radiology				
Calcification	Usually absent	Calcific tendonitis	Chondrocalcinosis	Usually absent
Erosion	May be characteristic	Severe damage Milwaukee shoulder	Often degenerative	May see marked destruction over short time
Crystals				
Type	Monosodium urate	Basic calcium phosphate	CPPD	May co-exist with gout
Shape	Needle	Single crystals not seen with LM	Small, rod-like	
Birefringence	Strong, negative	Not birefringent	Weak, positive	
Synovial fluid				
Appearance	Clear/Turbid			Turbid
Viscosity	Reduced			Reduced
WCC/ml	10000–20000			>25000
Neutrophils	~80%			~95%

The incidence of CyA related gout in renal transplant recipients is estimated at 10%, and is increased by concurrent diuretic use.[37] Potential factors causing CyA induced hyperuricaemia are decreased renal function and tubular dysfunction in handling of urate.

Symptoms can be severe with early tophi. An unusual pattern of gouty arthropathy with sacroilitis and enthesopathy has been described in transplant recipients.[38]

Prophylactic therapy may include probenecid or low dose colchicine if renal function is normal. Low dose allopurinol can be used if the dose of azathioprine is reduced and the patient monitored carefully.[37] Concomitant use of allopurinol and azathioprine may lead to leucopaenia. Non-steroidal anti-inflammatories (NSAIDs) and colchicine can be used with caution in acute attacks, if renal function is acceptable. Intra-articular corticosteroid is often used as the treatment of choice. Simultaneous joint aspiration allows synovial fluid to be examined under polarized light for crystals, and cultured for bacteria and fungi. The presence of urate crystals in the aspirate does not exclude co-existent infection.

Hydroxyapatite

Basic calcium phosphate crystals (BCP) found in pathological tissues and fluid include carbonate-substituted apatite, octacalcium phosphate, and tricalcium phosphate. Periarticular deposits tend to cause acute inflammatory episodes such as calcific rotator cuff tendinitis, whereas intra-articular BCP is more often associated with chronic, non-inflammatory degeneration, for example Milwaukee shoulder.[37]

Hyperphosphataemia occurs with reduced glomerular filtration, and is further increased by secondary hyperparathyroidism in chronic renal failure. Crystals deposit when the calcium-phosphate solubility product exceeds 14 mmol/L. Radiographs in periarticular disease show soft tissue calcification adjacent to joints with no erosions and normal joint space.[1]

Most acute disease responds to anti-inflammatory agents, but disease may be resistant or recurrent. Colchicine may be equally effective.[39] Resistant episodes can be treated with needle aspiration or injection of corticosteroids. If unsuccessful, arthroscopic calcium removal and bursectomy has been suggested.[40]

In Milwaukee shoulder, NSAIDs and physical therapy are used. Intra-articular corticosteroids are often unhelpful with mild, transient pain relief. There is often severe radiographic damage. Prevention of this form of crystal deposition in CRF is by dietary phosphate restriction, dialysis, and phosphate binding agents. Parathyroidectomy can be considered if these measures fail.[1]

Pseudogout (pyrophosphate)

Calcium pyrophosphate deposition (CPPD) is less common in renal disease than urate or BCP deposition, and is rare in dialysis patients. There is an association with Bartter's syndrome, and deposition can lead to acute synovitis.[1]

Disease results from deposition of crystals in articular cartilage. Clinical manifestations include an acute monoarticular or pauciarticular arthritis known as pseudogout, and a chronic arthritis resembling degenerative joint disease.

The natural history of attacks is more variable than gout, and prolonged symptoms may be due to the common association between CPPD disease and osteoarthritis. Predisposing factors include hyperparathyroidism, age, trauma, meniscectomy, hypomagnesaemia, hypothyroidism, hypophosphataemia, and haemochromatosis. However, treatment of the underlying condition may not alter the course of the arthritis. Rarely, joint infection may coexist with CPPD crystals.

Oral colchicine has been shown to be effective as a prophylactic measure, but not as an acute treatment. Intravenous colchicine in CPPD disease has been shown to be effective, but patient comorbidity may preclude its use. Intra-articular corticosteroids are the mainstay of therapy and reduce symptom duration as compared with NSAIDs.[41] Adrenocorticotrophic hormone (ACTH) has been used with some success in acute pseudogout, as well as in gout.[42]

Sepsis

Infectious complications in renal transplant recipients are common, with agents including opportunistic organisms, such as mycobacteria and fungi, as well as common pathogens. Impaired host defences secondary to underlying renal disease or immunosuppression, and pre-existing joint damage are potential contributors to septic arthritis post-transplant.[43] Frequency of septic arthritis has been documented at less than 1%,[44] however this rises to 19% in those who have a joint replacement after organ transplant.[45]

Gram–negative joint infections in this group have been associated with concurrent urinary tract infection.[46] Other potential sources of infection should also be considered. Sepsis usually occurs in a single joint, most often within 18 months of transplant. A history of intra-articular corticosteroid injection, or infection in the joint prior to transplant, should raise the index of suspicion.

Gout and infection may co-exist,[47] and thorough assessment of the synovial fluid is the definitive means of distinguishing between the two.

Acute bone pain syndrome

There are several reports in the literature of bone pain in renal transplant recipients on CyA,[48–51] with prevalence calculated at 19%.[51]

Symptoms can develop up to two years post-renal transplant, and usually disappear within 2–6 weeks of stopping the drug.[52] Pain is usually reported to be bilateral, acute in onset and episodic with a deep aching sensation, lasting several hours at a time. It usually affects the knees and ankles but can affect other areas including wrists, shoulder and thighs, and is often worse at night or when lying flat. The pain appears generally related to higher serum levels of CyA, and reducing the dose may improve symptoms.[53,52] Examination is usually normal, and there are no consistent investigation abnormalities.[49]

NSAIDs and other analgesics are reported to be ineffective, with some patients requiring intravenous opiates to control pain.[48] Our group has documented a patient with psoriatic arthritis on CyA who required opiate analgesia prior to the syndrome being recognized. The patient's symptoms resolved within days of discontinuing the CyA. Nifedipine has provided complete relief of symptoms in 21 out of 22 patients in a prospective study.[51]

The pathophysiology is unclear, but a vascular aetiology has been suggested in view of the good response to calcium channel blockers. This syndrome has also been described with tacrolimus.[54]

Reflex sympathetic dystrophy (RSD)

RSD has been described, usually occurring 2–3 months after renal transplant. Incidence has been described as between 2% and 2.5%.[55] Patients present with symmetrical pain in the ankles and knees, and difficulty walking. Upper limb symptoms are rare. Physical findings include periarticular soft tissue swelling and vasomotor changes, and investigations show patchy osteoporosis on radiographs and increased epiphyseal uptake of 99 mTc with a periarticular distribution. Patients tend to be on CyA therapy with blood levels greater than 200 ng/ml, and symptoms improve when doses of CyA are reduced and blood levels fall. Treatment with calcitonin and calcium channel blockers has been shown to be effective.[56] The efficacy of corticosteroids in the treatment of uncomplicated RSD has been demonstrated.[57] It is possible that this may protect against the development of a full RSD pattern. Given the similar features between RSD and acute bone pain syndrome, it may be that acute bone pain syndrome is a part of the spectrum of RSD and that signs are masked by concurrent corticosteroid use.

Acknowledgement

Radiographs supplied courtesy of Dr P O'Connor, Department of Radiology, The Leeds Teaching Hospitals NHS Trust.

References

1. Ferrari R. Rheumatological manifestations of renal disease. *Current Opinion in Rheumatology* 1996; 8: 72–6.
2. Schmidt H., Stracke H., Schatz H. *et al.* Osteocalcin serum levels in patients following renal transplantation. *Klin Wochenschr* 1989; 67: 297–303.
3. Cundy T. and Kanis J.A. Rapid suppression of plasma alkaline phosphatase activity after renal transplantation in patients with renal osteodystrophy. *Clin Chim Acta* 1987; 164: 285–91.
4. Briner V.A., Landman J., Brunner F.P. and Thiel G. Cyclosporin A-induced transient rise in plasma alkaline phosphatase in kidney transplant patients. *Transplant Int* 1993; 6: 99–107.

5. Coen G., Mazzaferro S. Bone Metabolism and its Assessment in Renal Failure. *Nephron* 1994; 67: 383–401.
6. Chazot C., Chazot I., *et al.* Functional study of hands among patients dialysed for more than ten years. *Nephrology, Dialysis, Transplantation* 1993; 8(4): 347–51.
7. Sethi D., Morgan T.C. *et al.* Dialysis arthropathy: a clinical, biochemical, radiological and histological study of 36 patients. *Quarterly J Med* 1990; 77(282): 1061–82.
8. Scheumann G.F., Holch M. *et al.* Pathological fractures and lytic bone lesions of the femoral neck associated with beta 2-microglobulin amyloid deposition in long-term dialysis patients. *Archive of Orthopaedic and Trauma Surgery* 1991; 10(2): 93–7.
9. Hardouin P., Flipo R.M. *et al.* Dialysis-related beta 2-microglobulinamyloid arthropathy. Improvement of clinical symptoms after a switch of dialysis membranes. *Clin Rheum* 1988; 7(1): 41–5.
10. Rodino M.A. and Shane E. Osteoporosis after organ transplantation. *Am J Med* 1998; 104: 459–69.
11. Grotz W.H., Mundinger F.A., Gugel B *et al.* Bone mineral density after kidney transplantation. *Transplantation* 1995; 59: 982–6.
12. Arlen D.J. and Adachi J.D. Are bisphosphonates useful in the management of corticosteroid-induced osteoporosis in transplant patients? *Journal of Nephrology* 1998; 11(5): 5–8.
13. Pichette V., Bonnardeaux A., Prudhomme L. *et al.* Long-term bone loss in kidney transplant recipients: A cross-sectional and longitudinal study. *Am J Kidney Diseases* 1996; 28: 105–14.
14. Grotz W.H., Mundinger A., Gugel B. *et al.* Bone fracture and osteodensitometry with dual energy X-ray absorptiometry in kidney transplant recipients. *Transplantation* 1994; 58: 912–5.
15. Nisbeth U., Lindh E., Ljunghall S. *et al.* Fracture frequency after kidney transplantation. *Transplant Proc* 1994; 26: 1764.
16. Epstein S., Shane E. and Bilezikian J.P. Organ transplantation and osteoporosis. *Current Opinion in Rheumatology* 1995; 7: 255–61.
17. Grotz W.H., Mundinger F.A., Rasenack J. *et al.* Bone loss after kidney transplantation: a longitudinal study in 115 graft recipients. *Nephrol Dial Transplant* 1995; 10: 2096–100.
18. Bourbigot B., Moal M.C. and Cledes J. Bone histology in renal transplant patients receiving cyclosporin. *Lancet* 1988; I: 1048–49.
19. Kelly P.J., Sambrook P.N. and Eisman J.A. Potential protection by cyclosporin against glucocorticoid effects on bone. *Lancet* 1989; II: 1388.
20. Movsowitz C., Schlosberg M., Epstein S. *et al.* Combined treatment with cyclosporin A and cortisone acetate minimises the adverse bone effects of either agent alone. *J Orthop Res* 1990; 8(5): 635–41.
21. Aubia J., Masramon J., Serrano S., Lloveras J. and Marinose L. Bone histology in renal transplant patients receiving cyclosporin. *Lancet* 1988; I: 1048.
22. Movsovitz C., Epstein S., Fallon M., Ismail F. and Thomas S. Cyclosporin-A in vivo produces severe osteopenia in the rat. *Endocrin* 1988; 123(5): 2571–77.
23. Shane E., Rivas M.D., Silverberg S.J., Kim T.S., Staron R.B. and Bilezikian J.P. Osteoporosis after cardiac transplantation. *Am J Med* 1993; 94: 257–64.
24. Cvetkovic M., Mann G., Romero D. *et al.* Deleterious effects of long term cyclosporin A, cyclosporin G, and FK506 on bone mineral metabolism in vivo. *Transplantation* 1994; 57: 1231–37.

25. Epstein S. and Shane E. Transplantation osteoporosis. In: Marcus R., Feldman D., Kelsey J., eds. *Osteoporosis*. New York: Academic Press; 1996; 947–57.

26. Shane E. and Epstein S. Immunosuppressive therapy and the skeleton. *Trends Endocrinol Metab* 1994; 4: 169–75.

27. Lukert B.P. Glucocorticoid-induced osteoporosis. In: Marcus R., Feldman D., Kelsey J., eds. *Osteoporosis*. New York: Academic Press; 1996, 801–20.

28. Lukert B. and Kream B.E. Clinical and basic aspects of glucocorticoid action in bone. In: Bilezikian J.P., Raisz L.G., Rodan G.A., eds. *Principles of Bone Biology*. New York: Academic Press; 1996, 533–48.

29. Le Parc J.M., Andre T., Helenon O. *et al.* Osteonecrosis of the hip in renal transplant recipients. Changes in functional status and magnetic resonance imaging findings over three years in three hundred and five patients. *Rev Rhum Engl Ed* 1996, 63(6): 413–20.

30. Lausten G.S., Lemser T., Jensen P.K. and Egfjord M. Necrosis of the femoral head after kidney transplantation. *Clinical Transplantation* 1998, 12: 572–4.

31. Nishiyama K. and Okinaga A. Osteonecrosis after renal transplantation in children. *Clin Orthop* 1993; 295: 168–71.

32. Mulliken B.D., Renfrew D.L., Brand R.A. and Whitten C.G. Prevalence of previously undetected osteonecrosis of the femoral head in renal transplant patients. *Radiology* 1994; 192: 831–34.

33. Kyd R.J. Bone and joint complications of maintenance haemodialysis and renal transplantation. *N Z Med J* 1979; 89(627): 4–7.

34. Grevitt M.P. and Spencer J.D. Avascular necrosis of the hip treated by hemiarthroplasty: results in renal transplant patients. *J Arthroplasty* 1995; 10: 205–11.

35. Deo S, Gibbons C.L., Emerton M. and Simpson A.H. Total hip replacement in renal transplant patients. *J Bone Joint Surg Br* 1995; 77(2): 299–302.

36. Devlin V.J., Einhorn T.A. *et al.* Total hip arthroplasty after renal transplantation. Long-term follow-up study and assessment of metabolic bone status. *J Arthroplasty* 1988; 3(3): 205–13.

37. Rosenthal A.K. and Ryan L.M. Treatment of refractory crystal-associated arthritis. *Rheumatic Diseases Clinic of North America* 1995; 21(1): 151–61.

38. Cohen M.R. and Cohen E.P. Enthesopathy and atvoical gouty arthritis following renal transplantation: a case control study. *Rev Rhum· (Engl. Ed.)* 1995; 62(2): 86–90.

39. Thompson G.R., Ting Y.M., Riggs G.A. *et al.* Calcific tendinitis and soft-tissue calcification resembling gout. *JAMA* 1968; 203: 464.

40. Ark J.W., Flock T.J., Flatow E.L. *et al.* Arthroscopic treatment of calcific tendinitis of the shoulder. *Arthroscopy* 1992; 8: 183.

41. O'Duffy J.D. Clinical studies of acute pseudogout attacks: Comments on prevalence, predispositions and treatment. *Arthritis Rheum* 1976; 19: 349.

42. Ritter J.M., Kerr L.D., Valeriano-Marcet J. *et al.* The use of parenteral ACTH for acute crystal-induced synovitis in patients with multiple medical problems. *Arthritis Rheum* 1992; S225–35.

43. Vincenti F., Amend W.J., Feduska N.J. and Salvatierra Ojr. Septic arthritis following renal transplant. *Nephron* 1982; 30(3): 253–6.

44. Bomalaski J.S., Williamson P.K. and Goldstein C.S. Infectious arthritis in renal transplant patients. *Arth Rheum* 1986; 29(2): 227–32.

45. Tannenbaum D.A., Matthews L.S. and Grady-Benson J.C. Infection around joint replacements in patients who have a renal or liver transplantation. *J Bone Joint Surg Am* 1997; 79(1): 36–43.

46. Chong T.K. and Holley J.L. Gram-negative arthritis with a simultaneous urinary tract infection in a renal transplant recipient. *Am J Nephrol* 1990; 10(3): 248–50.
47. Sinnott J.T. 4th, Holt D.A. Cryptococcal pyarthrosis complicating gouty arthritis. *South Med J* 1989; 82(12): 1555–6.
48. Gauthier V.J. and Barbosa L.M. Bone pain in transplant recipients responsive to calcium channel blockers. *Ann Intern Med* 1994; 121: 863–65.
49. Lucas V.P. and Ponge T.D., Plougastel-Lucas M.L. *et al.* Musculoskeletal pain in renal-transplant recipients. *NEJM* 1991; 325(20): 1449–50.
50. Stevens J.M., Hilson A.J. and Sweny P. Post-renal transplant distal limb bone pain. *Transplantation* 1995; 60(3): 305–7.
51. Barbosa L.M., Gauthier V.J. and Davis C.L. Bone pain that responds to calcium channel blockers. A retrospective and prospective study of transplant recipients. *Transplantation* 1995; 59(4): 541–4.
52. Lucas V., Hourmant M., Soulillou J.P., Rossard A. and Prost A. Epiphyseal bone pain caused by cyclosporin A in 28 patients with renal transplantation. *Rev Rhum Mal Osteoartic* 1990; 57(1): 79–84.
53. Bouteiller G., Lloverass J.J., Condouret J., Durroux R. and Durrand D. Painful pol-yarticular syndrome probably induced by cyclosporin in three patients with a kidney transplant and one with a heart transplant. *Rev Rheum Mal Osteoartic* 1989; 56(11): 753–5.
54. Villaverde V., Cantalejo M., Balsa A. and Mola E.M. Leg bone pain syndrome in a kidney transplant patient treated with tacrolimus (FK506). *Ann Rheum Dis* 1999; 58: 653–4.
55. Munoz-Gomez J., Collado A., Gratacos J. *et al.* Reflex sympathetic dystrophy syn-drome of the lower limbs in renal transplant patients treated with Cyclosporin A. *Arthritis Rheum* 1991 May; 34(5): 625–30.
56. Grandtnerova B., Spisiakova D., Lepej J. and Markova I. Reflex sympathetic dystro-phy of the lower limbs after kidney transplantation. *Transpal Int* 1998; 11(S1): S331–3.
57. Munoz-Gomez J., Collado A., Gratacos J. *et al.* Reflex sympathetic dystrophy syn-drome of the lower limbs in renal transplant patients treated with cyclosporin A. *Arthritis Rheum* 1991; 34: 625–30.

Index